Study Guide to Accompany

Maternal and Child Health Nursing

Care of the Childbearing and Childrearing Family

Sixth Edition

Prepared by

JOYCE YOUNG JOHNSON, PhD, RN

EDNA BOYD-DAVIS, RN, BSN, MN

MARYANN FOLEY, RN, BSN

Wolters Kluwer | Lippincott Williams & Wilkins
Health

Philadelphia · Baltimore · New York · London
Buenos Aires · Hong Kong · Sydney · Tokyo

Product Manager: Helene Caprari
Manufacturing Manager: Karin Duffield
Production Services: Aptara, Inc.

9 8 7 6 5 4 3 2

ISBN: 978-1-6054-7024-5

Care has been taken to confirm the accuracy of the information presented and to describe generally accepted practices. However, the author, editors, and publisher are not responsible for errors or omissions or for any consequences from application of the information in this book and make no warranty, expressed or implied, with respect to the currency, completeness, or accuracy of the contents of the publication. Application of this information in a particular situation remains the professional responsibility of the practitioner; the clinical treatments described and recommended may not be considered absolute and universal recommendations.

The author, editors, and publisher have exerted every effort to ensure that drug selection and dosage set forth in this text are in accordance with the current recommendations and practice at the time of publication. However, in view of ongoing research, changes in government regulations, and the constant flow of information relating to drug therapy and drug reactions, the reader is urged to check the package insert for each drug for any change in indications and dosage and for added warnings and precautions. This is particularly important when the recommended agent is a new or infrequently employed drug.

Some drugs and medical devices presented in this publication have Food and Drug Administration (FDA) clearance for limited use in restricted research settings. It is the responsibility of the health care provider to ascertain the FDA status of each drug or device planned for use in his or her clinical practice.

LWW.com

Preface

This *Study Guide* originally written by Joyce Young Johnson, PhD, RN and Edna Boyd-Davis, RN, BSN, MN, was revised by Maryann Foley, RN, BSN, to accompany the sixth edition of *Maternal and Child Health Nursing*, by Adele Pillitteri. The Study Guide is designed to help you practice and retain the knowledge you have gained from the textbook, and it is structured to integrate that knowledge and give you a basis for applying it in your nursing practice. The following types of exercises are provided in each chapter of the Study Guide.

ASSESSING YOUR UNDERSTANDING

The first section of each Study Guide chapter concentrates on the basic information of the textbook chapter and helps you to remember key concepts, vocabulary, and principles.

- Fill in the Blanks

  Fill in the Blanks exercises test important chapter information, encouraging you to recall key points.

- Labeling

  Labeling exercises are used where you need to remember certain visual representations of the concepts presented in the textbook.

- Match the Following

  Matching questions test your knowledge of the definition of key terms.

- Sequencing

  Sequencing exercises ask you to remember particular sequences or orders, for instance, testing processes and prioritizing nursing actions.

- Short Answers

  Short answer questions will cover facts, concepts, procedures, and principles of the chapter. These questions ask you to recall information as well as demonstrate your comprehension of the information.

APPLYING YOUR KNOWLEDGE

The second section of each Study Guide chapter consists of case study—based exercises that ask you to begin to apply the knowledge you have gained from the textbook chapter and reinforced in the first section of the Study Guide chapter. A case study scenario based on the chapter's content is presented, and then you are asked to answer some questions, in writing, related to the case study. The questions cover the following areas:

- Assessment
- Planning Nursing Care
- Communication
- Reflection

PRACTICING FOR NCLEX

The third and final section of the Study Chapters helps you practice NCLEX-style questions while further reinforcing the knowledge you have been gaining and testing for yourself through the textbook chapter and the first two sections of the Study Guide chapter. In keeping with the NCLEX, the questions presented are multiple-choice and scenario-based, asking you to reflect, consider, and apply what you know and to choose the best answer out of those offered.

ANSWER KEYS

The answers for all of the exercises and questions in the Study Guide are provided at the back of the book, so you can assess your own learning as you complete each chapter.

We hope you will find this Study Guide to be helpful and enjoyable, and we wish you every success in your studies toward becoming a nurse.

Contents

A Framework for Maternal and Child Health Nursing

CHAPTER OVERVIEW

Chapter 1 presents an overview of maternal and child health nursing. The use of nursing process, nursing research, and nursing theory in the provision of quality care is discussed. The standards of maternal and child health nursing practice, the changing discipline, and the varied roles assumed by nurses in maternal and child health nursing are also explored.

LEARNING OBJECTIVES

After mastering the contents of this chapter, you should be able to do the following:

1. Identify the goals and philosophy of maternal and child health nursing.

2. Describe the evolution, scope, standards, and professional roles for nurses in maternal and child health nursing.

3. Describe family-centered care and ways that maternal and child health nursing could be made more family centered.

4. Define common statistical terms used in the field, such as infant and maternal mortality.

5. Identify legal and ethical issues important to maternal and child health nursing.

6. Use critical thinking to identify areas of care that could benefit from additional research or application of evidence-based practice.

7. Discuss the interplay of nursing process, evidence-based practice, and nursing theory as they relate to the future of maternal and child health nursing practice.

8. Integrate knowledge of trends in maternal and child health care with the nursing process to achieve quality maternal and child health nursing care.

KEY TERMS

case manager
certified nurse-midwife
clinical nurse specialist
client advocacy
evidence-based practice
fertility rate
genetic nurse counselor
maternal and child health nursing

mortality rate
neonate
nurse practitioner
nursing research
puerperium
scope of practice

MASTERING THE INFORMATION

FILL IN THE BLANKS

Supply the missing term or the information requested.

1. The _____ _____ _____ is an advanced practice nurse who is skilled in the care of the newborn, both ill and well.

2. The nurse must understand the _____ of practice, which is the range of services and care that may be provided by the nurse based on state requirements.

3. Health _____ involves actions to prevent further complications from an illness.

4. Teaching and role-modeling are essential components involved with health _____.

MATCHING

Match the terms in Column I with a definition, example, or related statement from Column II. Place the letter corresponding to the answer in the space provided.

Column I

1. ____ Guidelines developed by the American Nurses Association and Association of Women's Health, Obstetric, and Neonatal Nurses

2. ____ Prompt diagnosis and treatment of illness using interventions that will return the client to wellness most rapidly.

3. ____ Controlled investigation of problems with implications for nursing practice.

4. ____ Care of a woman before conception and through pregnancy, and care of the child prenatally, from birth and the neonatal period, and from infancy through adolescence

5. ____ The 6-week period following childbirth; the "fourth trimester"

6. ____ Use of a combination of research, clinical expertise, and patient preferences to guide decision making for practice

7. ____ Education of clients to be aware of good health through teaching and role modeling

8. ____ The promotion and maintenance of optimal family health to ensure cycles of optimal childbearing and childrearing.

Column II

a. Maternal and child nursing

b. Health promotion

c. Nursing research

d. Primary goal of maternal and child health nursing

e. Health restoration

f. Standards of maternal and child health nursing practice

g. Puerperium

h. Evidence-based practice

SHORT ANSWER

Supply the missing term or the information requested.

1. Discuss two of six trends in maternal and child health nursing care and the associated implications for nurses.

   _____

   _____

2. Explain the effect that shorter hospital stays will have on client care planning for a child during the postoperative period, particularly on client and family teaching.

   _____

   _____

3. Discuss methods of promoting empowerment of parents and children in the health care setting.

   _____

   _____

APPLYING YOUR KNOWLEDGE

CASE STUDY

Chin Won, age 26, presents at the community health center in her last trimester of pregnancy for her initial prenatal care visit. She is found to have an elevated blood pressure and excessive swelling in her legs and feet. The fetus appears small on the sonogram.

1. Explain how things could have been different if Chin Won had sought prenatal care during her first trimester.

_____

_____

_____

2. What measures might the nurse take to ensure that Chin Won's care is family centered?

_____

_____

_____

3. What cultural aspects would be important to assess when planning Chin Won's care throughout the pregnancy and puerperium?

_____

_____

_____

CRITICAL INQUIRY EXERCISE

1. Write a brief statement on your opinion regarding termination of pregnancy when the woman is at risk from the pregnancy and the fetus is healthy.

2. Prepare a plan for establishing an environment in which a hospitalized child can maintain a sense of parenting and family security. Include discussions of room appearance, visiting arrangements, care schedule, and input into care activities.

CRITICAL EXPLORATION

Examine the policy at a local maternal–child care facility regarding the procedure a nurse must follow if she suspects that a woman and her children are victims of an abusive male family member.

PRACTICING FOR NCLEX

MULTIPLE-CHOICE QUESTIONS

Circle the letter that corresponds to the best answer for each question.

1. When describing maternal mortality to a group of student, the instructor would define this term as the number of
   a. fetal deaths occurring as a result of maternal negligence during pregnancy.
   b. maternal deaths per 100,000 live births due to a direct result of the reproductive process.
   c. pregnancies per 1000 women that result in maternal death.
   d. fetal deaths (fetus weight over 500 g) per 1000 live births resulting in maternal death.

2. A newly admitted client expresses a wish to continue taking the herbal medicine she brought from home to help relieve her abdominal pain. Which response would be most appropriate?
   a. "You shouldn't believe in alternative thera-pies; they don't work as well as modern medications."
   b. "The doctor won't like it if you take any medication other than that prescribed."
   c. "You can take the herbal medication, but only after you've taken the prescribed med-ications I give you."
   d. "We have to check this herbal medicine to be sure it doesn't interfere with prescribed medications."

3. Which of the following represents an important implication for nursing related to the regionalization of pediatric care?
   a. Being away from home represents a fun adventure to children, so the nurse must ensure that the child takes health care seriously.
   b. Having the family members in a different city will allow for better bonding between the child and the hospital staff.
   c. Regionalization allows the nurse to isolate the child from parental overprotectiveness, which might slow development.
   d. The nurse has the responsibility to see that children and parents feel as welcome in the regional center as they would in a small hospital.

4. Since health care consumers are increasingly discriminating in their demands, which of the following would be most effective in facilitating consumer empowerment by the maternal–child health nurse?

   a. Allow minimal input from the client and family members into the planning of care to prevent excessive interference.

   b. Keep family members informed and help them make decisions about their child's care.

   c. Limit family visitation to prevent collaboration with the client and discovery of minor errors in care.

   d. Remind the client and family members that in the hospital setting, the nurse is in charge.

5. Which statement best reflects the description of an expanded role for nurses in maternal–child health?

   a. Clinical nurse specialists are prepared at the baccalaureate degree level and are capable of independent care of children.

   b. If a pediatric nurse practitioner (PNP) determines that a child has a major illness, the PNP can independently prescribe appropriate medication.

   c. Nurse-midwives can assume full responsibility for the care and management of women with uncomplicated pregnancies.

   d. Pediatric nurse practitioners are registered nurses who are usually prepared at the associate degree level.

ALTERNATE FORMAT QUESTIONS

Multiple-Answer Multiple-Choice Questions

Circle the letter(s) corresponding to the appropriate answer(s). Select all that apply.

1. When discussing the leading causes of neonatal infant mortality, which of the following would the nurse expect to include?

   a. Prematurity.

   b. Low birth weight.

   c. Congenital anomalies.

   d. Gestational diabetes.

   e. Malnutrition.

2. Which of the following are examples of the implications for nursing as related to the trends and concerns regarding health care costs?

   a. The average American cannot afford to hire a nurse practitioner instead of a physician to provide less expensive but more comprehensive family health care.

   b. Nurses must become more cost conscious about supplies and services and help reduce cost while maintaining quality care.

   c. Health care is less expensive today because most families have begun to participate in health promotion activities using primary care nurses.

   d. Lack of financial ability to pay is a major reason for women not seeking and obtaining prenatal care.

   e. Access to support from governmental programs has eliminated most of the problems associated with absence of prenatal care.

Sociocultural Aspects of Maternal and Child Health Nursing

CHAPTER OVERVIEW

Chapter 2 provides the student with a fundamental understanding of culture and implications for diversity in maternal and child nursing. It explores the various socioeconomic and cultural influences to assist the student in identifying behaviors that are culture-specific while respecting the individuality of all persons. A case study is presented to assist the student in planning for nutrition as it relates to culture. The critical thinking exercises examine sociocultural issues to be considered when formulating the plan of care.

LEARNING OBJECTIVES

After mastering the contents of this chapter, you should be able to do the following:

1. Describe ways that sociocultural influences affect maternal and child health nursing.

2. Identify National Health Goals related to sociocultural considerations that nurses can help the nation achieve.

3. Use critical thinking to analyze how sociocultural aspects of care affect family functioning and health and develop ways to make nursing care more family centered.

4. Assess a family for sociocultural influences that might influence the way it responds to childbearing and childrearing.

5. Formulate nursing diagnoses related to culturally influenced aspects of nursing care.

6. Develop outcomes to assist families who have specific cultural needs to thrive in their community.

7. Plan and implement nursing care that respects the sociocultural needs and wishes of families.

8. Implement nursing care to assist a family adapt to today's changing sociocultural environment.

9. Evaluate expected outcomes for achievement and effectiveness of care.

10. Identify areas of care related to sociocultural considerations that could benefit from additional nursing research or application of evidence-based practice.

11. Integrate sociocultural aspects of care with nursing process to achieve quality maternal and child health nursing care.

KEY TERMS

acculturation	minority
assimilation	mores
cultural values	norms
culture	prejudice
discrimination	stereotyping
diversity	taboos
ethnicity	transcultural nursing
ethnocentrism	

MASTERING THE INFORMATION

FILL IN THE BLANKS

Supply the missing term or the information requested.

1. The term _____ commonly refers to people who speak Spanish as their primary language.

2. _____ avoid making direct eye contact with another individual during a conversation as a form of respect.

3. Three taboos that are universal are _____, incest, and cannibalism.

4. _____ refers to the belief that people are different based on their physical or cultural traits.

MATCHING

Match the terms in Column II with a definition, example, or related statement from Column I. Place the letter corresponding to the answer in the space provided.

Column I

1. ___ Individual perception that one's own culture is superior to all others.

2. ___ A view of the world and a set of traditions that a specific social group uses and transmits to the next generation.

3. ___ A cultural group into which one was born.

4. ___ Expectation of a set of behavioral characteristics from a group without regard to the individual characteristics of group members.

5. ___ The care of patients that is guided by cultural aspects and respects individual differences.

6. ___ The usual values of a group.

Column II

a. Culture
b. Transcultural nursing
c. Mores
d. Stereotyping
e. Ethnocentrism
f. Ethnicity

TRUE OR FALSE

Indicate if the following statements are true or false by placing a "T" or "F" in the space provided.

___ 1. The predominant culture in the United States stresses that everyone should be employed productively (the Protestant work ethic).

___ 2. Some families may use trusted family members as a reference for health care rather than a physician.

APPLYING YOUR KNOWLEDGE

CASE STUDY

Tatiana Ochoa is a 30-year-old Mexican-American woman in her second trimester of pregnancy. She is visiting the clinic for a prenatal examination. The nurse finds that Mrs. Ochoa is anemic.

1. What approach will the nurse use to assess the source of Mrs. Ochoa's anemia?

_____

_____

_____

2. What actions would be appropriate for the nurse to do to facilitate adequate nutritional intake to correct the anemia yet allow Mrs. Ochoa to consume the diet she prefers?

_____

_____

_____

CRITICAL INQUIRY EXERCISE

1. Some hospitals have taken an active role to include cultural sensitivity in the care of patients and their families. Research the hospitals in your area to identify those who have telephone service agreements to assist families with language interpretation.

2. Collaborate with your classmates to create a mock nursing care plan for patients of this ethnic orientation who may be experiencing problems attending appointments or making the appointments on time.

CRITICAL EXPLORATION

Select a patient you are caring for in the clinical setting and create a nursing care plan for him or her, including an assessment of the family and the community. State the nursing diagnosis found in making your assessment, and provide the appropriate nursing orders.

PRACTICING FOR NCLEX

MULTIPLE-CHOICE QUESTIONS

Circle the letter that corresponds to the best answer for each question.

1. Which of the following phrases best describes assimilation as related to sociocultural differences?
   a. An adoption of the most dominant culture's values and influences.
   b. A loss of cultural expression as the customs of a dominant culture are taken on.
   c. A family tradition practiced in future generations.
   d. Placement of "labels" on groups of people according to their ethnic backgrounds.

2. A nurse overhears another group of nurses talking. One of the group states, "Men are never any good at diapering babies." The nurse interprets this statement as an example of
   a. discrimination.
   b. stereotyping.
   c. acculturation.
   d. ethnocentrism.

3. In the 1800s, large numbers of immigrants came to the United States from many different countries and gave up their native country's traditions and values. Which of the following is the common explanation for the actions of these immigrants?
   a. The immigrants found the American culture and beliefs to be equal or superior to their own.
   b. The immigrants feared the Americans and participated in the American culture to avoid cruelty and punishment.
   c. The immigrants joined the giant American "melting pot."
   d. Immigrants who did not take on the American culture were placed in lower socioeconomic groups.

ALTERNATE FORMAT QUESTIONS

Multiple-Answer Multiple-Choice Questions

Circle the letter(s) corresponding to the appropriate answer(s). Select all that apply.

1. Which of the following strategies would be helpful in recognizing cultural influences on pain management?
   a. Using an assessment tool.
   b. Appreciating that people do not always express pain the same way.
   c. Recognizing that the communication of pain is acceptable within all cultures.
   d. Understanding that the meaning of pain varies between cultures.
   e. Developing an awareness of your personal values and beliefs.

2. Members of a nuclear family in most cultures include
   a. mother.
   b. father.
   c. grandfather.
   d. grandmother.
   e. children.
   f. aunts.
   g. uncles.

The Childbearing and Childrearing Family

CHAPTER OVERVIEW

Chapter 3 provides a description of the family and how the family is the focus of modern nursing practice. The many types of families are presented, with family tasks and life cycles described according to Duvall and Miller (1990). The importance of providing nursing care that addresses families at their level of understanding, as indicated by their stage of development, is well demonstrated. This chapter challenges the student to use the family and community assessment tools to assist him or her in determining the relation of the family to the community. The student is instructed to use outcome identification when formulating a nursing plan of care to promote healthy families.

LEARNING OBJECTIVES

After mastering the content in this chapter, you should be able to do the following:

1. Describe family structure, function, and roles, and ways that these are changing.

2. Identify National Health Goals related to the family and specific ways that nurses can help the nation achieve these goals.

3. Use critical thinking to analyze additional ways that nursing care can be more family centered or that family members can be better integrated into maternal–child health care.

4. Assess a family for structure and healthy function.

5. Formulate nursing diagnoses related to family health.

6. Develop expected outcomes to help a family achieve optimal health.

7. Plan health teaching strategies, such as helping a family modify its lifestyle to adjust to a pregnancy, accommodate an ill child, or face a major life event such as loss of a job.

8. Implement nursing care, such as teaching a family more effective wellness behaviors.

9. Evaluate outcome criteria for achievement and effectiveness of nursing care to be certain that expected outcomes have been achieved.

10. Identify areas of care related to family nursing that could benefit from additional nursing research or the application of evidence-based practice.

11. Integrate knowledge of family nursing with nursing process to promote quality maternal and child health nursing care.

KEY TERMS

ecomap	family theory
family	genogram
family nursing	polygamy
family of orientation	polygyny
family of procreation	

MASTERING THE INFORMATION

FILL IN THE BLANKS

Supply the missing term or the information requested.

1. Parents may receive remuneration for the care of the child; care is theoretically temporary; children in these families may feel very insecure. This type of family is called a _____ family.

2. Members are related by social values, are free choice-oriented, and/or may follow a charismatic leader. This type of family is called a _____ family.

3. How well a family works together and meets any crisis depends on its structure and _____.

4. Homosexual unions in which children may be added to the family by artificial insemination or adoption. This type of family is called a _____ family.

5. A family of orientation is the family one is born into, and a family of _____ is one the person establishes.

MATCHING

Match the terms in Column II with a definition, example, or related statement from Column I. Place the letter corresponding to the answer in the space provided.

Column I

1. ____ An important nursing role is health education concerning well-child care. The nurse should also assess the parents' ability to care for an infant with health problems.

2. ____ Accidents involving children are a major health concern, and growth and development needs and safety considerations are increased.

3. ____ Older family members are more likely to suffer from chronic and disabling conditions than are younger members.

4. ____ Members of the family work to obtain a mutually satisfying relationship, relate well to their families, and plan for parenthood.

5. ____ Accidents, homicide, and suicide are the major causes of death. The nurse has an important role in facilitating communication between family members and spends time counseling them on safety, proper care of and respect for firearms, and drug abuse.

Column II

a. Family with an adolescent
b. Early childbearing family
c. Family with a preschool child
d. The family in retirement
e. Marriage

APPLYING YOUR KNOWLEDGE

CASE STUDY

The nurse is counseling a family who is anticipating the adoption of a 6-year-old boy. The family is currently in the marriage stage of growth and development.

1. What rationale should the nurse use to formulate an approach when advising this family to visit a health care facility soon after the adopted child has arrived in the home?

2. What are some common factors that exist with parents who adopt children that may cause the parents to be less resilient when adjusting their lives to the presence of a new baby?

3. Why would it be extremely important for the adoptive parents to tell the child of his adoption as early as possible?

4. The adoption has been final for 6 months, and the family visits the community health center for a well-child preschool checkup. The parents state that the child exhibited defiant and hostile behaviors after being told of his adoption. How would the nurse analyze this behavior and give an explanation to the parents?

_____

_____

_____

CRITICAL INQUIRY EXERCISE

1. Identify a patient in your clinical setting and use the family assessment tool to identify the various systems in his or her community.

2. Use the results to create an ecomap (diagram depicting the relationship between the family and the community).

CRITICAL EXPLORATION

Select a patient you are caring for in the clinical setting and create a nursing care plan for him or her, including an assessment of the family and the community. State the nursing diagnosis found in making your assessment, and provide the appropriate nursing orders.

PRACTICING FOR NCLEX

MULTIPLE-CHOICE QUESTIONS

Circle the letter that corresponds to the best answer for each question.

1. Which of the following would be representative of a goal related to achieving healthy family and community life?
   a. Maintain the baseline positive for blood lead level.
   b. Work with families with financial management.
   c. Lower the amount of physical abuse directed toward women.
   d. Support gay rights activists.

2. Which of the following best describes family nursing?
   a. Concentrates on the family as the client.
   b. Concentrates on the individual as the client.
   c. Concentrates on the family point of view.
   d. Concentrates on the individual's point of view.

3. Which of the following is a characteristic of the single-parent family?
   a. Provides support to family members because of its small size.
   b. Involves reconstitution support and increased security.
   c. Provides increased opportunities for self-reliance.
   d. Uses family resources to provide temporary psychosocial comfort.

ALTERNATE FORMAT QUESTIONS

Multiple-Answer Multiple-Choice Questions

Circle the letter(s) corresponding to the appropriate answer(s). Select all that apply.

1. According to Duvall and Miller (1990), which of the following tasks would be considered essential for a family?
   a. Physical maintenance.
   b. Socialization of family members.
   c. Recommendations for marriage counseling.
   d. Allocation of resources.
   e. Division of labor.

2. When describing a dyad family unit to a group of students, which of the following would the nurse include?
   a. Husband.
   b. Wife.
   c. Male child.
   d. Grandmother.
   e. Man.
   f. Woman.

3. When preparing an oral presentation for a local community group about the factors that have impacted the patterns of family life, which of the following would the nurse include?

   a. Reduced mobility of families.

   b. Increased dual-earning families.

   c. Drop in numbers of single-parent families.

   d. Constancy of cultural values and characteristics.

   e. Reduced government-aid programs.

   f. Rise in technological innovations.

The Childbearing and Childrearing Family in the Community

CHAPTER OVERVIEW

Chapter 4 discusses the usual health concerns associated with pregnancy and childhood that may necessitate home care nursing. It also addresses the appropriate nursing actions required to identify and assist a client in the home setting. Medication therapy is reviewed and nursing implications related to the administration of medications and patient/family teaching are outlined. The use of the nursing process to plan and provide appropriate care and teaching to assist the patient and family in providing care and avoiding complications is discussed.

LEARNING OBJECTIVES

After mastering the content in this chapter, you should be able to do the following:

1. Describe a healthy community and usual nursing and client concerns when home care is required during pregnancy or childhood.

2. Identify National Health Goals related to home care during pregnancy or childhood that nurses can help the nation achieve.

3. Use critical thinking to analyze how home care influences family functioning, and develop ways to make home nursing care more family centered.

4. Assess a pregnant woman or child and their community for likely success for home care.

5. Formulate nursing diagnoses related to care of a child or pregnant client at home.

6. Identify expected outcomes for a family requiring home care.

7. Plan nursing care appropriate to meet the needs of a home care client such as suggesting ways to keep in contact with significant others.

8. Implement nursing care to meet the needs of a pregnant woman or child on home care, such as teaching techniques of intravenous therapy.

9. Evaluate expected outcomes for effectiveness and achievement of care.

10. Identify areas of home care nursing that could benefit from additional nursing research or application of evidence-based practice.

11. Integrate knowledge of home care with nursing process to achieve quality maternal and child health nursing care.

KEY TERMS

community
direct care
home care
hospice care

indirect care
perinatal home care
skilled home nursing care

MASTERING THE INFORMATION

FILL IN THE BLANKS

Supply the missing term or the information requested.

1. The nurse should plan visits at times that are convenient for the family in order not to disrupt _____.

2. Pregnant women and children receiving home care need to be re-evaluated approximately every _____ days to see if their high-risk level has changed.

3. Care in the home in which a nurse plans and supervises care given by others is called _____ care.

4. When obtaining the health history and performing a physical exam in the client's home environment, the nurse must provide _____ and maintain _____.

5. If the home situation becomes unsafe while the nurse is visiting, the nurse should _____ immediately.

6. When providing care in the home, the nurse performs _____ before touching a client for assessment.

MATCHING

Match the terms in column I with a definition, example, or related statement from Column II. Place the letter corresponding to the answer in the space provided.

Column I

1. ____ Total parenteral nutrition
2. ____ Perinatal home care
3. ____ Postvisit planning
4. ____ Skilled home nursing care
5. ____ Enteral nutrition

Column II

a. Provision or supervision of care of a pregnant woman in the home by a home or community health care agency.

b. A method of supplying complete nutrition and fluid to women with hyperemesis gravidarum that may be administered in the home setting.

c. Nursing care provided in the home that includes physician-prescribed procedures such as a dressing changes.

d. Documentation, communication, and evaluation of client's future needs.

e. Nutrition commonly delivered by way of a feeding tube.

SHORT ANSWER

Supply the missing term or the information requested.

1. Discuss how nurses can be instrumental in helping the nation achieve National Health Goals related to prevention of preterm birth.

_____
_____

2. Describe the situations in which home care commonly is used for children.

_____
_____

APPLYING YOUR KNOWLEDGE

CASE STUDY

Peg Waters, age 32, is admitted onto your unit. She is pregnant with her first child. Her husband is present and they both appear anxious because Peg has gone into labor in her 34th week of gestation.

1. Her preterm labor has been halted and Peg is to be discharged home with follow up by a home care nurse. Peg states, "I don't know how I'm going to manage staying at home and not working." What would the nurse's best response be, and why?

_____
_____
_____

2. What key points would be essential for the home care nurse to address when visiting Peg?

_____

_____

_____

CRITICAL INQUIRY EXERCISE

1. What key points would you address in a teaching plan for an adolescent who is on home care because she is experiencing preterm labor in her 32nd week of gestation? How would this plan differ for a 28-year-old woman and a 38-year-old woman?

2. You are supervising a home care assistant caring for a pregnant client. What are some areas you would discuss with the assistant before the first client visit?

CRITICAL EXPLORATION

Accompany a home health care nurse on one or more visits to a home-bound preterm labor patient. What are the major assessments and interventions made by the nurse? What changes would you make in the patient's regimen, if any, based on your observations?

PRACTICING FOR NCLEX

MULTIPLE-CHOICE QUESTIONS

Circle the letter that corresponds to the best answer for each question.

1. When planning a home visit, the nurse should do which of the following?
   a. Keep his or her schedule, destination, and travel route confidential to protect client privacy.
   b. Learn the location of public phones in the neighborhood.
   c. Drop in to visit the client on occasion to observe the family in a realistic state.
   d. Drive straight home if he or she suspects someone is following him or her.

2. Disadvantages of home care for an ill child include which of the following?
   a. Care is done in the client's home.
   b. Family members are included in the plan of care.
   c. The family is required to assume a greater responsibility for monitoring.
   d. Family interactions, values, and priorities are more obvious than in a health care setting.

3. Which of the following is accurate instruction the nurse might need to provide to the pregnant woman receiving home care?
   a. To promote elimination, the woman should avoid high-fiber foods.
   b. When monitoring uterine contractions, the woman should count and time the contractions for 10 minutes.
   c. The woman should alternate arms with each reading when monitoring her blood pressure.
   d. Serial fundal height measurements should be taken at the same location each time.

4. Jackie's husband states he wants to help his wife who is being treated at home for preterm labor. You could instruct him to do which of the following?
   a. Walk with Jackie two times each day to help her maintain adequate exercise to prevent thrombus formation.
   b. Restrict Jackie's intake of fluids to four glasses daily to prevent pulmonary edema.
   c. Remind Jackie to monitor fetal movements once a week to watch for fetal hyperactivity.
   d. Assume responsibility for child care and household duties to help Jackie maintain strict bed rest.

ALTERNATE FORMAT QUESTIONS

Multiple-Answer Multiple-Choice Questions

Circle the letter(s) corresponding to the appropriate answer(s). Select all that apply.

1. When visiting a client in the home, which of the following would be a priority assessment?
   a. Health history.
   b. Political views.
   c. Mental status.
   d. Activities and rest pattern.
   e. Professional goals.
   f. Transportation to follow-up appointments.

2. A nurse is planning a visit to the home of a child and his family. When assessing the home environment, which of the following would be essential to determine?
   a. Presence of telephone.
   b. Safety of house for home care.
   c. Color scheme of the child's room.
   d. Evidence of rodents in the home.
   e. Adequacy of water and heat.
   f. Refrigeration facilities.

3. Which of the following would be most effective to ensure a home care nurse's safety when traveling and making home visits?
   a. Using a shortcut through an alley.
   b. Carrying a large backpack with supplies.
   c. Walking determinedly with confidence.
   d. Parking vehicle in a well-lighted busy area.
   e. Locking valuables in the trunk on arrival at the home.
   f. Entering by using the front door.

The Nursing Role in Reproductive and Sexual Health

CHAPTER OVERVIEW

Chapter 5 reviews the anatomy and physiology of the reproductive system. It addresses sexuality as it relates to each stage of growth and development in the lives of human beings. The nurse's role in providing sex education to children, adolescents, and adults is illustrated through teaching concepts in this chapter. A case study is included to assist the student in researching information about the current national health concerns and goals.

LEARNING OBJECTIVES

After mastering the content in this chapter, you should be able to do the following:

1. Describe anatomy and physiology pertinent to reproductive and sexual health.

2. Identify National Health Goals related to reproductive health and sexuality that nurses can help the nation achieve.

3. Use critical thinking to analyze ways in which clients' reproductive and sexual health can be improved for healthier childbearing and adult health within a family-centered framework.

4. Assess a couple for anatomic and physiologic health, biologic gender, gender role, gender identity, and readiness for childbearing.

5. Formulate nursing diagnoses related to reproductive and sexual health.

6. Identify appropriate outcomes for reproductive and sexual health education.

7. Plan nursing care related to anatomic and physiologic readiness for childbearing or sexual health, such as helping adolescents discuss concerns in these areas.

8. Implement nursing care related to reproductive and sexual health, such as educating middle schoolchildren about menstruation.

9. Evaluate expected outcomes for achievement and effectiveness of care.

10. Identify areas of care in relation to reproductive and sexual health that could benefit from additional nursing research or application of evidence-based practice.

11. Integrate knowledge of reproductive health and sexuality with nursing process to achieve quality maternal and child health nursing care.

KEY TERMS

adrenarche
andrology
anteflexion
anteversion
aspermia
bicornuate uterus
biologic gender
culdoscopy
cystocele
dyspareunia
erectile dysfunction
gender identity
gender role
gonad
gynecology
gynecomastia

laparoscopy
menarche
menopause
menorrhagia
metrorrhagia
oocyte
premature ejaculation
rectocele
retroflexion
retroversion
thelarche
transsexual
transvestite
vaginismus
voyeurism

MASTERING THE INFORMATION

FILL IN THE BLANKS

Supply the missing term or the information requested.

1. The _____ is the body organ that produces cells necessary for reproduction.

2. _____ is the stage of life at which menstrual cycles cease.

3. _____._____ is the initiation of breast development influenced by estrogen.

MATCHING

Match the terms in Column II with a definition, example, or related statement from Column I. Place the letter corresponding to the answer in the space provided.

Column I

1. ____ Inner sense a person has of being male or female.

2. ____ Ridge of tissue formed by the posterior joining of the labia minora and the labia majora.

3. ____ Structure located bilateral to the urinary meatus; supplies lubrication to external genitalia during coitus.

4. ____ Sexual fulfillment with members of the same sex.

5. ____ Structure contains four parts: interstitium, isthmus, ampulla, and infundibula.

6. ____ A pad of adipose tissue located over the symphysis pubis.

7. ____ Term used to denote chromosomal sexual development.

8. ____ Structure that serves to support and protect the reproductive and other pelvic organs.

9. ____ Structure that accommodates the growing fetus during pregnancy.

10. ____ Elastic semicircle of tissue that covers the opening of the vagina.

11. ____ Small, rounded organ of erectile tissue at the forward function of the labia minora; sensitive to touch and temperature and is the center of sexual arousal.

Column II

a. Fallopian tubes
b. Uterus
c. Homosexual
d. Mons veneris
e. Clitoris
f. Fourchette
g. Biologic gender
h. Pelvis
i. Hymen
j. Skene's glands
k. Gender identity

TRUE OR FALSE

Indicate if the following statements are true or false by placing a "T" or "F" in the space provided.

Mrs. Bell telephones the nurse in a well health care center because she would like information regarding ovulation. She states that she has a 28-day menstrual cycle and would like to know when she should expect ovulation to occur. In advising Mrs. Bell the nurse would know that

____ 1. Ovulation occurs at the midpoint of this woman's menstrual cycle.

____ 2. Basal body temperature is affected by the production of progesterone and is lowered just prior to ovulation.

APPLYING YOUR KNOWLEDGE

CASE STUDY

As a summer student taking an independent study course, you are a mentor for a group of prospective college students. These students are matriculating in a post-high school program for persons pursuing health careers. To complete their curriculum, you must address the following principles of reproductive and sexual health.

1. State the primary role of the nurse in the promotion of reproductive health.

_____

_____

_____

2. Describe four physiologic functions that explain how the activity of the hypothalamus influences the menstrual cycle.

_____

_____

_____

3. Summarize the physiological changes that occur in older adults that may alter the ability of both male and female to be sexually active.

_____

_____

_____

4. Identify National Health Goals related to reproductive and sexual health and how the nurse may support the nation to achieve these goals.

_____

_____

_____

CRITICAL INQUIRY EXERCISE

Create a teaching plan to be used in a group setting for teenage girls. Describe how conception takes place using the sequel approach from the point of ovulation.

CRITICAL EXPLORATION

Visit a public health department and assess the approach the nurse uses to teach about reproductive health care to patients who are requesting birth control measures for the first time.

PRACTICING FOR NCLEX

MULTIPLE-CHOICE QUESTIONS

Circle the letter that corresponds to the best answer for each question.

1. The nurse is counseling 11-year-old Mandy and her mother in an ambulatory health care setting. The mother is communicating concerns to the nurse with regard to anticipatory guidance about menstruation. Mandy has not reached menarche. The family appears receptive and interested about the importance of health care. The nurse would know that including menstruation as a part of health education on this visit would be important because
   a. menopausal changes that could be a threat to Mandy's health may be occurring.
   b. menarche should have occurred at age 9.
   c. Mandy is in jeopardy for experiencing regular cyclic hormonal changes.
   d. menstruation is considered to be an initiation to sexuality and womanhood.

2. Some couples experience sexual dysfunction. When the female does not experience an orgasm because the male ejaculates before he desires, the dysfunction is referred to as
   a. dyspareunia.
   b. premature vaginismus.
   c. premature ejaculation.
   d. failure to achieve orgasm.

3. During the assessment, a female patient reports that she is experiencing pain during sexual intercourse. She has a history of endometriosis and vaginal infection. The nurse documents the patient's complaint as which of the following?
   a. Dyspareunia.
   b. Premature vaginismus.
   c. Sadomasochism.
   d. Fetishism.

ALTERNATE FORMAT QUESTIONS

Multiple-Answer Multiple-Choice Questions

Circle the letter(s) corresponding to the appropriate answer(s). Select all that apply.

1. An instructor is preparing a class for a group of students about the male reproductive structures. The instructor is planning to describe the secretion by the seminal vesicles as being high in which of the following?
   a. Sugar.
   b. Protein.
   c. Electrolytes.
   d. Prostaglandins.
   e. Acids.

2. After teaching a group of students about the structures associated with the female reproductive system, the nurse determines that the teaching was successful when the students identify which structures?
   a. Labia minora
   b. Vas deferens.
   c. Ovaries.
   d. Labia majora.
   e. Seminal vesicles.

3. Which of the following events would occur during the excitement phase of the sexual response cycle?
   a. Increased clitoral size.
   b. Mucosal fluid on vaginal walls.
   c. Testicular elevation.
   d. Scrotal thinning.
   e. Vaginal widening.
   f. Ejaculation of semen.

Assisting the Family With Reproductive Life Planning

CHAPTER OVERVIEW

Chapter 6 discusses the methods available for reproductive life planning. These methods are presented with their physiologic actions and the impact on future pregnancies. The chapter examines the process of ovulation and potential side effects of an ovulation-suppressing agent. The principles of therapeutic communication when counseling the family who seeks health care on reproductive life planning are also discussed. Case studies are provided to assist the student in learning why specific methods of reproductive life planning are recommended over other available methods.

LEARNING OBJECTIVES

After mastering the content in this chapter, you should be able to do the following:

1. Describe common methods of reproductive life planning and the advantages, disadvantages, and risk factors associated with each.

2. Identify National Health Goals related to reproductive life planning that nurses can help the nation achieve.

3. Use critical thinking to analyze ways that family-centered reproductive life planning can be accomplished.

4. Assess clients for reproductive life planning needs.

5. Formulate nursing diagnoses related to reproductive life planning concerns.

6. Identify expected outcomes for couples desiring reproductive life planning.

7. Plan nursing care related to reproductive life planning, such as helping a client select a suitable reproductive planning method.

8. Implement nursing care related to reproductive life planning, such as educating adolescents about the use of condoms as a safer sex practice as well as to prevent unwanted pregnancy.

9. Evaluate expected outcomes for achievement and effectiveness of care.

10. Identify areas related to reproductive life planning that could benefit from additional nursing research or application of evidence-based practice.

11. Integrate knowledge of reproductive life planning with nursing process to achieve quality maternal and child health nursing care.

KEY TERMS

abstinence
barrier method
basal body temperature
cervical cap
coitus
coitus interruptus
condom
contraceptive
diaphragm
elective termination of
   pregnancy
fertile days
fertility awareness

intrauterine device
laparoscopy
natural family
   planning
reproductive life
   planning
spermicide
transdermal contra-
   ception
tubal ligation
vaginal ring
vasectomy

MASTERING THE INFORMATION

FILL IN THE BLANKS

Supply the missing term or the information requested.

1. _____ prevents pregnancy by collecting the spermatozoa before they can be deposited in the vagina.

2. A _____ is a circular rubber disk that fits over the cervix to form a barrier against the entrance of spermatozoa.

3. A vaginal ring surrounds the cervix and continually releases a combination of _____ and _____ .

MATCHING

Match the terms in Column II with a definition, example, or related statement from Column I. Place the letter corresponding to the answer in the space provided.

Column I

1. ____ Excision and blocking of the vas deferens to prevent passage of the spermatozoa.

2. ____ Production of antibodies against Rh-positive blood.

3. ____ A result of an accidental injection of saline solution into a blood vessel.

4. ____ Removal of the uterine lining by suction or a syringe.

5. ____ Contraceptive method with a 0% failure rate.

Column II

a. Hypernatremia
b. Menstrual extraction
c. Isoimmunization
d. Vasectomy
e. Abstinence

SHORT ANSWER

Supply the missing term or the information requested.

1. Describe three physiologic functions that suppress ovulation when "the pill" is used as a method of contraception.

   _____

   _____

2. Describe how the "minipill" differs from the traditional oral contraceptive.

   _____

   _____

3. Discuss the use of intrauterine devices (IUDs), spermicides, and condoms by adolescents as methods of reproductive life planning.

   _____

   _____

APPLYING YOUR KNOWLEDGE

CASE STUDY 1

1. Friday, April 20, marks 1 week since Mrs. Nugent gave birth to a 6-lb, 7.5-oz son. She has elected to use an oral contraceptive as her reproductive life planning method after his delivery. The physician prescribes an oral contraceptive to be taken for 21 days. Mrs. Nugent tells the nurse she is not clear about when to take her pills.

1. What instructions should the nurse give Mrs. Nugent on starting the use of this oral contraceptive?

   _____

   _____

   _____

2. How often should Mrs. Nugent take the pills, and when should she expect her menstrual flow to begin?

_____

_____

_____

3. What are some suggestions that the nurse can offer Mrs. Nugent to help her remember to take her pill?

_____

_____

_____

CASE STUDY 2

2. Ms. Jordan brings her 16-year-old daughter Tammy to the physician's office. Tammy experienced menarche 2 months ago and Ms. Jordan suspects she is sexually active. Ms. Jordan is requesting an oral contraceptive as a method for reproductive life planning for her daughter.

1. What permanent damage may occur if use of the oral contraceptive begins before the cycle is regulated?

_____

_____

_____

2. Explain the relationship between oral contraception and the potential for alteration in skeletal growth with adolescent girls.

_____

_____

_____

CASE STUDY 3

3. Mrs. Patterson, age 40, married and the mother of three children, is visiting the health care center to electively terminate her pregnancy at 8 weeks of gestation. She visits the community health care facility to be counseled on the procedure. As she is being examined, she asks the nurse if terminating her pregnancy would reflect negatively on her as a patient.

1. What are some very important guidelines that the nurse must remember when responding to Mrs. Patterson?

_____

_____

_____

2. Mrs. Patterson is administered a laminaria for dilation of the cervix. Why would Mrs. Patterson be routinely placed on antibiotic therapy with this procedure?

_____

_____

_____

CRITICAL INQUIRY EXERCISE

1. Prepare a nursing care plan to provide health education and counseling for a patient who will be undergoing an elective tubal ligation. Focus on the future implications of the procedure.

2. Prepare a teaching plan for an adolescent who is pregnant and has expressed a desire to learn about contraceptives. The plan should address safer sex and a suitable method of reproductive life planning.

CRITICAL EXPLORATION

1. Use the teaching plan that you constructed for the above exercise to teach a teen group in a community health care setting about safer sex and reproductive life planning.

2. Survey the retail market for condoms that are self-lubricated and treated with nonoxynol-9. Present your findings when counseling the adolescent in a clinical setting.

PRACTICING FOR NCLEX

MULTIPLE-CHOICE QUESTIONS

Circle the letter that corresponds to the best answer for each question.

1. A woman is scheduled for a tubal ligation involving the use of carbon dioxide to raise the abdominal wall. The nurse identifies this as a
   a. culdoscopy.
   b. laparoscopy.
   c. hysterectomy.
   d. minilaparotomy.

2. The nurse is teaching a woman about using oral contraceptives. The nurse would instruct the woman to take the first pill on which day of the week after the start of menstrual flow?
   a. Sunday.
   b. Monday.
   c. Wednesday.
   d. Saturday.

3. When counseling an adolescent girl who expresses a desire to begin using the oral contraceptive method of reproductive life planning, the nurse would determine that oral contraceptives would be an appropriate choice if the adolescent has been experiencing menses for at least how long?
   a. 1 year.
   b. 2 years.
   c. 3 years.
   d. 4 years.

4. A woman is receiving medoxyprogesterone acetate (Depo-Provera) for contraception demonstrates understanding of this agent when she identifies which of the following as a possible side effect?
   a. Thrombophlebitis.
   b. Weight gain.
   c. Excessive menstrual flow.
   d. Osteoporosis.

ALTERNATE FORMAT QUESTIONS
Multiple-Answer Multiple-Choice Questions

Circle the letter(s) corresponding to the appropriate answer(s). Select all that apply.

1. After teaching a group of young women about the possible side effects of oral contraceptives, the nurse determines that the teaching has been successful when the group identifies which of the following?
   a. Nausea.
   b. Weight loss.
   c. Headache.
   d. Breast tenderness.
   e. Alternating cycles.

2. When the pill is used for contraception, which of the following occur to suppress ovulation?
   a. Suppression of follicle-simulating hormone.
   b. Interference with progesterone secretion.
   c. Increase in amount of cervical mucus.
   d. Decrease in cervical mucus permeability.
   e. Suppression of luteinizing hormone.

3. A woman who is 16 weeks pregnant comes to the clinic for an elective termination of pregnancy. Which of the following methods would be appropriate for this woman?
   a. Menstrual extraction.
   b. Dilatation and curettage.
   c. Dilatation and vacuum extraction.
   d. Prostaglandin induction.
   e. Saline induction.
   f. Hysterotomy.

The Nursing Role in Genetic Assessment and Counseling

CHAPTER OVERVIEW

Chapter 7 presents an overview of basic principles and concepts related to genetic assessment and counseling. The inheritance of disease and types of genetic defects are discussed. The role of nurses in genetic counseling and the care of clients with genetic disorders are explored.

LEARNING OBJECTIVES

After mastering the content in this chapter, you should be able to do the following:

1. Describe the nature of inheritance, patterns of recessive and dominant Mendelian inheritance, and common chromosomal aberrations that cause physical or cognitive disorders.

2. Identify National Health Goals related to genetic disorders that nurses can help the nation achieve.

3. Use critical thinking to analyze ways that nurses can make genetic assessment or education more family centered.

4. Assess a family for their adjustment to the probability of inheriting a genetic disorder.

5. Formulate nursing diagnoses related to genetic disorders.

6. Establish expected outcomes that meet the needs of the family undergoing genetic assessment and counseling.

7. Plan nursing care related to a potential alteration in genetic health, such as assisting with an amniocentesis.

8. Implement nursing care such as counseling a family with a genetic disorder.

9. Evaluate expected outcomes for achievement and effectiveness of care.

10. Identify areas related to genetic assessment that could benefit from additional nursing research or application of evidence-based practice.

11. Integrate knowledge of genetic inheritance with nursing process to achieve quality maternal and child health nursing care.

KEY TERMS

alleles	genotype
chromosomes	heterozygous
cytogenetics	homozygous
dermatoglyphics	karyotype
genes	meiosis
genetics	nondisjunction
genome	phenotype

MASTERING THE INFORMATION

FILL IN THE BLANKS

Supply the missing term or the information requested.

1. Health professionals have a legal and _____ obligation to share genetic information with the involved couple and no one else.

2. Genetic counseling will inform a couple about the genetic disorder and the chances that their child might _____ it.

3. A person's _____ refers to his or her actual gene composition.

MATCHING

Match the terms in Column II with a definition, example, or related statement from Column I. Place the letter corresponding to the answer in the space provided.

Column I

1. ____ Expression of genetic material allowing identification whether chromosomal material has come from the male or female parent.

2. ____ Specific point on a chromosome, marking the location of a missing or abnormal gene.

3. ____ A woman agreeing to undergo artificial insemination by the male partner's sperm and to bear a child for the couple.

4. ____ Material of heredity, strands of genes in the nucleus of body cells.

5. ____ When paired with other genes, these genes always be expressed.

6. ____ Ability to be passed from one generation to the next.

7. ____ Visual inspection of the chromosome pattern.

8. ____ Having two like genes for a trait.

9. ____ An outward appearance or expression of the genes.

Column II

a. Genetic disorder

b. Chromosomes

c. Phenotype

d. Imprinting

e. Homozygous

f. Surrogate

g. Dominant gene

h. Genetic marker

i. Karyotyping

SHORT ANSWER

Supply the missing term or the information requested.

1. Discuss the merits of genetic testing for a couple at risk for having a child with an incurable genetic disease.

_____

_____

2. Differentiate between the chance of inheriting a disease if both parents are heterozygous for the trait and the disease is autosomal dominantly inherited, and the chance of inheritance if the disease is autosomal recessively inherited.

_____

_____

3. Discuss two of the four main purposes of genetic counseling.

_____

_____

4. Discuss why genetic counseling might be ineffective after the diagnosis of the pregnancy or immediately after the birth of a child with a defect.

_____

_____

APPLYING YOUR KNOWLEDGE

CASE STUDY

Bell and Bennie Johnson, both 32 years old, have been married for 1 year and want to have a baby. Bell has come for a complete physical and states she is concerned that she is too old for a healthy pregnancy. While doing the history, the nurse discovers Bell has a brother with Duchenne muscular dystrophy (DMD).

1. What is the significance of X-linked inheritance in determining the chances that Bell will have a baby with DMD if Bell is a carrier?

_____

_____

_____

2. If Bell gives birth to a child with DMD, what nursing actions would be appropriate to help Bennie and Bell in planning for the future needs of their family and the child? Would it be appropriate for the nurse to approach family members, explain the genetic defect, and encourage them to support the couple? Why or why not?

_____

_____

_____

CRITICAL INQUIRY EXERCISE

1. Write a brief statement on your opinion regarding the use of amniocentesis to determine if a fetus is without defects and if the couple should continue or terminate the pregnancy.

2. How might testing to determine the gender of an infant become an ethical dilemma? What are your thoughts regarding the use of modern technology to determine the gender of a child when a gender-specific genetic disorder is possible? When no disorder is likely?

CRITICAL EXPLORATION

Attend a genetic counseling session and write a short report on the content discussed and reactions noted from the couple.

PRACTICING FOR NCLEX

MULTIPLE-CHOICE QUESTIONS

Circle the letter that corresponds to the best answer for each question.

1. If "large feet" is a recessive trait and one parent is heterozygous for the trait and the other parent is homozygous for the trait, what are the chances that a child of this union will have large feet?

a. 25% (one in four).
b. 50% (two in four).
c. 75% (three in four).
d. 100% (four in four).

2. Which of the following individuals must be heterozygous for the recessive disease trait?
a. Adam, who has no symptoms of the disease but has a child with the disease.
b. Barbara, who displays no symptoms and has no children with the disease.
c. Peter, who has symptoms of the disease and has an affected child.
d. Wendy, who has symptoms of the disease but has no affected child.

3. Which of the following couples would benefit most from referral for immediate genetic counseling?
a. Tom, age 50, and Alice, age 42, who have just discovered they are going to have a baby.
b. Jim and Melissa, who have just had an infant with cystic fibrosis.
c. John and Jean, who want to have a baby but only want a male child.
d. Pete, who has hemophilia, and DeeDee, married for a year and want to have a child.

4. What role would be most appropriate for the nurse involved with genetic counseling?
a. Assess the options available to a couple and select the best ones to present for the couple to choose from.
b. Inform the couple of the procedures they may undergo in genetic screening and in genetic counseling.
c. Instruct parents on the need for an immediate abortion if both persons have the trait for a dominant disease.
d. Limit the information provided to the couple about the genetic defect to avoid influencing their decision.

5. To determine if a disorder occurred by chance or is carried by family members, a nurse should collect which of the following data?
a. A history of the couple's sexual pattern during the time of conception.
b. As complete a family history of infant deaths or abnormalities as possible.

c. A prenatal history of nausea and reports of back pain in the last trimester.

d. Physical assessment of the infant's eye and hair color.

6. Nursing measures that may be implemented when preparing a woman for amniocentesis should include which of the following?

    a. Determining that the woman is in her fifth to eighth week of pregnancy.

    b. Discussing the 10% risk of possible spontaneous miscarriage.

    c. Supporting her as she is beginning to accept the pregnancy and bond with the fetus.

    d. Explaining that the procedure involves scanning with no invasive measures.

ALTERNATE FORMAT QUESTIONS

Multiple-Answer Multiple-Choice Questions

Circle the letter(s) corresponding to the appropriate answer(s). Select all that apply.

1. Couples who undergo genetic counseling and are informed that they have a genetic abnormality in the family and might have a child with a genetic defect may experience which of the following behaviors?

    a. Loss of self-esteem.

    b. Blame.

    c. Embarrassment.

    d. Joy.

    e. Anger.

    f. Depression.

2. After teaching a class on various types of genetic disorders, the instructor determines that the class has understood the information when they identify which of the following as examples of autosomal recessive disorders?

    a. Marfan syndrome.

    b. Huntington disease.

    c. Tay–Sachs disease.

    d. Cystic fibrosis.

    e. Hemophilia.

3. Which of the following would be important for the nurse to keep in mind when caring for a couple undergoing genetic testing, counseling, and therapy?

    a. The couple is mandated to participate in screening.

    b. Signed informed consent is necessary for any genetic screening procedure.

    c. Results are provided to the couple after several validations for accuracy.

    b. The couple are the only ones to whom the results are given.

    c. The couple is strongly encouraged to undergo an abortion for a defect.

Nursing Care of the Subfertile Couple

CHAPTER OVERVIEW

Chapter 8 presents an overview of clients with fertility problems. The underlying physiologic and psychological bases for subfertility problems are discussed. The use of the nursing process to address the needs of clients coping with subfertility is explored.

LEARNING OBJECTIVES

After mastering the content in this chapter, you should be able to do the following:

1. Describe common causes of subfertility in both men and women.

2. Identify National Health Goals related to subfertility that nurses can help the nation achieve.

3. Use critical thinking to analyze ways that a fertility assessment can be more family centered.

4. Describe common assessments necessary to detect subfertility.

5. Formulate nursing diagnoses related to subfertility.

6. Identify appropriate outcomes for the subfertile couple.

7. Plan nursing interventions to meet the needs of a couple with a diagnosis of subfertility.

8. Assist with interventions associated with the diagnosis of subfertility or measures to promote fertility, such as health teaching.

9. Evaluate outcomes for achievement and effectiveness of care.

10. Identify areas of nursing care related to fertility that could benefit from additional nursing research or application of evidence-based practice.

11. Integrate knowledge about subfertility with the nursing process to achieve quality maternal and child health nursing care.

KEY TERMS

anovulation
cryptorchidism
endometriosis
erectile dysfunction
in vitro fertilization
pelvic inflammatory
    disease
sperm count
sperm motility
spermatogenesis
sterility
subfertility
therapeutic insemination
varicocele

MASTERING THE INFORMATION

FILL IN THE BLANKS

Supply the missing term or the information requested.

1. A uterine endometrial _____ may result in symptoms of bleeding and clot passage after the procedure.

2. A woman who is allergic to iodine and is scheduled for a hysterosalpingography is considered to be at risk for an _____ reaction.

3. Undescended testes, also called _____ may lead to lowered sperm production.

MATCHING

Match the terms in Column II with a definition, example, or related statement from Column I. Place the letter corresponding to the answer in the space provided.

Column I

1. ___ The inability to conceive a child or sustain a pregnancy to childbirth.

2. ___ The production of sperm cells.

3. ___ Introduction of a thin, hollow, lighted tube through the abdomen to examine the ovaries and uterus.

4. ___ A test for ovulation involving monitoring a monthly graph to determine when ovulation occurs.

5. ___ The inability to conceive because of a known condition.

6. ___ Enlargement of a testicular vein may result in subfertility due to venous congestion.

7. ___ Absent ova production.

8. ___ Radiographic examination of the fallopian tubes using a radiopaque medium to evaluate tubal patency.

9. ___ The couple cannot conceive a child at present but has had a previous viable pregnancy.

10. ___ Implanation of uterine nodules to locations outside the uterus.

Column II

a. Anovulation
b. Hysterosalpinogography
c. Basal body temperature
d. Endometriosis
e. Infertility
f. Laparoscopy
g. Secondary subfertility
h. Spermatogenesis
i. Sterility
j. Varicocele

SHORT ANSWER

Supply the missing term or the information requested.

1. Depending on a couple's motivations for fertility testing, their reaction to study results may vary from _____ to _____ for children never to be born.

2. A _____ _____ is a woman who agrees to be impregnated by a man's sperm and carry the child for him and his partner.

3. When vaginal pH is _____ , sperm motility is limited or destroyed.

4. _____ _____ is the instillation of sperm into the uterus to aid conception.

5. _____ _____ fertilization involves exposing an egg to sperm outside the woman's body and transferring the embryo.

APPLYING YOUR KNOWLEDGE

CASE STUDY

Marilyn and Palo Jaketes have been married for 3 years. For the past year they have had unprotected sex an average of three or four times per week in an effort to conceive. They have come to the clinic for assessment and counseling.

1. How might the ages of Mr. and Mrs. Jaketes affect their fertility evaluation and possible solutions for subfertility?

2. What cultural beliefs might the Jaketes have that should be considered when discussing measures to facilitate fertility? How might cultural beliefs affect their choice of alternatives to childbirth?

CRITICAL INQUIRY EXERCISE

1. Prepare a teaching plan for an infertile couple that outlines various options.

2. When might adoption be an unacceptable option for a couple?

CRITICAL EXPLORATION

Explore the facilities in your city to which you might refer clients with subfertility problems (e.g., sperm or egg banks, clinics, and adoption agencies).

PRACTICING FOR NCLEX

MULTIPLE-CHOICE QUESTIONS

Circle the letter that corresponds to the best answer for each question.

1. Which of the following is true about fertility studies?
   a. Fertility studies should be undertaken more quickly with younger women.
   b. If a couple is very anxious, studies should not be delayed regardless of the couple's age.
   c. Initial testing involves primarily the partner who is suspected of being infertile.
   d. Women under 30 years of age should be referred for evaluation after 6 months of subfertility.

2. Diane has been told she has blocked fallopian tubes. Which of the following fertility options should the nurse help her to explore?
   a. Hormonal therapy.
   b. Therapeutic insemination.
   c. In vitro fertilization.
   d. Gamete intrafallopian transfer.

3. Which of the following suggestions would be most appropriate to give to a couple to aid conception?
   a. Having coitus every day will increase chances for fertility.

   b. Douching should be done before coitus to promote sperm mobility.
   c. Male-superior position is best because it places sperm near the cervix.
   d. The woman should ambulate immediately after coitus to mobilize the egg toward sperm.

ALTERNATE FORMAT QUESTIONS

Multiple-Answer Multiple-Choice Questions

Circle the letter(s) corresponding to the appropriate answer(s). Select all that apply.

1. Which of the following would be most appropriate to include when teaching a man to increase his sperm count.
   a. Increase frequency of coitus.
   b. Wear clothing that does not restrict or overheat the scrotum.
   c. Avoid frequent use of hot baths.
   d. Increase alcohol intake.
   e. Increase sport activities.

2. When discussing the benefits associated with childless living with a couple who is subfertile, which of the following would the nurse include?
   a. Career growth.
   b. Pursuit of hobbies.
   c. Antisocial behaviors.
   d. Personal contributions to society.
   e. Continuance of education.

3. Which of the following tests might be used to assess the patency of a woman's fallopian tubes?
   a. Hysterosalpingography.
   b. Basal body temperature monitoring.
   c. Antisperm antibody testing.
   d. Sonohysterography.
   e. Endometrial biopsy.
   f. Hysteroscopy.

CHAPTER 9

The Growing Fetus

CHAPTER OVERVIEW

The development of the fetus is a complex phenomenon that originates from the union of an ovum and a sperm. When united, the ovum and the sperm form a single cell called the zygote. This chapter allows the student to explore all the stages of fetal development, enabling him or her to help the childbearing family understand the changes that take place during pregnancy. The student is also challenged to learn nursing principles necessary to conduct fetal monitoring and convey findings to the members of the childbearing family.

LEARNING OBJECTIVES

After mastering the content in this chapter, you should be able to do the following:

1. Describe the growth and development of a fetus by gestation week.

2. Identify National Health Goals related to fetal growth that nurses can help the nation achieve.

3. Use critical thinking to analyze ways to make care family centered, even at this early point in life.

4. Assess fetal growth and development through maternal and pregnancy landmarks.

5. Formulate nursing diagnoses related to the needs of a fetus.

6. Establish expected outcomes to meet the needs of a growing fetus.

7. Plan nursing care that promotes healthy fetal growth and development such as nutrition counseling.

8. Implement nursing care to help ensure both a safe fetal environment and a safe pregnancy outcome.

9. Evaluate expected outcomes for achievement and effectiveness of care.

10. Identify areas of fetal health that could benefit from additional nursing research or application of evidence-based practice.

11. Integrate knowledge of fetal growth and development with nursing process to achieve quality maternal and child health nursing care.

KEY TERMS

age of viability	foramen ovale
amniocentesis	hydramnios
amniotic membrane	implantation
cephalocaudal	McDonald's rule
chorionic membrane	meconium
chorionic villi	nonstress test
decidua	oligohydramnios
embryo	organogenesis
estimated date of birth	surfactant
fertilization	trophoblast
fetoscopy	umbilical cord
fetus	zygote

MASTERING THE INFORMATION

FILL IN THE BLANKS

Supply the missing term or the information requested.

1. The second fetal membrane lining the chorionic membrane is the _____ _____ membrane.

2. _____ occurs when the fetus is unable to swallow.

3. Fusion of the chromosomal material of the ovum and spermatozoon form a _____.

MATCHING

Match the terms in Column II with a definition, example, or related statement from Column I. Place the letter corresponding to the answer in the space provided.

Column I

1. ____ Three-part organ (basalis, capsularis, and vera) that is discarded following the birth of a child.

2. ____ Hormone found in the bloodstream shortly after conception and prior to first missed menstrual period.

3. ____ Transvaginal aspiration of fluid from the extraembryonic cavity in early pregnancy.

4. ____ Aspiration of amniotic fluid from the pregnant uterus for examination.

5. ____ A method of determining that the fetus is growing in utero by measuring fundal (uterine) height.

6. ____ A developmental pattern that proceeds from head to tail.

7. ____ Contact between the blastocyst and the uterine endothelium occurring approximately 8 to 10 days after fertilization.

8. ____ A gelatinous mucopolysaccharide that gives the umbilical cord body and prevents pressure on the vein and arteries.

9. ____ Important function in transporting oxygen and nutrients to the fetus from the placenta and returning waste products from the fetus to the placenta.

10. ____ A phospholipid substance that decreases alveolar surface tension on expiration.

Column II

a. Implantation
b. Amniocentesis
c. Surfactant
d. Decidua
e. Umbilical cord
f. McDonald's rule
g. Wharton's jelly
h. Human chorionic gonadotropin
i. Cephalocaudal
j. Coelocentesis

CHRONOLOGICAL ORDER

Assign the correct gestational age to the description and then place in order from the being to ending of fetal life.

Weeks of gestations descriptions of fetus

1. _____ Heart has septum and valves. Facial features are definitely discernible.

2. _____ Average weight is 1600 g; assumes delivery position; store iron.

3. _____ Additional deposits of subcutaneous fat and lanugo start to diminish.

4. _____ Average weight is 1200 g; lung alveoli begin maturing with surfactant.

5. _____ Formation of lanugo; liver and pancreas are functioning; fetus demonstrate swallowing reflex.

6. _____ Quickening experienced by the mother; beginning of vernix caseosa.

7. _____ Nail beds forming on toes and fingers; tooth buds present; heart sounds audible by Doppler instrument.

8. _____ Average weight is 550 g; passive antibody transfer from mother to fetus.

SHORT ANSWER

Supply the missing term or the information requested.

1. Explain how nutrients are exchanged from the mother to the fetus during pregnancy.

   _____

   _____

APPLYING YOUR KNOWLEDGE

CASE STUDY

Mrs. Menendez is 44 years of age and at 28 weeks' gestation. She is admitted to the hospital after experiencing acute abdominal pain for several days. The physician orders a biophysical profile procedure to determine the well-being of the fetus.

1. How many parameters are to be considered in the biophysical profile and what is the highest potential score for each parameter?

   _____

   _____

   _____

2. Explain the reliability of the biophysical profile as an assessment tool.

   _____

   _____

   _____

3. What major roles does the nurse play in obtaining the information for a biophysical profile?

   _____

   _____

   _____

CRITICAL INQUIRY EXERCISE

1. Construct a diagram to illustrate how a couple may use the woman's body metabolic temperature as an indicator to predict ovulation. Demonstrate how coitus occurring 1 to 2 days before ovulation, as well as after ovulation, can result in fertilization.

2. Use colorful markers to draw a diagram of fetal circulation. Ask your instructor to allot you a portion of your laboratory class time to present your diagram. Name all anatomical structures of fetal circulation and discuss their functions.

CRITICAL EXPLORATION

Formulate a nursing care plan expected outcome that addresses adequate fetal oxygenation throughout gestation. Then visit a health clinic on a day that several prenatal patients are scheduled to be seen. Note all of the implementations and procedures of the health care provider that can be viewed as actions to accomplish your goal.

PRACTICING FOR NCLEX

MULTIPLE-CHOICE QUESTIONS

Circle the letter that corresponds to the best answer for each question.

1. Beverly is being seen on her first prenatal visit at the health care clinic in her community. She reports that the first day of her last menstrual period was May 7, 2009. As calculated by Nagele's rule, Beverly's EDC will be
   a. New Year's Day 2010 (1-1-10).
   b. Valentine's Day 2010 (2-14-10).
   c. Veterans Day 2010 (11-12-10).
   d. April Fool's Day 2010 (4-1-10).

2. Mr. and Mrs. Mitchell are expecting their first child. On their visit to the physician's office for a scheduled appointment, they are jubilant over the pregnancy and curious about the health care procedures. As the nurse prepares Mrs. Mitchell for her assessment, she uses the Doppler to listen for the fetal heart tone. The nurse will expect the heart tone to be in a normal range of
   a. 110 to 120.
   b. 120 to 160.
   c. 170 to 180.
   d. 180 to 200.

3. The nurse is preparing Mrs. Mitchell for an ultrasound. Which action would be most appropriate?
   a. Instruct her to empty her bladder.
   b. Have her drink 8 oz of water every 15 minutes for 1.5 hours before the test.
   c. Shave her abdomen.
   d. Place Mrs. Mitchell in semi-Fowler's position with legs elevated.

4. A pregnant woman's partner asks the nurse to explain why his wife needs an ultrasound. The nurse would respond appropriately by stating that

   a. "An ultrasound is a common examination to monitor how the infant is growing and moving and to check for any complications."

   b. "The ultrasound test is used to measure the length and weight of your baby and to detect any chromosome abnormalities."

   c. "The ultrasound test is given to every pregnant woman; the reason why is complicated, but we'll let you know if the results are abnormal."

   d. "The doctor will explain the test to you, but I can tell you that we are checking to see if there are any problems with the pregnancy."

5. Mrs. Morrell complained of discomfort after having had an amniocentesis procedure. She is at 20 weeks' gestation and is 45 years old. Which of the following symptoms would prompt immediate action?

   a. Lab results reveal abnormal chromosome cells.

   b. Amniotic fluid contains fetal urine.

   c. Mrs. Morrell reports moderate vaginal bleeding.

   d. Mrs. Morrell describes symptoms of Braxton Hicks contractions.

ALTERNATE FORMAT QUESTIONS

Multiple-Answer Multiple-Choice Questions

Circle the letter(s) corresponding to the appropriate answer(s). Select all that apply.

1. Which of the following structures are derived from the ectoderm germ layer?

   a. Sebaceous glands.

   b. Brain.

   c. Bladder.

   d. Heart.

   e. Skin.

   f. Sense organs.

2. The nurse would explain which of the following when teaching a pregnant woman about the information obtained with a biophysical profile? Select all that apply.

   a. Fetal breathing.

   b. Fetal movement.

   c. Fetal tone.

   d. Amniotic fluid volume.

   e. Fetal heart rate reactivity.

   f. Lecithin/sphingomyelin ratio.

3. Which of the following hormones are produced by the placenta?

   a. Follicle-stimulating hormone.

   b. Human chorionic gonadotropin.

   c. Estrogen.

   d. Human chorionic somatomammotropin.

   e. Progesterone.

   f. Testosterone.

Psychological and Physiologic Changes of Pregnancy

CHAPTER OVERVIEW

Chapter 10 addresses the psychological and physical changes a woman and her partner experience during pregnancy. Although the physiologic changes of pregnancy are dynamic and extensive, they are considered an extension of normal physiology. The nurse uses this concept when preparing teaching plans and developing plans of care. At the completion of this chapter the student will be knowledgeable about the interplay of these changes, enabling the student to understand how to promote pregnancy as an extension of wellness in the family and throughout the pregnancy and early parenthood.

LEARNING OBJECTIVES

After mastering the content in this chapter, you should be able to do the following:

1. Describe common psychological and physiologic changes that occur with pregnancy and the relationship of the changes to pregnancy diagnosis.

2. Identify National Health Goals related to preconception counseling and prenatal care that nurses can help the nation achieve.

3. Use critical thinking to analyze how the physiologic and psychological changes of pregnancy affect family functioning, and develop ways to make nursing care more family centered.

4. Assess a woman for the psychological and physiologic changes that occur with pregnancy.

5. Formulate nursing diagnoses related to the psychological and physiologic changes of pregnancy.

6. Identify expected outcomes for a family's psychological and physical adaptation to pregnancy.

7. Plan nursing care related to the changes and diagnosis of pregnancy, such as helping a woman plan to arrange for adequate rest.

8. Implement nursing care, such as health teaching related to the expected changes of pregnancy.

9. Evaluate outcome criteria for the achievement and effectiveness of care.

10. Identify areas of nursing care related to the psychological and physiologic changes of pregnancy that could benefit from additional nursing research or application of evidence-based practice.

11. Integrate knowledge of the psychological and physiologic changes of pregnancy with nursing process to achieve quality maternal and child health nursing care.

KEY TERMS

ballottement	linia nigra
Braxton Hicks contractions	melasma
	Montgomery's tubercles
Chadwick's sign	multipara
couvade syndrome	operculum
diastasis	polyuria
Goodell's sign	primigravida
Hegar's sign	quickening
lightening	striae gravidarum

MASTERING THE INFORMATION

FILL IN THE BLANKS

Supply the missing term or the information requested.

1. _____ is a term used to describe the woman who has had one or more than one birth.

2. _____ describes a woman in her first pregnancy.

3. Softening of the cervix in pregnancy is called _____.

MATCHING

Match the terms in Column II with a definition, example, or related statement from Column I. Place the letter corresponding to the answer in the space provided.

Column I

1. ___ Positive test for hCG hormone in urine
2. ___ Palpation of fetal movements
3. ___ Quickening
4. ___ Chadwick's sign
5. ___ Striae gravidarum
6. ___ Auscultation of fetal heart sounds
7. ___ Fetal outline felt by examiner
8. ___ Breast changes
9. ___ Braxton Hicks contractions
10. ___ Sonographic evidence of fetal outline
11. ___ Ballottement.

Column II

a. Presumptive sign of pregnancy
b. Probable sign of pregnancy
c. Positive sign of pregnancy

SHORT ANSWER

Supply the missing term or the information requested.

1. What can the nurse do to help achieve the National Health Goals for women during pregnancy?

2. You are caring for a pregnant client in the third trimester. What is one reason that you would advise her to lie in the lateral recumbent position while sleeping?

3. What explanation would the nurse give to an expectant mother who has glucose in her urine but has tested negative for gestational diabetes?

4. Explain why it is important that pregnancy be diagnosed as early as possible and how this diagnosis may affect the woman's lifestyle and health status.

APPLYING YOUR KNOWLEDGE

CASE STUDY

Dove Whitewater, age 44, has come to the clinic for a pregnancy test. She is alone, appears very anxious, and has an obvious swelling around her abdominal area. She states she has been nauseous for the past 5 months and usually eats only a light lunch since food makes her sick in the morning and at night.

1. What emotions might Dove reveal when her pregnancy is confirmed?

2. Dove states she might decide to terminate her pregnancy. What would your response be?

_____

_____

_____

CRITICAL INQUIRY EXERCISE

1. Develop a teaching plan that would give anticipatory guidance with reference to the acceptance of pregnancy. How might this plan be different for a single woman than for a married woman?

2. Explain how some psychological changes of pregnancy can be caused or aggravated by the physiologic changes of pregnancy.

CRITICAL EXPLORATION

1. Perform assessments on three pregnant women in the first, second, and third trimesters. Record findings from your interviews that describe the psychological tasks of accepting the pregnancy, accepting the baby, and preparing for parenthood.

2. Assess a client in the second trimester of pregnancy who is experiencing Braxton Hicks contractions. Explain the differences between these and labor contractions.

PRACTICING FOR NCLEX

MULTIPLE-CHOICE QUESTIONS

Circle the letter that corresponds to the best answer for each question.

1. Helga, age 21, is pregnant with her first child. She is in her second trimester and complains of problems with drooling. You would explain that
   a. she should be admitted to the hospital to assess the cause of this unusual symptom.
   b. this symptom shows a deficiency of sodium and indicates she should increase her salt intake.
   c. drooling is the body's way of eliminating excess fluid to prevent high blood pressure.
   d. the drooling is called "hyperptyalism" and is due to her increased hormone levels.

2. John, age 33, has just found out his girlfriend Ceilie is 4 months pregnant. Which of the following might indicate that a teaching plan is needed?
   a. John has not expressed pleasure or displeasure regarding the pregnancy.
   b. John refers to the fetus as "it" when talking to Ceilie about the pregnancy.
   c. John expresses great concern that if Ceilie breastfeeds she will ruin her figure.
   d. John says he hopes Ceilie will exercise more so she might have an easy vaginal delivery.

3. Which of the following most accurately reflects the psychological tasks associated with pregnancy?
   a. During the first trimester women begin "nest-building" activities.
   b. During the second trimester "quickening" contributes to acceptance of the baby.
   c. During the third trimester the father-to-be usually begins the process of accepting the pregnancy.
   d. During the first trimester the father-to-be begins preparing for parenthood.

4. Which of the following is a positive example of reworking developmental tasks?
   a. The father-to-be begins to fantasize about being a carefree bachelor.
   b. A pregnant adolescent states she understands why her mother made her come home before dark.
   c. The father-to-be states his partner does not care for him since her pregnancy.
   d. A 42-year-old mother-to-be role-plays life before pregnancy.

5. Which of the following might indicate a problem in adjustment to pregnancy?
   a. A pregnant woman whose mother was abusive to her refuses to think about or discuss it.
   b. The pregnant woman reports an increase in sexual desire and greater enjoyment of sex.
   c. The father-to-be reports that his pregnant wife has frequent mood swings.
   d. The pregnant woman shows difficulty making decisions at work and at home.

ALTERNATE FORMAT QUESTIONS

Multiple-Answer Multiple-Choice Questions

Circle the letter(s) corresponding to the appropriate answer(s). Select all that apply.

1. Which of the following changes in the gastrointestinal system are associated with pregnancy?
   a. Displacement of the stomach and intestines.
   b. Constipation.
   c. Flatulence.
   d. Increased appetite.
   e. Hyperptyalism.
   f. Diarrhea.

2. Which of the following are changes in the endocrine system as a result of pregnancy?
   a. Formulation of the placenta as an endocrine gland.
   b. An increase in the parathyroid's size.
   c. Decrease in thyroid hormone production.
   d. Decrease in thyroid gland size.
   e. Production of oxytocin by the pituitary gland.

3. Which of the following characterize the psychological changes associated with the second trimester of pregnancy?
   a. Narcissism.
   b. Acceptance of the baby.
   c. Ambivalence.
   d. Introversion.
   e. Nest-building.

Assessing Fetal and Maternal Health: Prenatal Care

CHAPTER OVERVIEW

When a woman visits a health care facility for the first prenatal visit, an assertive effort should be made by the health care providers to validate the pregnancy, determine the woman's health status and risk for complications, and initiate strategies that will encourage the woman and her family to establish positive behavior patterns of health promotion during the pregnancy and throughout their lives. This chapter allows the student to review the anatomic structures of the female body and demonstrate knowledge of how to appropriately intervene to provide nursing care, education, and guidance from the first visit throughout the mother's pregnancy. Although most signs indicating complications occur toward the end of pregnancy, women need to know what these are early on so that prompt intervention can occur. A case study is included to help the student integrate therapeutic communication skills and nursing actions when assisting the patient with her first prenatal visit that includes a pelvic examination.

LEARNING OBJECTIVES

After mastering the content in this chapter, you should be able to do the following:

1. Describe the areas of health assessment commonly included in prenatal visits.

2. Identify National Health Goals related to prenatal care that nurses can help the nation achieve.

3. Use critical thinking to analyze ways to ensure that prenatal care is family centered.

4. Assess a pregnant woman's health status and readiness for pregnancy.

5. Formulate nursing diagnoses related to women's health status during pregnancy.

6. Identify expected outcomes to help ensure a safe pregnancy.

7. Plan nursing care, such as preparing a woman for a pelvic examination or fundal measurement.

8. Implement nursing care, such as establishing a risk score for pregnancy.

9. Evaluate expected outcomes for achievement and effectiveness of care.

10. Identify areas of prenatal care that could benefit from additional nursing research or application of evidence-based practice.

11. Integrate knowledge of pregnancy health assessment with nursing process to achieve quality maternal and child health care.

KEY TERMS

chloasma
conjugate vera
diagonal conjugate
erosion
gravida
ischial tuberosity
lithotomy position
multigravida

multipara
nulligravida
para
primigravida
primipara
speculum
true conjugate

MASTERING THE INFORMATION

FILL IN THE BLANKS

Supply the missing term or the information requested.

1. A(n) _____ pelvis has a well-rounded inlet and a wide pubic arch.

2. In a(n) _____ pelvis, the transverse diameter is narrow and anteroposterior diameter of the inlet is larger than normal.

3. A(n) _____ pelvis has an oval-shaped inlet and is smoothly curved.

4. In a(n) _____, the pubic arch forms an acute angle, narrowing lower dimensions of the pelvis.

MATCHING

Match the terms in Column I with a definition, example, or related statement from Column II. Place the letter corresponding to the answer in the space provided.

Column I

1. ___ Endocervical

2. ___ Cervical os

3. ___ Posterior vaginal fornix

Column II

a. Place applicator just below the cervix, rolling gently to obtain secretions. Place on laboratory slide.

b. Use a wet saline applicator and insert it through the speculum into the os of the cervix. Rotate clockwise and counterclockwise. Place on laboratory slide.

c. Press uneven end of supplied spatula on the os, rotate, and scrape cells in a circular motion. Place on laboratory slide.

TRUE OR FALSE

Indicate if the following statements are true or false by placing a "T" or "F" in the space provided.

1. ___ The cervical os is observed as round and small in a nulligravida client.

2. ___ Petroleum lubricant should be used on the speculum when viewing the cervix.

3. ___ When a client is infected with a Chlamydia infection, the vaginal mucosa appears extremely inflamed with a greenish-yellow discharge.

4. ___ A platypelloid pelvis accommodates childbirth with fewer difficulties than do the other three types of pelvis.

5. ___ The purpose of a prenatal visit is to establish a baseline of present health and minimize the risk of possible complications.

APPLYING YOUR KNOWLEDGE

CASE STUDY

Mrs. Goldstein is scheduled in the prenatal clinic for a pelvic examination. She will need to be prepared for the examination of several internal and external reproductive organs.

1. What position should Mrs. Goldstein assume once she is on the examination table?

_____

_____

_____

2. Name the instruments that the nurse should have available for the examination.

_____

_____

_____

3. How may a support person be of assistance to Mrs. Goldstein?

_____

_____

_____

CRITICAL INQUIRY EXERCISE

1. Diagram the four types of pelvis on a poster. Illustrate to your class how the anatomy of the pelvis may accommodate or hamper the fetus as it progresses through the birthing process.

2. Determine four assessment criteria that would reveal findings that could help determine that a pregnant woman is at high risk for the HIV infection.

CRITICAL EXPLORATION

Visit a prenatal health care setting and select a patient in the third trimester of her pregnancy who has been counseled and diagnosed as having a pelvis incompetent for delivery. Use your diagram as a tool to help the family understand the information discussed during counseling concerning the structure of the expectant mother's pelvis.

PRACTICING FOR NCLEX

MULTIPLE-CHOICE QUESTIONS

Circle the letter that corresponds to the best answer for each question.

1. A pregnant client has delayed her first prenatal visit, coming to the clinic only after she starts to experience edema of the feet and hands. The nurse takes a history and performs a physical examination. The client's response to one of the nurse's questions is, "This is my third pregnancy. I miscarried twice, the first time I was 8 weeks pregnant and the last time I was 26 weeks." The nurse correctly records Mrs. Barton's pregnancy status as
   a. Gravida 2 P0.
   b. Gravida 2 P1.
   c. Gravida 3 P1.
   d. Gravida 3 P0.

2. During the examination of a pregnant client, while lying in the lithotomy position the client complains of dizziness and nausea. What would be an appropriate nursing action to relieve the client's discomfort?
   a. Administering an antiemetic ordered by the physician.
   b. Offering small sips of ginger ale.

   c. Assisting the client to a side-lying position temporarily.
   d. Discontinuing the examination.

3. Diplopia was noted during the assessment of a pregnant client. This condition is described as
   a. elevated pigmentation of the skin.
   b. double vision.
   c. facial edema.
   d. gingivitis.

4. Which of the following injectable vaccines would be safe to administer to a pregnant client?
   a. Varicella.
   b. Measles.
   c. Mumps.
   d. Polio.

5. A pregnant client is in her 33rd week of gestation. The nurse would assist the client in scheduling her next appointment in
   a. 1 month.
   b. 3 weeks.
   c. 2 weeks.
   d. 1 week.

ALTERNATE FORMAT QUESTIONS
Multiple-Answer Multiple-Choice Questions

Circle the letter(s) corresponding to the appropriate answer(s). Select all that apply.

1. A nurse is teaching a pregnant woman about possible signs indicating complications that need to be reported immediately. Which of the following would the nurse include in the teaching?
   a. Vaginal bleeding.
   b. Fever.
   c. Vomiting once a day.
   d. Abdominal pain.
   e. Stress incontinence.

2. A woman comes to the clinic for a follow prenatal visit. She is 16 weeks pregnant. Which of the following would be done?
   a. Blood pressure measurement.
   b. Clean-catch urine specimen.
   c. Maternal serum level for alpha-fetoprotein.
   d. Glucose screening.
   e. Anti-Rh titer.

3. Which of the following actions would be most helpful for improving prenatal care services?

   a. Ensuring privacy for all assessments being completed.

   b. Scheduling appointments within 24 hours of first calling the setting.

   c. Using waiting room time by providing education.

   d. Recording pregnancy information so the woman can read it.

   e. Encouraging women to participate in decision-making about care.

Promoting Fetal and Maternal Health

CHAPTER OVERVIEW

Chapter 12 provides an overview of nursing care related to health promotion during pregnancy and the prevention of fetal exposure to teratogens. The general self-care needs of the pregnant woman, common discomforts encountered during pregnancy, and preparations for labor are reviewed. The use of the nursing process to plan and provide appropriate teaching for the woman throughout pregnancy is explored.

LEARNING OBJECTIVES

After mastering the content in this chapter, you should be able to do the following:

1. Describe health behaviors important for a healthy pregnancy outcome.

2. Identify National Health Goals related to a healthy pregnancy lifestyle that nurses can help the nation achieve.

3. Use critical thinking to analyze ways to promote both individualized and family-centered prenatal care.

4. Assess a woman for healthy practices and concerns during pregnancy.

5. Formulate nursing diagnoses related to a healthy pregnancy.

6. Identify expected outcomes to promote a healthy pregnancy such as encouraging daily exercise.

7. Plan health-promotion strategies to limit exposure to teratogens or reduce the minor discomforts of pregnancy.

8. Implement care to promote positive health practices during pregnancy.

9. Evaluate outcomes for achievement and effectiveness of care.

10. Identify areas of prenatal care that could benefit from additional nursing research or the application of evidence-based practice.

11. Integrate knowledge of health-promotion strategies with the nursing process to achieve quality maternal and child health nursing care.

KEY TERMS

cytomegalovirus	Sims' position
fetal alcohol syndrome	teratogen
leukorrhea	toxoplasmosis

MASTERING THE INFORMATION

FILL IN THE BLANKS

Supply the missing term or the information requested.

1. Assessment of the pregnant woman concentrates on screening for the presence of _____ in the pregnant woman's environment and any abnormalities that might be occurring with the pregnancy.

2. Breast tenderness is a common discomfort during the _____ trimester.

3. _____ are varicosities of the rectal veins.

MATCHING

Match the terms in Column I with a definition, example or related statement from Column II. Place the letter corresponding to the answer in the space provided.

Column I

1. ___ Braxton Hicks contractions

2. ___ Cytomegalovirus

3. ___ Fetal alcohol syndrome

4. ___ Leukorrhea

5. ___ Palmar erythema

6. ___ Headache

7. ___ Pelvic radiation

8. ___ Modified Sims' position

9. ___ Teratogen

10. ___ Toxoplasmosis

Column II

a. Whitish, viscous vaginal discharge.

b. A possible result of expanding blood volume that puts pressure on cerebral arteries.

c. Any factor, chemical or physical, that adversely affects the fertilized ovum, the embryo, or the fetus.

d. A protozoan infection spread through contact with cat stool.

e. Laterally lying with the abdomen on the bed and the top leg forward.

f. A member of the herpes family that can cause extensive fetal damage.

g. Infant who is small for gestational age, with mental retardation and characteristic craniofacial deformity.

h. Symptom occurring in early pregnancy, probably caused by increased estrogen levels.

i. Uterine cramps that may begin at the 8th to 12th week of pregnancy.

j. Necessary avoidance by all women of childbearing age except during the first 10 days of menstrual cycle.

SHORT ANSWER

Supply the missing term or the information requested.

1. What major intervention is associated with health promotion during pregnancy?

_____

_____

2. For each of the following activities, discuss one concept that should be discussed with the pregnant woman: bathing, breast care, perineal hygiene, dressing, sexual activity, exercise, sleep, and travel.

_____

_____

3. Describe five categories of potentially teratogenic drugs.

_____

_____

4. Discuss two instructions the nurse should provide to a pregnant woman who will be working related to all jobs, jobs requiring standing or walking, and jobs that require physical exertion.

_____

_____

5. Discuss how maternal stress may have a teratogenic effect.

_____

_____

APPLYING YOUR KNOWLEDGE

CASE STUDY

Ginene Varez, 31 years of age, visits your clinic for her first prenatal checkup. She is in her first trimester of pregnancy. She complains of skipping heartbeats, headache, and nausea, and states she is worried that the "tension" of her job as an accountant in a perfume factory will have a negative effect on her baby. Her blood pressure and pulse are in the normal range.

1. What would you explain to Ginene about a common physical change of pregnancy that has likely resulted in both the headache and heart palpitations?

_____

_____

_____

2. What measures would you suggest to help Ginene reduce anxiety from her job?

_____

_____

_____

CRITICAL INQUIRY EXERCISE

1. Prepare a teaching plan for a working woman that addresses methods for maintaining adequate nutrition and rest.

2. What are some realistic ways a pregnant woman can minimize exposure to common teratogens in the environment?

CRITICAL EXPLORATION

Observe the initial prenatal visit for women in each of the following age groups: 12 to 17, 25 to 30, and 35 to 40. Note the differences and similarities in instructions given regarding activities and rest, and nutritional needs.

PRACTICING FOR NCLEX

MULTIPLE-CHOICE QUESTIONS

Circle the letter that corresponds to the best answer for each question.

1. Bobby has been experiencing severe constipation during her eighth month of pregnancy. An appropriate goal or outcome for Bobby would be to
   a. become accustomed to the constipation and accept it as unavoidable.
   b. consume a diet containing high fiber, fruit, and extra amounts of fluid.
   c. have a bowel movement every other day to avoid daily straining activity.
   d. refrain from taking her iron supplement since it probably caused the problem.

2. When planning a teaching strategy for a pregnant woman, the nurse should do which of the following?
   a. Give information about how the woman can manage the specific problems she identifies as relevant in her life.
   b. Omit information related to minor pains of pregnancy to prevent the woman from developing hypochondria.
   c. Provide information to the woman in a group session with other pregnant women so she can have someone to discuss it with.
   d. During the first prenatal visit, teach a woman all the measures necessary for health promotion throughout the pregnancy.

3. Bonnie, 6 months pregnant, is commuting 2 to 3 hours by car to school for a 6-week session. The nurse should discuss which of the following with Bonnie about travel?
   a. Dangers related to wearing lap seatbelts during the early months of pregnancy.
   b. Methods of relieving stiffness and muscle aches and improving circulation during the drive.
   c. The importance of taking motion sickness medications to lessen the nausea from driving.
   d. The need to call her doctor and drive home immediately if she experiences premature labor or any danger signs of pregnancy.

4. Sheila, 7 months pregnant, reports feeling her heart skipping a beat sometimes. The nurse recognizes these as heart palpitations and identifies which of the following as an appropriate outcome? Sheila will
   a. demonstrate moving slowly from one position to another.
   b. lie supine when sleeping to keep pressure on her vena cava.
   c. plan a diet menu that includes high vitamin C content.
   d. verbalize intent to limit fluids to lower her heart's workload.

5. Dee is in her second month of pregnancy and complains of abdominal pain. Which action by the nurse would be most appropriate?

   a. Encourage Dee to put strong direct pressure on her fundus and hold it for 15 minutes whenever she feels this pain.

   b. Inform Dee that abdominal pain is expected at this stage of her pregnancy and she should learn to adjust to it.

   c. Inquire about the specific nature and location of the pain Dee reported, since it could indicate a complication.

   d. Tell Dee to lie on her side at night to relieve the pressure on her intestinal tract and stomach.

6. Which of the following would the nurse expect to assess less commonly in early pregnancy?

   a. Braxton Hicks contractions.

   b. Frequency of urination.

   c. Ankle edema.

   d. Varicosities.

7. Tina is a heavy smoker (two packs per day) and is pregnant. Which of the following measures undertaken by Tina would indicate that a teaching plan for her had been most effective?

   a. She limited her cigarette smoking to one pack per day during her last months of pregnancy.

   b. She decreased her smoking by two cigarettes per day until she had stopped completely.

   c. She stated she will smoke only filtered cigarettes while she is pregnant.

   d. She voiced understanding that she will use nicotine gum and stop smoking immediately.

ALTERNATE FORMAT QUESTIONS
Multiple-Answer Multiple-Choice Questions

Circle the letter(s) corresponding to the appropriate answer(s). Select all that apply.

1. Which of the following are common discomforts experienced during the first trimester of pregnancy?

   a. Hemorrhoids.

   b. Breast tenderness.

   c. Diarrhea.

   d. Menstrual "spotting."

   e. Frequent urination.

2. Which of the following would be viewed as signs of beginning labor.

   a. Depression.

   b. Rupture of membrane.

   c. Contractions.

   d. Slight elevation in temperature.

   e. Lightening.

3. A nurse would assess a pregnant woman for maternal infections that may cause fetal harm including which of the following?

   a. Rubella.

   b. Toxoplasmosis.

   c. Cytomegalovirus.

   d. Herpes simplex.

   e. Strep throat.

   f. Rhinovirus.

Promoting Nutritional Health During Pregnancy

CHAPTER OVERVIEW

Chapter 13 provides an overview of the nutritional needs of a woman throughout pregnancy. The nutritional guidelines for pregnancy are reviewed. Promoting nutrition in women with special needs is also addressed. The use of the nursing process to plan and provide appropriate teaching related to nutritional health during pregnancy is explored.

LEARNING OBJECTIVES

After mastering the content in this chapter, you should be able to do the following:

1. Discuss the recommendations for healthy nutrition during pregnancy.

2. Identify National Health Goals related to nutrition and pregnancy that nurses can help the nation achieve.

3. Use critical thinking to analyze the effects of different life situations on nutrition patterns to create ways nutritional health can be both improved and family centered.

4. Assess a woman for nutritional adequacy during pregnancy.

5. Formulate nursing diagnoses related to nutritional concerns during pregnancy.

6. Develop expected outcomes to assist a pregnant woman achieve optimal nutrition during pregnancy.

7. Plan health-teaching strategies, such as ways to increase folic acid and calcium intake to promote optimal nutritional intake during pregnancy.

8. Implement nursing care that encourages healthy nutritional practices during pregnancy.

9. Evaluate expected outcomes for achievement and effectiveness of care.

10. Identify areas related to nutrition and pregnancy that could benefit from additional nursing research or application of evidence-based practice.

11. Integrate nutrition knowledge with nursing process to achieve quality maternal and child health nursing care.

KEY TERMS

body mass index
complete protein
Hawthorne effect
heartburn (pyrosis)
hypercholesterolemia
hyperplasia
hypertrophy
incomplete
    protein
lactase
obese
overweight
pica
underweight

MASTERING THE INFORMATION

FILL IN THE BLANKS

Supply the missing term or the information requested.

1. A weight gain of _____ to _____ kg is currently recommended as an average weight gain in pregnancy.

2. Pregnant women who are vegetarians may lack vitamin _____, vitamin _____, and _____ in their diet.

3. Underweight women may need to increase their caloric intake by _____ to _____ calories above the calories ordinarily specified during pregnancy.

MATCHING

Match the terms in Column I with a definition, example, or related statement from Column II. Place the letter corresponding to the answer in the space provided.

Column I

1. ____ Complete protein
2. ____ Hyperplasia
3. ____ Incomplete protein
4. ____ Lactase
5. ____ Linoleic acid
6. ____ Obese
7. ____ Phenylketonuria
8. ____ Pica
9. ____ Complementary proteins
10. ____ Pyrosis

Column II

a. A fatty oil that cannot be manufactured in the body from other sources.
b. Foods containing fewer than eight of the essential amino acids.
c. An abnormal craving for nonfood substances.
d. A food containing all eight essential amino acids.
e. An increase in the number of cells formed.
f. Foods that when cooked together provide all eight amino acids.
g. A burning sensation along the esophagus caused by decreased gastric motility.

h. For a woman weighing over 200 pounds, having a body mass index over 30, or being 50% above ideal body weight.
i. The enzyme needed to break down milk sugar into glucose and galactose.
j. An inability to convert an essential amino acid into tyrosine.

SHORT ANSWER

Supply the missing term or the information requested.

1. Discuss the relationship between maternal dietary intake and fetal growth and development.

2. What factors may cause a woman to have decreased nutritional stores during pregnancy?

3. Discuss two types of food that should be avoided in pregnancy. Why should these foods be avoided?

4. Indicate the sources of the following substances and their significance for the pregnant woman: protein, calcium, fat, folic acid, iodine, iron.

APPLYING YOUR KNOWLEDGE

CASE STUDY

Ellen, age 16, is in her second trimester of pregnancy. She is at the clinic for her initial prenatal visit.

1. What are the most important initial assessments you would make before discussing nutritional needs with Ellen?

2. What nutritional intake behaviors do most adolescents exhibit that might make it difficult to promote adequate nutrition for Ellen and her fetus?

_____

_____

_____

3. Compare the dietary instructions you might provide for a pregnant adolescent like Ellen with those for a pregnant woman over age 40.

_____

_____

_____

CRITICAL INQUIRY EXERCISE

1. Prepare a 24-hour recall history using your own nutritional intake. Assess your dietary intake for adequacy. What changes would be necessary if you were pregnant?

2. What are five common foods served at fast-food restaurants that could be eaten to meet nutritional requirements? What are five foods that would be poor nutritional choices for the pregnant woman?

CRITICAL EXPLORATION

Perform a diet history on a pregnant adolescent woman and develop a teaching plan that addresses the nutritional needs of pregnancy.

PRACTICING FOR NCLEX

MULTIPLE-CHOICE QUESTIONS

Circle the letter that corresponds to the best answer for each question.

1. Which of the following measures undertaken by a pregnant woman would indicate that a teaching plan on nutrition during pregnancy had been effective?

a. Plans a diet limiting protein intake to minimize metabolic waste during her last months of pregnancy.

b. Remains slim during the first 5 months of her pregnancy and small during the final months of pregnancy.

c. States she understands that, although she is obese, she should not diet to lose weight but should avoid eating empty calories.

d. Voices understanding that she should take over-the-counter vitamin and mineral preparations twice daily to supplement her diet.

2. Pam is a 23-year-old single mother who has a 15-month-old and a 3-month-old who was premature; she had a miscarriage before the birth of her 3-month-old. Her diet history revealed that she likes to eat fish and chicken. Pam should be considered at nutritional risk because of her

a. prior pregnancies.

b. risky age group.

c. single marital status.

d. unusual food preferences.

3. A woman with phenylketonuria should do which of the following?

a. Avoid pregnancy, since it would aggravate her condition.

b. Avoid food restrictions of any kind during her pregnancy.

c. Return to a low-phenylalanine diet before becoming pregnant.

d. Increase her intake of phenylalanine if she will breastfeed.

4. Which of the following would be an appropriate nursing intervention to help a woman with nausea and vomiting maintain adequate nutritional intake?

a. Advise her to take daily laxatives to stimulate peristalsis and food digestion.

b. Encourage her to eat meals before going to bed, when nausea is less severe.

c. Suggest she eat foods that are high in fat to increase caloric intake.

d. Teach her to refrain from eating for at least 6 hours prior to bedtime.

ALTERNATE FORMAT QUESTIONS

Multiple-Answer Multiple-Choice Questions

Circle the letter(s) corresponding to the appropriate answer(s). Select all that apply.

1. Which of the following foods would be most appropriate for the nurse to suggest a pregnant client consume if that client is experiencing low hemoglobin levels?

   a. Eggs.

   b. Vegetable oils.

   c. Milk.

   d. Green leafy vegetable.

   e. Organ meats.

2. Bonnie, 3 months pregnant, has reported for her first prenatal visit. The nurse should instruct her to do which of the following?

   a. Eat foods rich in protein, iron, and other nutrients to provide an additional 300 calories each day.

   b. Increase her intake of carbohydrates such as breads and sweets to prevent protein metabolism.

   c. Eat small and frequent meals to increase absorption and decrease nausea.

   d. Eat whenever she feels hungry because her body will let her know when she needs nutrients and extra calories.

   e. Limit intake of amino acids to prevent development of diabetic ketoacidosis.

3. A pregnant woman is experiencing pyrosis. Which of the following instructions would be most helpful?

   a. Eating small more frequent meals rather than larger ones.

   b. Sleeping on her left side with two pillows.

   c. Waiting at least 2 hours after eating before attempting to lie down.

   d. Consuming increased amounts of tuna and swordfish.

   e. Avoiding the intake of oils, such as olive oil in the diet.

Preparing a Family for Childbirth and Parenting

CHAPTER OVERVIEW

Chapter 14 addresses the woman and family who are preparing for the birth of a child. Physical and psychological readiness is addressed in terms of exercises and psychological techniques for pain control. The nursing interventions during the laboring process in the various types of birth settings are presented. The chapter presents a case study that describes principles pertinent to providing guidance to parents who may choose to participate in an alternative birth method.

LEARNING OBJECTIVES

After mastering the content in this chapter, you should be able to do the following:

1. Describe common preparations for childbirth and parenting including common settings for birth.

2. Identify National Health Goals related to preparation for parenthood that nurses can help the nation achieve.

3. Use critical thinking to analyze ways that birth can be made more family centered through the use of prepared childbirth classes and alternative birth settings.

4. Assess a couple for readiness for childbirth in regard to choice of birth attendant, preparation for labor, and setting.

5. Formulate nursing diagnoses related to preparation for childbirth and parenting.

6. Identify expected outcomes for a couple preparing for childbirth and parenting.

7. Plan nursing care such as teaching exercises for strengthening abdominal and perineal muscles for childbirth.

8. Implement nursing care such as supporting a woman during labor by the Lamaze method of childbirth or helping a couple select and prepare for an alternative birth setting such as the home.

9. Evaluate outcome criteria for achievement and effectiveness of care.

10. Identify areas related to preparation for childbirth that could benefit from additional nursing research or application of evidence-based practice.

11. Integrate the principles of prepared childbirth with nursing process to achieve quality maternal and child health nursing care.

KEY TERMS

alternative birthing
  centers (ABCs)
birthing bed
birthing chairs
birthing room
cleansing breath
conditioned reflexes

consciously controlled
  breathing
conscious relaxation
distraction
doula
effleurage

gating control theory of pain perception

labor-delivery-recovery-postpartum room (LDRP)

Leboyer method

psychoprophylactic vaginal birth after cesarean birth (VBAC)

e. Positioning the feet flat on the floor while stretching the perineal muscles.

f. Method of childbirth based on the premise that fear lead to tension, which leads to pain.

MASTERING THE INFORMATION

FILL IN THE BLANKS

Supply the missing term or the information requested.

1. Encouraging progressive breathing, including conscious relaxation, is called _____.

2. _____ is light abdominal massage in conjunction with breathing exercises.

3. _____ exercises are used with repetition to strengthen the floor of the perineum.

4. Prevention of pain during birth by use of the mind is called the _____ method.

MATCHING

Match the terms in Column I with a definition, example, or related statement from Column II. Place the letter corresponding to the answer in the space provided.

Column I

1. ___ Imagery

2. ___ Dick-Read method

3. ___ Conditioned reflex

4. ___ Tailor sitting

5. ___ Squatting

6. ___ Bradley method

Column II

a. Measure that maintains blood supply to the lower limbs while stretching the perineum.

b. A physical response prompted by hearing a word or phrase.

c. Method of childbirth based on the belief that birth is a natural process that should include the husband during the entire birthing process.

d. Intense focusing on an object ("sensate focus") to keep sensory input from reaching the cortex of the brain.

SHORT ANSWER

Supply the missing term or the information requested.

1. Describe the physiology of the following techniques of the gate control theory.

   a. Distraction

   _____

   _____

   b. Reduction of anxiety

   _____

   _____

2. Identify the advantages and disadvantages for the following birth settings.

   a. Hospital

      i. Advantages

      _____

      _____

      ii. Disadvantages

      _____

      _____

   b. Alternative birth center

      i. Advantages

      _____

      _____

      ii. Disadvantages

      _____

      _____

   c. Home birth

      i. Advantages

      _____

      _____

      ii. Disadvantages

      _____

      _____

APPLYING YOUR KNOWLEDGE

CASE STUDY

Mrs. Virion, age 22, is interested in delivering her baby at home.

1. What factors would cause a woman to be considered a good candidate for a home birth?

_____

_____

_____

2. What is considered to be the main advantage of a home birth?

_____

_____

_____

3. State the expected outcomes when teaching Mrs. Virion how to perform the following exercises: abdominal contraction, pelvic floor contractions, and pelvic rocking.

_____

_____

_____

CRITICAL INQUIRY EXERCISE

1. Develop a teaching plan for the techniques of perineal exercises. Include a proposed time schedule for implementing the exercises for a woman who works from 8 AM to 5 PM.

2. Outline the main features of the popular Lamaze method of birthing. What behavioral characteristics would you look for in the family who would be most appropriate for this method?

CRITICAL EXPLORATION

1. Attend a prenatal class at a well-baby health clinic. Present an overview of childbirth methods and education principles; discuss the ultimate goal of childbirth. Then provide the names of some referral sources to the mothers so they may obtain more information on childbirth and parenting education.

2. Interview a couple who has recently become aware of their pregnancy. Discuss several alternative settings for the birth and emphasize the advantages and disadvantages of each.

PRACTICING FOR NCLEX

MULTIPLE-CHOICE QUESTIONS

Circle the letter that corresponds to the best answer for each question.

1. Effleurage, a technique used to displace pain, is described as
   a. light abdominal massage.
   b. focusing on an object to block sensory input.
   c. the prophylaxis method.
   d. the psychosexual method.

2. In consciously controlled breathing methods, level 5 behaviors are defined as
   a. slow chest breathing at a rate of 6 to 12 breaths per minute.
   b. shallow, continuous chest panting at about 60 breaths per minute.
   c. pant-blow rhythm intermittently with forceful exhalations.
   d. light breathing with rib cage expansion up to 40 breaths per minute.

3. Flexing the lumbar spine can relieve backaches during pregnancy and early labor. This exercise is called
   a. Kegel exercising.
   b. pelvic rocking.
   c. squatting.
   d. tailor sitting.

ALTERNATE FORMAT QUESTIONS

Multiple-Answer Multiple-Choice Questions

Circle the letter(s) corresponding to the appropriate answer(s). Select all that apply.

1. Which of the following would be most appropriate to do for the birth environment in preparation for the Leboyer method?
   a. Spraying the birthing room just before delivery with insecticides to reduce the microorganism counts.
   b. Raising the temperature of the room slightly just before the birth.
   c. Keeping the birthing room as cool as the hospital delivery room to reduce the chance of bacteria growth.

d. Darkening the room after the birth and assessment to lessen the impact of the environmental change on the newborn.

e. Adjusting the room to operate as a negative pressure room to insure protection from environmental infections.

2. Which of the following instructions would be most appropriate to help a pregnant woman avoid orthostatic hypertension?

a. Sitting upright on awakening for several minutes before standing.

b. Holding her breath while exercising.

c. Hyperextending her lower back.

d. Getting up slowly from the floor after exercising.

e. Rolling from side to side during exercise.

3. When instructing a pregnant woman about exercises to strengthen muscles in preparation for labor and birth, which of the following would be included?

a. Extend the heel rather than pointing your toes.

b. Never practice second stage pushing.

c. Put one leg on top of the other with tailor sitting.

d. Wait until you are in your third trimester before doing the exercises.

e. Rise from the floor slowly to avoid dizziness.

Nursing Care of a Family During Labor and Birth

CHAPTER OVERVIEW

Chapter 15 provides an overview of the components and process of labor and discusses nursing care of the woman and her family in labor. Problems and concerns that may manifest during each stage of labor are reviewed. The use of the nursing process to plan and provide care throughout the stages of labor is explored.

LEARNING OBJECTIVES

After mastering the content in this chapter, you should be able to do the following:

1. Describe common theories explaining the onset of labor and the role of passenger, passage, and powers in labor.

2. Identify National Health Goals related to safe labor and birth that nurses can help the nation achieve.

3. Use critical thinking to analyze ways that nurses can make labor and birth more family centered.

4. Assess a family in labor, identifying the woman's readiness, stage, and progression.

5. Formulate nursing diagnoses related to the physiologic and psychological aspects of labor and birth.

6. Establish expected outcomes to meet the needs of a family throughout the labor process.

7. Plan nursing interventions to meet the needs and promote optimal outcomes for a woman and her family during labor and birth.

8. Implement nursing care for a family during labor such as teaching about the stages of labor.

9. Evaluate expected outcomes for achievement and effectiveness of care.

10. Identify areas related to labor and birth that could benefit from additional nursing research or application of evidence-based practice.

11. Integrate knowledge of nursing care in labor with nursing process to achieve quality maternal and child health nursing care.

KEY TERMS

attitude	Leopold's maneuvers
breech presentation	lie
cardinal movements	molding
of labor	pathologic retraction
cephalic presentation	ring
crowning	physiologic retraction
dilatation	ring
effacement	position
engagement	ripening
episiotomy	station
fetal descent	transition

MASTERING THE INFORMATION

FILL IN THE BLANKS

Supply the missing term or the information requested.

1. As the fetal head moves from above to below, the level of the ischial spines, the station, or degree of engagement moves from _____ to _____ stations.

2. The first division of the first stage of labor is the _____ division.

3. The softening of the cervix, which occurs in preparation for labor, is called _____.

MATCHING

Match the terms in Column I with a definition, example, or related statement from Column II. Place the letter corresponding to the answer in the space provided.

Column I

1. ____ Attitude
2. ____ Crowning
3. ____ Amnioinfusion
4. ____ Effacement
5. ____ Engagement
6. ____ Fontanelle
7. ____ Labor
8. ____ Molding
9. ____ Physiologic retraction ring
10. ____ Power
11. ____ Braxton Hicks

Column II

a. Occurs when the presenting part of the fetus has settled into the pelvis at the level of the ischial spines.

b. The shortening and thinning of the cervical canal.

c. Membrane-covered spaces at the junction of the main fetal skull suture lines.

d. The degree of flexion the fetus assumes or the relation of the fetal parts to each other.

e. The change in shape of the fetal skull produced by the force of the uterine contractions pressing the vertex against the closed cervix.

f. A series of events by which uterine contractions expel the fetus and placenta from the woman's body.

g. A ridge of the inner uterine surface representing the boundary between the thick active and thinner inactive portions of the uterus.

h. The addition of a sterile fluid into the pregnant uterus.

i. Irregular uterine cramps, which may signal the impending onset of true labor.

j. Supplied by the fundus of the uterus and supplemented by abdominal muscles; results in the expulsion of the fetus from the uterus.

k. The appearance of the presenting part of the fetus at the opening in the vagina.

Additional Matching Exercises

Column I

1. ____ The occiput of the fetus points to the left anterior quadrant in a vertex position.

2. ____ The triangular fontanelle points toward the right anterior pelvic quadrant.

3. ____ The fetal anus of a breech presentation is pointed toward the right maternal pelvis.

4. ____ The fetal chin is facing left across the pelvic midsection.

5. ____ The fetal shoulder is located in the right lower posterior pelvic area.

Column II

a. Right scapuloposterior (RAP)
b. Left occipitotransverse (LOT)
c. Left mentotransverse (LMT)
d. Right occipitoanterior (ROA)

e. Left occipitoanterior (LOA)

f. Right sacroanterior (RSaA)

SHORT ANSWER

Supply the missing term or the information requested.

1. Following rupture of the membranes, _____ should be taken every hour because of the possibility of infection.

2. During the process of labor, the fetus passes from the _____ through the _____ and _____ to the _____ _____.

3. Three of the six signs of impending labor are _____, _____, and _____.

4. The four integrated concepts contributing to the success of labor include: _____ (fetus), _____ (woman's pelvis), _____ (uterine factors), and _____(woman's feelings).

5. The four methods by which the fetal position, presentation, and lie are established are combined abdominal _____ and _____, _____ _____, auscultation of _____ _____ _____, and _____.

6. Discuss three of the factors that may influence the beginning of labor.

_____

_____

7. Discuss the role of diaphoresis in temperature regulation during labor.

_____

_____

8. Describe the resulting effect when a body part other than the vertex presents.

_____

_____

9. Describe the process and purpose of Leopold's maneuvers.

_____

_____

10. Discuss the psychological responses of a woman to labor and the nurse's role.

_____

_____

11. Compare and contrast the changes occurring in the maternal pulse and blood pressure with changes occurring in the fetal pulse and blood pressure during contractions.

_____

_____

12. Discuss the role that the father or a significant other might play in the labor experience.

_____

_____

13. Indicate the significance of each of the following abnormal fetal heart rate patterns: fetal tachycardia, fetal bradycardia, late deceleration, variable pattern, and sinusoidal pattern.

_____

_____

APPLYING YOUR KNOWLEDGE

CASE STUDY

Effie is a 21-year-old primipara who has completed natural childbirth classes with her coach, her husband. She is admitted at noon to the birthing room after 3 hours of active labor at home. She is dilated 3 cm and 80% effaced. Her sister is with her, and she is concerned about causing her husband to miss time at work needlessly early. He is a low-paid hourly worker, and they are a one-income family.

1. What would you explain to Effie about the progression of her labor, and how would you advise her regarding contacting her husband?

_____

_____

_____

2. How could you support Effie, or teach the family to support Effie, if her husband was not present during the second stage of her labor?

_____

_____

_____

3. How would your support for Effie differ if she were a woman who had previously had a difficult delivery?

_____

_____

_____

CRITICAL INQUIRY EXERCISE

1. Prepare a teaching plan for a woman in labor that addresses methods for maintaining a maximum state of comfort during the first and second stages of labor.

2. Briefly explain how you would support a woman who has decided to put her baby up for adoption through the labor process. How would your support measures differ, if at all, for an adolescent girl?

CRITICAL EXPLORATION

Chart the progression of a woman in the active phases of labor on commercial graph forms or using square-ruled graph paper. Note if the progression appears normal or abnormal by comparison with the chart presented in your text.

PRACTICING FOR NCLEX

MULTIPLE-CHOICE QUESTIONS

Circle the letter that corresponds to the best answer for each question.

1. Bobby has been experiencing regular, coordinated contractions with cervical dilation moving from 4 to 6 cm in the last half-hour, and her membranes are still intact. Bobby is in which stage of labor?

   a. Latent phase of the second stage of labor.

   b. Active phase of the first stage of labor.

   c. Placental stage or the third stage of labor.

   d. Second stage of labor.

2. When planning comfort measures to help the woman in active labor tolerate her pain, the nurse must consider which of the following?

   a. Early labor contractions are usually regular, coordinated, and very painful.

   b. If properly prepared, women will require no pain medication.

   c. Pain medication given during the latent phase of labor is not likely to impair contractions.

   d. The active phase of labor can be a time of true discomfort and high anxiety.

3. Sheila is in her first stage of labor and the nurse notices a prominent and observable abdominal indentation that she recognizes as a pathologic retraction ring. The nurse should respond to these findings by doing which of the following?

   a. Inform Sheila that this indentation is normal, to decrease her anxiety.

   b. Instruct Sheila to lie on her right side to prevent pressure on her abdomen.

   c. Recognize this as an indication that labor is almost complete.

   d. Report this danger sign to the physician immediately.

4. Frances is admitted in active labor. The nurse locates fetal heart sounds in the upper left quadrant of her abdomen. The nurse would recognize which of the following?

   a. Frances will probably deliver very quickly and without problems.

   b. This indicates that the fetus is probably in the breech position.

   c. The fetus is in the most common anterior fetal position.

   d. This position is referred to as being left anteriopelvic.

5. While interviewing a woman in labor, which information would be least important to obtain?

   a. Whether the pregnancy was planned.

   b. The use of drugs or medications during pregnancy.

c. Maternal concerns regarding fetal health.

d. If the woman's mother has come with her.

6. When timing the length of a contraction, the nurse would do which of the following?

   a. Ask the woman when the beginning of the contraction is felt, then time the interval from this point until the woman states the contraction has subsided.

   b. Gently palpate the abdomen for the beginning of the tightening of the uterus; time the interval from this point until the uterine tightening subsides.

   c. Lightly touch the abdomen and time the interval from the beginning of the uterine tensing to the beginning of the next tensing.

   d. Note the upward slopes of the contraction on the monitor graph and measure from one upward slope to the next upward slope.

7. Which of the following is very important when performing fetal monitoring?

   a. Informing the mother and significant others that the fetal heart rate will vary during the labor process.

   b. Instructing the mother that she must lie supine to obtain the most accurate readings of fetal status.

   c. Keeping the monitor strap on the woman's abdomen tightly and securely fitted despite maternal discomfort.

   d. Maintaining a continuous watch on the monitor, since it is the primary source of data on maternal—fetal status.

8. When preparing a pregnant client for internal electronic fetal monitoring, which of the following would the nurse need to keep in mind?

   a. There is little restriction on maternal ambulation.

   b. It can be applied before rupture of the membranes.

   c. A clearer printout of the fetal heart rate is provided.

   d. It cannot be initiated if the fetal head is engaged.

9. Which assessment finding would lead the nurse to suspect fetal distress?

   a. Fetal heart rate acceleration occurring with fetal movement.

   b. Early decelerations occurring during contractions late in labor.

   c. Serial fetal blood pH levels of 7.10 to 7.15.

   d. Fetus is positioned in the left occipitoanterior area.

10. If variable deceleration is noted on the fetal heart monitor, the nurse should do which of the following?

    a. Limit oral and intravenous fluids to decrease maternal fluid volume and decrease circulatory overload.

    b. Prepare a needle and large syringe so that excess amniotic fluid causing the problem can be removed.

    c. Remove oxygen, if present, and instruct the mother to breathe slowly, since this is a sign of hyperventilation.

    d. Turn the mother to a different position to relieve pressure on the umbilical cord and restore circulation.

11. If a woman will be placing her baby up for adoption, which of the following nursing measures should be implemented during labor?

    a. Avoid discussing the baby during the health history to minimize the woman's anxiety.

    b. Support the woman as needed by accepting the decisions she makes regarding holding the baby.

    c. Protect the woman from visitors and family members who might try to change her mind.

    d. Take the baby away as soon as possible after birth to prevent bonding from occurring.

12. After the placenta is delivered, the nurse may have which of the following responsibilities?

    a. Administering intramuscular oxytocin to facilitate uterine contractility.

    b. Monitoring for blood loss greater than 60 cc indicative of gross hemorrhage.

    c. Noting if the placenta makes a Schultze presentation, which is a sign of a major complication.

    d. Pushing down on the relaxed uterus to aid in the removal of the placenta.

13. Immediately after episiotomy repair, the nurse would do which of the following?

    a. Cleanse the woman's anal area, then perineum and vulva, to remove any fecal incontinence or vaginal secretions.

    b. Monitor the woman for shaking and complaints of chill sensations, which may indicate an adverse reaction to medications.

    c. Palpate the uterine fundus for size, consistency, and position, and take vital signs to obtain baseline data.

    d. Remove all coverings except a clean, light hospital gown to prevent the development of postpartal fever.

14. Which of the following outcomes would be appropriate for the woman in labor without a support person? The client will

    a. reunite with her child's father before labor is complete.

    b. verbalize that she felt supported during the labor process.

    c. indicate that she was comfortable going through labor alone.

    d. state the labor process was a smooth, rewarding experience.

15. Which of the following signs could indicate maternal distress during labor?

    a. Maternal heart rate of 90 to 100 beats per minute during labor.

    b. Uterine contractions less frequent and intense as labor progresses.

    c. Reports of feeling the need to have a bowel movement.

    d. Contractions lasting for approximately 60 to 90 seconds.

ALTERNATE FORMAT QUESTIONS

Multiple-Answer Multiple-Choice Questions

Circle the letter(s) corresponding to the appropriate answer(s). Select all that apply.

1. When teaching a pregnant woman about a vaginal birth after cesarean birth (VBAC), which information would be most appropriate to include?

    a. Instructions regarding the labor process are not needed.

    b. The woman may respond as if this is her first labor experience.

    c. The outcome of VBAC is usually without complications.

    d. Women usually prefer cesarean birth to vaginal delivery.

    e. The woman may need oxytocin to help strengthen uterine contractions.

2. Which assessment findings would lead the nurse to suspect that a pregnant woman is in the transition phase of the first stage of labor?

    a. Cervix is dilated 9 cm.

    b. Contractions occur every 2 minutes.

    c. Contractions last about 30 seconds.

    d. Cervix is dilated 3 cm.

    e. Women resists being touched.

3. Passage of the fetus through the birth canal involves different position changes. Place the position changes below in the sequence that they occur.

    a. Internal rotation.

    b. Descent.

    c. Flexion.

    d. External rotation.

    e. Extension.

    f. Expulsion.

Hot Spot Questions
Using the illustration, indicate the term or phrase that describes the fetal position that is occurring.

1.

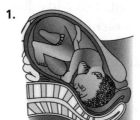

    a. Extension.

    b. Internal rotation.

2.

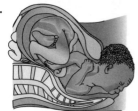

a. Extension.

b. Flexion.

Using the illustration, indicate the location of the fetal head when it is engaged.

3.

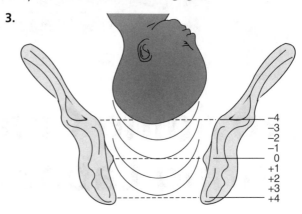

16

Providing Comfort During Labor and Birth

CHAPTER OVERVIEW

Chapter 16 provides an overview of the physiology and perception of pain during labor and principles of pain management, including pharmacologic methods and support of the woman's chosen technique for relaxation and prepared childbirth. The use of the nursing process to plan and provide comfort for the woman throughout labor and delivery is explored.

LEARNING OBJECTIVES

After mastering the content in this chapter, you should be able to do the following:

1. Describe the physiologic basis of contractions during labor and how analgesia, anesthesia, and alternative therapies can be used to promote a woman's comfort during labor and birth.

2. Identify National Health Goals related to analgesia and anesthesia and childbirth that nurses can help the nation achieve.

3. Use critical thinking to analyze ways to maintain family-centered care when analgesia and anesthesia are used in childbirth.

4. Assess the degree and type of discomfort a woman is experiencing during labor and birth, including her ability to cope with it effectively.

5. Formulate nursing diagnoses related to the effect of pain or pain management during labor and birth.

6. Establish expected outcomes to meet the needs of a woman experiencing discomfort during labor and birth.

7. Plan nursing interventions to promote comfort during labor and birth such as teaching about relaxation or breathing exercises.

8. Implement common complementary and pharmacologic measures for pain management during labor and birth.

9. Evaluate expected outcomes for effectiveness and achievement of care.

10. Identify areas related to promoting comfort during labor that could benefit from additional nursing research or application of evidence-based practice.

11. Integrate knowledge of pain management during labor and birth with the nursing process to achieve quality maternal and child health nursing care.

KEY TERMS

analgesia
anesthesia
doula
endorphins
epidural anesthesia
pain

pressure anesthesia
pudendal nerve block
transcutaneous electrical nerve stimulation (TENS)

MASTERING THE INFORMATION

MATCHING

Match the terms in Column I with a definition, example, or related statement from Column II. Place the letter corresponding to the answer in the space provided.

Column I

1. ___ Aspiration

2. ___ Endorphin

3. ___ Spinal anesthesia

4. ___ General anesthesia

5. ___ Pain

6. ___ Meperidine hydrochloride (Demerol)

7. ___ Pudendal nerve block

8. ___ Regional anesthesia

9. ___ Transcutaneous electrical nerve stimulation (TENS)

10. ___ Intrathecal narcotics

Column II

a. Injection of anesthetic at the level of the ischial spine; allows for low forceps delivery and episiotomy repair.

b. A synthetic narcotic with sedative and antispasmodic action.

c. Opiate-like substance produced naturally by the body to reduce pain.

d. Minimal fetal effects when compared with systemic anesthetics; leaves the uterus capable of optimal postpartal contraction.

e. A subjective symptom; any sensation of discomfort.

f. Blockage of afferent fibers, preventing pain from traveling to the spinal cord synapses from the uterus; also effective with extreme back pain.

g. A local anesthetic agent injected into the third lumbar space.

h. An injection of medication into the spinal canal by way of a catheter.

i. Inhalation of vomitus that may cause occlusion of the airway.

j. Not a preferred method of pain control in childbirth; requires maternal intubation and increases the risk of aspiration.

SHORT ANSWER

Supply the missing term or the information requested.

1. The use of pain control drugs during labor and delivery and the associated risks of fetal bradycardia and maternal hypotension must be weighed against the alternative risk to the mother. What would this risk be?

_____

_____

2. How can nurses help the nation meet the goals of reducing maternal and fetal deaths related to analgesia and anesthesia administered during labor and birth?

_____

_____

3. During uterine contractions of labor, the two major sources of pain are _____ and _____.

4. During the first stage of labor, pain relief must either be _____ or block the synapse sites at spinal column level _____ through _____.

5. Discuss the significance of informing a woman about the use of drugs and the ultimate effect of the various pain relief measures.

_____

_____

6. Explain how knowledge regarding the labor and delivery process might have an impact on the pain experienced during labor.

_____

_____

7. Discuss the importance of timing in the administration of pain relief medications during labor.

_____

_____

8. Discuss the role that a significant other might play in facilitating pain relief during the labor experience.

_____

_____

APPLYING YOUR KNOWLEDGE

CASE STUDY

Alice and Mike are in the birthing room performing breathing exercises during her third hour of true labor. This is their first pregnancy and birth. Alice is dilated 4 cm. Mike appears nervous but is enthusiastic and caring in his coaching.

1. What impact could Mike's nervousness have on Alice and the progress of her labor? What nursing actions would be indicated to address his nervousness?

_____

_____

_____

2. Alice has asked about the risks of using a narcotic analgesic to relieve her pain now. What information would you give her regarding the benefits and disadvantages of analgesic agents at this stage in her labor?

_____

_____

_____

3. What information would you give Alice and Mike about pain control during the second and third phases of labor?

_____

_____

_____

CRITICAL INQUIRY EXERCISE

1. Prepare a pain management plan for a woman in labor that includes two nonpharmacologic pain relief measures and two medical pain relief methods, with nursing implications for monitoring and prevention of drug-related complications.

2. Prepare a checklist of the priority assessments and related nursing actions for managing pain in each stage of labor.

CRITICAL EXPLORATION

Monitor a woman through the entire labor process. Note the methods used by the woman and the health care team to maintain a maximum state of comfort during the first and second stages of labor.

PRACTICING FOR NCLEX

MULTIPLE-CHOICE QUESTIONS

Circle the letter that corresponds to the best answer for each question.

1. Barbara, a primipara, has been experiencing regular contractions with cervical dilation at 2 cm. Barbara could use which of the following pain relief measures safely?
   a. Acetylsalicylic acid.
   b. Breathing exercises.
   c. Narcotic analgesic.
   d. Pressure anesthesia.

2. When planning comfort measures to help the woman in active labor cope with her pain, the nurse must consider which of the following?
   a. Early labor contractions are usually regular, coordinated, and very painful.
   b. Proper preparation for labor typically results in the need for less medication to manage their pain.
   c. Pain medication given during the latent phase of labor is not likely to impair contractions.
   d. The transition phase of labor represents a time of minimum pain and discomfort.

3. Which of the following actions should the nurse take when administering meperidine (Demerol) to a woman in labor?
   a. Administer a dose of naloxone (Narcan) with the medication to boost the antianxiety effects.
   b. Inject the medication into the woman's subcutaneous tissue.
   c. Monitor the newborn for sedation for 3 to 4 hours after the drug is administered.
   d. Reassure the woman that this drug does not cross the placenta.

4. Which of the following would be most helpful for a pregnant woman in labor who has known heart disease?
   a. An epidural block.
   b. General anesthesia.
   c. Narcotic analgesics.
   d. Patient-controlled analgesia.

5. Which of the following measures could a nurse take to facilitate comfort in the labor process?

a. Apply a sanitary pad to decrease discomfort from vaginal secretions.

b. If membranes are ruptured and the fetus is not engaged, encourage ambulation.

c. Smooth the wrinkles from bed linen and remove sticky bedclothes.

d. Tell the woman to remain as still as possible throughout the labor process to decrease stimulation.

ALTERNATE FORMAT QUESTIONS

Multiple-Answer Multiple-Choice Questions

Circle the letter(s) corresponding to the appropriate answer(s). Select all that apply.

1. Which of the following drug types most likely would produce a fetal effect.

a. Drugs with a molecular weight above 1000.

b. Drugs with a molecular weight below 600.

c. Drugs that strongly bind to protein.

d. Fat-soluble drugs.

e. Drugs administered to a woman with a premature fetus.

f. Drugs that cause systemic maternal hypotension.

2. Which of the following outcomes indicate that pain management during labor has been effective. Select all that apply.

a. The woman reports pain now level 1 down from a level 8.

b. The fetal heart rate is reduced from 160 to 110.

c. The woman reports being more relaxed.

d. The contractions decrease in frequency and become less intense.

e. The woman's blood pressure is reduced from 130/76 to 100/40 mm Hg.

f. The woman's pushing efforts are increased.

3. Which of the following drugs would most likely be administered intrathecally for pain relief during labor?

a. Meperidine.

b. Morphine.

c. Fentanyl citrate.

d. Nalbuphine.

e. Butorphanol.

Nursing Care of the Postpartal Family

CHAPTER OVERVIEW

Chapter 17 presents an overview of the physiologic and psychological care of the postpartal woman and her family. The physiologic changes that occur after childbirth and the emotional effects of childbirth on the entire postpartal family are discussed. The use of the nursing process to plan and provide care for the postpartal family is explored.

LEARNING OBJECTIVES

After mastering the content in this chapter, you should be able to do the following:

1. Describe the psychological and physiologic changes that occur in a postpartal woman.

2. Identify National Health Goals related to the postpartal period that nurses can help the nation achieve.

3. Use critical thinking to analyze ways that postpartum nursing care can be more family centered.

4. Assess a woman and her family for physiologic and psychological changes after childbirth.

5. Formulate nursing diagnoses related to physi-ologic and psychological transitions of the postpartal period.

6. Identify expected outcomes for a postpartal woman and family related to the changes during this period.

7. Plan nursing care such as measures to aid uterine involution or encourage bonding.

8. Implement nursing care to aid the progression of physiologic and psychological transitions occurring in a postpartal woman and family such as teaching about breastfeeding.

9. Evaluate outcome criteria for the achievement and effectiveness of care.

10. Identify areas related to care of the postpartal family that could benefit from additional nursing research or application of evidence-based practice.

11. Integrate knowledge of the physiologic and psychological changes of the postpartal period with the nursing process to achieve quality maternal and child health nursing care.

KEY TERMS

afterpains	lochia
diastasis recti	postpartal depression
en face position	rooming-in
engorgement	sitz bath
engrossment	taking-hold phase
Homans' sign	taking-in phase
involution	uterine atony
letting-go phase	

MASTERING THE INFORMATION

FILL IN THE BLANKS

Supply the missing term or the information requested.

1. _____ exercises consists of contracting and relaxing the muscles of the perineum.

2. The pink or brownish vaginal drainage noted around the fourth postpartal day is called _____.

3. _____ refers to contraction of the uterus after birth causing intermittent cramping.

MATCHING

Match the terms in Column I with a definition, example, or related statement from Column II. Place the letter corresponding to the answer in the space provided.

Column I

1. ___ Uterine tone assessment
2. ___ An empty bladder
3. ___ Primary engorgement
4. ___ Hydronephrosis
5. ___ 2200 to 2300 kcal, high-protein diet
6. ___ Early ambulation
7. ___ Sitz bath
8. ___ Immediate maternal-child contact
9. ___ Oral contraception
10. ___ Follow-up examination visit

Column II

a. Measure necessary to promote tissue healing.
b. Intervention that reduces risk of perineal infection and promotes comfort.
c. A feeling of tenseness of breast tissue on day 3 or 4 postpartum.
d. An increase in size of the ureters occurring during pregnancy.
e. Activity that can be resumed possibly 2 to 3 weeks postpartum.
f. Measure important for detecting potential for postpartum hemorrhage.
g. Activity occurring 4 to 6 weeks after delivery.
h. Measure to decrease constipation and urinary retention.
i. Measure that prevents uterine displacement and promotes accurate assessment of uterine tone.
j. Measure important to facilitate bonding.

Additional Matching Exercises

Match the terms in Column I with a definition, example, or related statement from Column II. Place the letter corresponding to the answer in the space provided. Use each letter only once, some letters may not be used.

Column I

1. ___ Thrombophlebitis
2. ___ Urinary retention
3. ___ Mastitis
4. ___ Hemorrhage

Column II

a. Inflammation of the lining of the blood vessel.
b. Major danger during the immediate postoperative period.
c. Urine residual greater than 100 cc after catherization.
d. Infection of the breast.

SHORT ANSWER

Supply the missing term or the information requested.

1. What is the term describing a time of reflection for a postpartal woman in which she is passive and wants to be ministered to?

2. What is the formation of breast milk called?

3. What is the term describing the incision of the perineum made during the second stage of labor?

4. Briefly compare and contrast the taking-in, taking-hold, and letting-go postpartal phases.

_____

_____

5. Explain the use of sitz bath and ice packs in the care of the postpartal woman who had an episiotomy.

_____

_____

6. Describe the physiologic changes that occur in the indicated structures during the postpartal period.

a. Fundus

_____

_____

b. Cervix

_____

_____

c. Vagina

_____

_____

APPLYING YOUR KNOWLEDGE

CASE STUDY

Rena Despande, age 30, has just given birth to her third daughter. Her husband, age 39, states he wanted a boy but is glad both his wife and the baby are healthy. The baby weighed 10 pounds and Rena had to have an episiotomy.

1. What effect might Rena's husband's hopes for a male child have on the couple's postpartal adjustments? What nursing actions might be implemented?

_____

_____

_____

2. Rena shows reluctance to touch her perineal area and resists discussing perineal care. What factors (including culture) might contribute to

Rena's discomfort with performing and discussing perineal care?

_____

_____

_____

CRITICAL INQUIRY EXERCISE

1. Write a teaching plan that could be used to prepare new parents for the emotional awnd physiologic changes occurring after childbirth.

2. What suggestions would you make to a woman who states she has "no time" to perform muscle-strengthening exercises because of childcare and home care responsibilities but says she really wants to get back in shape?

CRITICAL EXPLORATION

1. During a pediatric clinical experience, perform postpartal assessments on two women and compare findings related to the physiologic and psychological status of each.

2. Interview a woman and her spouse (if possible) during the immediate postpartal period. Attempt to identify signs that the following are being experienced: abandonment, disappointment, or postpartal blues.

PRACTICING FOR NCLEX

MULTIPLE-CHOICE QUESTIONS

Circle the letter that corresponds to the best answer for each question.

1. Mrs. Peters states that her newborn daughter Millie is so thin and has so little hair. The nurse could best help Mrs. Peters by

a. recognizing that Mrs. Peters is feeling jealous and emphasizing that she does not have to find fault with the child to make herself feel attractive.

b. acknowledging Mrs. Peters' statements, explaining that the child will grow a lot during the first months, and then pointing out many of the baby's good features and behaviors.

c. asking Mrs. Peters if she was thin as a child and discussing the many dangers of being an underweight, malnourished newborn.

d. discussing postpartal blues with Mrs. Peters and the fact that negative observations and thoughts are common during this time.

2. The nurse, in planning to help a woman adjust to her new baby, must consider which of the following?

a. The mother will require little assistance since parental love is instinctive.

b. The more difficult the labor process, the stronger the mother's bond with her child.

c. It may be natural for the mother to be hesitant initially when touching the child.

d. Holding the child immediately after birth is overwhelming to a new mother and should be avoided.

3. Mrs. Jones has a 4-year-old son at home and is concerned about his reaction to the new baby. The nurse might do which of the following to best assist this postpartal family?

a. Instruct Mrs. Jones to write her son a letter and include a picture of the new baby.

b. Encourage Mrs. Jones to have another family member spend a lot of time with her son.

c. Arrange for the son to visit with Mrs. Jones and the baby as soon as possible.

d. Discuss the dangers of sibling rivalry with Mrs. Jones and encourage strict discipline.

4. When examining a postpartal woman, the nurse should immediately report

a. a fundus that is palpated 2 cm below the umbilicus on the second postpartal day.

b. a fundus that cannot be located by palpation on the ninth postpartal day.

c. a soft, spongy uterine fundus noted during the first hour postpartum.

d. red, bloody vaginal discharge on the perineal pad on the first day postpartum.

5. During the postpartal period, the new mother may experience an alteration in urinary elimination related to loss of bladder sensation. Which of the following data would indicate this problem?

a. A resonant sound noted on percussion of the lower abdominal area.

b. A firm fundus located 1 cm below the umbilicus on the first postpartal day.

c. Complaints of pain at the episiotomy site, particularly after ambulation.

d. Urinary output greater than 1500 mL during a 24-hour period.

6. The nurse could encourage which of the following measures to decrease the sense of abandonment experienced by the woman and her mate during the postpartal period?

a. The couple should plan extensive time with the new baby to increase their sense of bonding and decrease jealousy.

b. The father should be encouraged to share in the care and feeding of the child to increase feelings of involvement.

c. Discussions of parenting should be avoided during the immediate postpartal period to minimize anticipatory resentment.

d. The mother should be warned that being jealous of the attention her child is receiving is a sign of postpartal psychosis.

7. Which of the following statements related to the client's nutritional status is a common finding or recommended measure during the postpartal period?

a. Breastfeeding mothers should limit caloric intake to prevent fat-cell buildup in newborns, which could lead to obesity.

b. Fluid intake is limited for 48 hours because of the high fluid volume retained in the body after delivery.

c. High intake of meats, fish, chicken, and dairy products should be encouraged to facilitate good tissue repair.

d. The mother will have little desire for food or fluids for 24 hours because of the gluconeogenesis that occurs postpartum.

8. Which of the following is an appropriate nursing diagnosis for a postpartal mother with an episiotomy during the first 5 days postpartum?

a. Anxiety related to vaginal scar formation and decreased body image.

b. Imbalanced nutrition: more than body requirements related to increased appetite.

c. Risk for infection related to lochia and decreased perineal skin integrity.

d. Self-care deficit related to poor opportunity for independence.

9. The postpartal mother asks the nurse when her body will return to "normal." The nurse should implement a teaching plan about postpartal body changes that includes which of the following information?

   a. A fast heart rate and thready pulse will occasionally be noted and should be expected.

   b. Menstrual flow will return within 6 to 10 weeks after delivery unless the mother is breastfeeding.

   c. Varicosities and vascular blemishes will disappear by the sixth postpartal week.

   d. The weight gained during pregnancy is usually retained regardless of dietary and exercise efforts.

10. Which of the following would be cause for concern if found during a postpartal assessment?

    a. Diaphoresis during the period immediately after delivery.

    b. Hair loss over the postpartal period.

    c. Pale coloring of the inner conjunctiva.

    d. Reports of slight breast tenderness.

11. The most appropriate method for assessing the uterine fundus would be to

    a. massage the uterus between the thumb and middle finger until firm, then use a ruler to measure location.

    b. palpate the fundus while the woman has a full bladder to facilitate detection of the uterus.

    c. place both hands below the symphysis pubis and push upward until the lower end of the fundus is located.

    d. support the lower segment of the uterus while palpating the fundus to prevent inversion.

12. Placing the infant at the breast to breastfeed has what effect on uterine tone?

    a. Breastfeeding stimulates lactation increasing uterine clot formation.

    b. Stimulation of the breast causes oxytocin release decreasing uterine tone.

    c. An infant breastfeeding can increase uterine pressure leading to uterine rupture.

    d. Uterine contraction is stimulated by the infant sucking on the breast.

13. Which of the following is the most appropriate outcome for the postpartal mother and family?

    a. Client demonstrates the procedure for self-examination of the breast, the fundus, and perineal area and states her intent to perform these exams.

    b. Client's temperature is 100.4°F to 101°F; no redness or discharge of any kind is noted during the first 48 hours after delivery.

    c. Client does not request pain medication for episiotomy pain and tolerates breast discomfort with minimal comment.

    d. Client prepares a menu including low-calorie foods and minimal intake of meats and bread or starchy food products.

14. The nurse is caring for 14-year-old Lisa, who has decided to give her baby up for adoption. Which of the following should the nurse keep in mind?

    a. Lisa would probably keep her baby if she were given encouragement.

    b. After the delivery Lisa may express a desire to keep her baby, or she may want to continue with the adoption.

    c. During the taking-in phase of the puerperium, the nurse should encourage Lisa to reconsider her decision to abandon her baby.

    d. Lisa should not hold, see, or touch her baby after the delivery to decrease her feelings of loss after giving the child away.

15. An appropriate goal for a postpartal client who complains of being exhausted and unable to sleep would be that the client

    a. abstains from performing self-care and rests instead.

    b. states she feels rested during the postpartal period.

    c. sleeps during the night in order to stay awake all day.

    d. sleeps 8 hours every night after discharge from the hospital.

16. Which of the following might lead the nurse to identify the nursing diagnosis of "Situational low self-esteem related to lack of knowledge regarding psychological changes during the postpartal period" for a postpartal client?

    a. She denies that she has feelings of abandonment or fatigue.

b. She performs grooming and infant care activities.

c. She states that she will not be jealous of her child any longer.

d. She verbalizes that she has conflicting feelings.

ALTERNATE FORMAT QUESTIONS

Multiple-Answer Multiple-Choice Questions

Circle the letter(s) corresponding to the appropriate answer(s). Select all that apply.

1. Data supporting a diagnosis of "risk for imbalanced fluid volume related to subinvolution" would include

   a. blood pressure of 90/62 mm Hg noted on the third day after delivery.

   b. firm uterine fundus located at standard measurement level.

   c. lochia saturating one perineal pad per hour 12 hours postpartum.

   d. pulse slow and bounding during the first postpartal day.

   e. Temperature of 100.0°F (37.8°C) 4 hours postpartum.

2. Which of the following nursing interventions would be appropriate when caring for a client with an episiotomy who has the nursing diagnosis "Pain related to perineal sutures"?

   a. Apply ice packs to the perineal incision site to decrease edema.

   b. Encourage the client to contract and relax perineal muscles.

   c. Instruct client to use petroleum jelly or mineral oil on the episiotomy as desired.

   d. Limit pain medication to prevent dependence on narcotic analgesics.

   e. Encourage sexual activity after 1 week to loosen sutures.

3. Which of the following characteristics indicate that lochia flow is normal.

   a. Lochia amount increases with strenuous exercise.

   b. Lochia contains no large clots.

   c. Lochia is absent during the first 1 to 3 weeks after a cesarean birth.

   d. Lochia is white for the first 1 to 3 days postpartum.

   e. Lochia has the same odor as menstrual blood.

Nursing Care of a Family With a Newborn

CHAPTER OVERVIEW

Chapter 18 reviews the nursing care associated with a newborn and the newborn's family. It focuses on newborn assessment and care. Nurses need to be able to evaluate findings obtained on assessment and intervene appropriately when these findings suggest underlying pathology. This chapter assists the student in recognizing "normal" findings and differentiating them from abnormal findings. Anticipatory guidance with regard to feeding, daily routines, and the characteristics of stools is addressed.

LEARNING OBJECTIVES

After mastering the content in this chapter, you should be able to do the following:

1. Describe the normal characteristics of a term newborn.

2. Identify National Health Goals related to newborn care that nurses could help the nation achieve.

3. Use critical thinking to analyze ways that the care of a term newborn can be more family centered.

4. Assess a newborn for normal growth and development.

5. Formulate nursing diagnoses related to a newborn or the family of a newborn.

6. Identify expected outcomes for a newborn and family during the first 4 weeks of life.

7. Plan nursing care to augment normal development of a newborn, such as ways to aid parent–child bonding.

8. Implement nursing care of a normal newborn, such as instructing parents on how to care for their newborn.

9. Evaluate outcome criteria for the achievement and effectiveness of care.

10. Identify areas related to newborn assessment and care that could benefit from additional nursing research or application of evidence-based practice.

11. Integrate knowledge of newborn growth and development and immediate care needs with the nursing process to achieve quality maternal and child health nursing care.

KEY TERMS

acrocyanosis
caput succedaneum
cavernous hemangioma
central cyanosis
cephalhematoma
conduction
convection
erythema toxicum
evaporation
hemangiomas

mongolian spot
natal teeth
neonatal period
neonate
nevus flammeus
physiologic jaundice
pseudomenstruation
radiation
strawberry
    hemangioma

jaundice
kernicterus
lanugo
meconium
milia

subconjunctival
hemorrhage
thrush
transitional stool
vernix caseosa

e. Infant attempting to refuse solid foods.

f. Yellowing of the skin as a result of the breakdown of fetal red blood cells.

g. Port-wine stain-hemangioma lesion level with skin.

h. Vascular tumor of the skin, elevated areas formed by immature capillaries and epithelial cells.

i. One or two dental eruptions present at birth.

j. Time from birth through the first 28 days.

MASTERING THE INFORMATION

FILL IN THE BLANKS

Supply the missing term or the information requested.

1. The time of birth through the first 28 days of life is termed the _____ _____.

2. The average heart rate for the neonate is _____.

3. Cyanosis in the infant's feet and hands during the first 24 hours after birth is termed _____.

MATCHING

Match the terms in Column I with a definition, example, or related statement from Column II. Place the letter corresponding to the answer in the space provided.

Column I

1. ___ Subconjunctival hemorrhage

2. ___ Physiologic jaundice

3. ___ Crede treatment

4. ___ Extrusion reflex

5. ___ Nevus flammeus

6. ___ Cremasteric reflex

7. ___ Strawberry hemangioma

8. ___ Brown fat

9. ___ Neonatal period

10. ___ Natal teeth

Column II

a. A special tissue found in mature newborns to conserve or produce body heat.

b. Prophylaxis against gonorrheal conjunctivitis for the newborn.

c. Pressure during birth causing a red spot on the sclera.

d. Movement upward of the testes when the inner aspect of the thing is stroked.

TRUE OR FALSE

Indicate if the following statements are true or false by placing a "T" or "F" in the space provided.

1. ___ Infants who do not void within 24 hours after birth could possibly have urethral stenosis.

2. ___ Murmurs heard when examining the neonate usually indicate cardiac anomalies and must be corrected surgically.

3. ___ An accelerated count of leukocytes in the newborn's serology test suggests a response to an infection.

4. ___ A circumcision prevents phimosis and reduces the incidence of urinary tract infections.

SHORT ANSWER

Supply the missing term or the information requested.

1. The average respiratory rate for the neonate is _____ breaths per minute.

2. The infant is vulnerable to heat instability and loses heat readily through four separate mechanisms: _____, _____, _____, and _____.

3. List the six criteria described by Brazelton that are used as the basis to evaluate the newborn's behavioral capacity.

_____

_____

4. Describe and contrast the stools of a bottlefed and breastfed infant.

_____

_____

5. Why would the nurse be concerned after learning that a neonate has not passed a stool by 24 hours after birth?

_____

_____

6. Identify the behaviors exhibited by the new-born in the following periods:

   a. First period of reactivity.

   _____

   _____

   b. Second period of reactivity.

   _____

   _____

7. Explain the principles of safety when placing a child in a car seat or car seat belt.

   _____

   _____

8. Discuss the potential adverse effects of elective surgery to the male infant's penis.

   _____

   _____

9. Explain why parents, visitors, and hospital personnel with cold sores should not care for the newborn infant.

   _____

   _____

APPLYING YOUR KNOWLEDGE

CASE STUDY

Mrs. Calland delivered (vaginally) a baby boy to-day. Baby boy Calland was evaluated to be 38 weeks gestation and weigh 3200 g. Mrs. Calland plans to breastfeed her baby. You are assigned as the nurse to take care of her and her baby.

1. Shortly after delivery, several reflexes were tested on the infant. Make a list of reflexes that were tested and explain which maneuvers were used to complete the tests.

   _____

   _____

   _____

2. Within 12 hours after birth the infant passed a sticky black stool. Explain why this should not alarm you.

   _____

   _____

   _____

3. On the day of discharge, baby boy Calland appears to have yellow skin and sclera. What lab test might be ordered at this time? What would be indicated if the results are higher than normal values?

   _____

   _____

   _____

CRITICAL INQUIRY EXERCISE

1. Formulate a nursing care plan that will focus on nursing care for a male infant who has difficulty maintaining an appropriate body temperature.

2. Develop a neonatal admission assessment form that might be used in a newborn nursery.

CRITICAL EXPLORATION

1. Identify a mother who has just given birth to her first child. Formulate a teaching plan that will focus on immediate care needs for the newborn in the home environment. Discuss this information with the mother and include the father of the child, if he is available.

2. Locate the resources in your community that help families obtain car seats when they cannot afford to buy one.

3. Identify a newborn infant who is more than 24 hours old. Perform the Brazelton Neonatal Behavioral Assessment and present your findings to the class.

PRACTICING FOR NCLEX

MULTIPLE-CHOICE QUESTIONS

Circle the letter that corresponds to the best answer for each question.

1. The nurse is performing the morning assessment of baby boy Lee born yesterday at 39 weeks gestation and weighing 3500 g. When assessing the chest comparatively to the head, the nurse would expect

   a. the chest circumference to be about 2 cm less than the head circumference.

   b. the chest and head circumference to be equal.

   c. the head circumference to be about 2 cm less than the chest circumference.

   d. the head circumference to be about 3 cm more than the chest circumference.

2. A neonate's temperature is slightly subnormal 1 hour after birth. Which action would be most appropriate?

   a. Take the infant to the mother for bonding and transfer of body heat after mom rests for an hour.

   b. Place a second stockinette on the infant's head.

   c. Administer a warm bath with temperature slightly higher than usual.

   d. Place the infant under a radiant warmer or in a heated isolette.

3. Which assessment finding would cause the nurse to notify the physician?

   a. Breast tissue slightly engorged.

   b. Heart rate of 170 beats per minute.

   c. Crepitus palpated at the clavicular area.

   d. Frog-like positioning of the lower extremities.

4. When assessing the neonate, which finding would the nurse interpret as a pathological disturbance?

   a. Heart rate of 130 beats per minute.

   b. Rhonchi auscultated over the lung area.

   c. Neonate's abdomen, not the chest, rises when breathing.

   d. Nonpalpable femoral pulses.

5. The nurse attempts to elicit the Moro reflex in a neonate by

   a. stroking the cheek near the corner of the mouth.

   b. loudly tapping the bassinet.

   c. placing a substance on the anterior portion of neonate's tongue.

   d. stroking the side of the foot to have the toes fan out.

ALTERNATE FORMAT QUESTIONS

Multiple-Answer Multiple-Choice Questions

Circle the letter(s) corresponding to the appropriate answer(s). Select all that apply.

1. Which interventions would be most appropriate to promote parental–newborn bonding?

   a. Let the mother rest for 1 to 2 hours after birth before initiating contact with the newborn.

   b. Leave an amulet or other "good luck charm" from the parents in the newborn's bassinet.

   c. Compliment the newborn whose parents are from Cambodia or Laos about their desire to "ward off spirits."

   d. During first period of activity, ask which parent wants to hold the newborn and place him or her in the parent's arms.

   e. Encourage parents to hold and provide care for newborn while still in the hospital.

2. A nurse is assessing a newborn. Which of the following would be considered normal findings?

   a. Central cyanosis.

   b. Harlequin sign.

   c. Lanugo.

   d. Palmar desquamation.

   e. Milia.

   f. Lack of ear recoil on bending.

3. When performing eye prophylaxis at birth, which of the following would the nurse do?

   a. Use a single-use tube or package of ointment.

   b. Ensure the newborn's face is slightly wet.

   c. Shade the newborn's eyes from the overhead lights.

   d. Open one eye at a time using pressure on the lower and upper lids.

   e. Squeeze the ointment along the upper conjunctival sac from the inner canthus outward.

   f. Close the newborn's eye and wait about 5 seconds before wiping away any excess ointment.

Nutritional Needs of a Newborn

CHAPTER OVERVIEW

Chapter 19 reviews the nutritional needs of the newborn. The nutrients in breast milk and commercially prepared formulas are evaluated and contrasted. The physiology of good nutrition is important for the growth and development of the newborn infant. After reading this chapter, the student should know how to assess and evaluate the mother's ability to feed the infant and the infant's response to nutritional intake. The chapter also enables the student to provide nursing care for the mother and infant using a nursing plan of care as a teaching tool.

LEARNING OBJECTIVES

After mastering the content in this chapter, you should be able to do the following:

1. Describe nutritional requirements for a term newborn.

2. Identify National Health Goals related to newborn nutrition that nurses can help the nation achieve.

3. Use critical thinking to assist parents with nutritional problem solving and be sure newborn nutrition is family centered.

4. Assess nutritional intake and feeding method of a newborn to determine adequate nutritional status.

5. Formulate nursing diagnoses related to newborn nutrition.

6. Identify outcomes for a newborn and parents related to nutrition.

7. Plan a method of infant feeding with a mother that will be satisfying for both her and her infant.

8. Help parents implement newborn feeding such as supporting a new mother while breastfeeding.

9. Evaluate expected outcomes for achievement and effectiveness of care.

10. Identify areas related to nutrition and newborns that could benefit from additional nursing research or application of evidence-based practice.

11. Integrate knowledge of normal newborn nutrition with nursing process to achieve quality maternal and child health nursing care.

KEY TERMS

areola	interferon
bifidus factor	lactiferous sinuses
colostrum	lactoferrin
engorgement	let-down reflex
fore milk	lysozyme
hind milk	prolactin

MASTERING THE INFORMATION

FILL IN THE BLANKS

Supply the missing term or the information requested.

1. _____ milk is produced by the alveolar cells of the _____ gland in the presence of the hormone prolactin.

2. The infant promotes continuous milk production by _____.

3. An infant that is 1.5 months old and weighs 5 kg would require ____ to ____ calories per kg of body weight every 24 hours for adequate growth.

MATCHING

Match the terms in Column I with a definition, example, or related statement from Column II. Place the letter corresponding to the answer in the space provided.

Column I

1. ____ Adrenocorticosteroid hormone
2. ____ Lactose
3. ____ Histidine
4. ____ Linoleic acid
5. ____ Lactiferous sinuses
6. ____ Oxytocin
7. ____ IgA
8. ____ Soap
9. ____ Casein
10. ____ Colostrum
11. ____ Nipple rolling
12. ____ Lysozyme
13. ____ Hind milk
14. ____ Lactoferrin
15. ____ Fluoride

Column II

a. Substance that finds large molecules of foreign proteins including viruses and bacteria; prohibits absorption through the gastrointestinal tract.

b. Substance that probably plays a role in assisting mammary glands to secrete milk.

c. Hormone of the posterior pituitary gland that aids in uterine contractions.

d. Previously a procedure used to help make nipples more protuberant.

e. An amino acid essential for infant growth found in human breast milk and cow's milk.

f. Substance contraindicated when breastfeeding; tends to cause the nipples to dry and crack.

g. Thin, watery, yellow fluid consisting of protein, sugar, fat, water, minerals, vitamins, and maternal antibodies.

h. Reservoirs for breast milk located behind nipple.

i. The protein in cow's milk.

j. Iron-binding protein in breast milk interfering with the growth of pathogenic bacteria.

k. Necessary mineral for building sound teeth and resistance to tooth decay.

l. An enzyme in breast milk that actively destroys bacteria by dissolving their cell membranes.

m. "New milk" formed after the let-down reflex.

n. Sugar nutrients found in breast milk that provide ready glucose for rapid brain growth.

o. A fatty acid not found in skim milk but is necessary for growth and skin integrity in infants.

TRUE OR FALSE

Indicate if the following statements are true or false by placing a "T" or "F" in the space provided.

1. ____ Infants who are fed by propping the bottles are in potential danger of aspirating fluids.

2. ____ Infants put to bed with a bottle of milk risk developing "baby bottle syndrome."

3. ____ If a woman is experiencing sore nipples from breastfeeding, she should use a hand pump to express the milk manually until the nipples have had a chance to heal.

4. ____ Colostrum is the primary constituent of breast milk during the first 3 months of feeding.

5. ____ Oxytocin is released by breastfeeding and stimulates contractions.

6. ___ The more often breasts are emptied, the more efficiently they will fill and continue to maintain a good supply of milk.

7. ___ Placing the breastfed infant over one shoulder and gently stroking his or her back is the best position for burping him or her.

8. ___ Sore nipples are a contraindication for breastfeeding.

SHORT ANSWER

Supply the missing term or the information requested.

1. What event allows progesterone levels to drop and stimulates the production of the prolactin?

   _____

   _____

2. Prolactin-releasing factor stimulates the _____ _____ gland, which responds with active production of _____.

3. Describe the three major types of breast milk that are produced.

   _____

   _____

APPLYING YOUR KNOWLEDGE

CASE STUDY

Ms. Jackson delivered an 8-lb, 6-oz baby girl about 1 hour before your arrival to the clinical site this morning. Your instructor has assigned you to Ms. Jackson for the next 2 days of your clinical rotation. Her prenatal record indicates that she was considering breastfeeding but had not decided at the time of birth. You will need to be prepared to answer her questions about breastfeeding.

1. Compare the advantages and disadvantages of breastfeeding for the infant and mother.

   _____

   _____

   _____

2. What are some appropriate measures to relieve breast engorgement?

   _____

   _____

   _____

3. State how the infant should be properly placed on the breast for feeding.

   _____

   _____

   _____

CRITICAL INQUIRY EXERCISE

1. Mrs. Jones' water supply is furnished by her private well. She will be preparing formula for her newborn infant. Outline the steps of sterilization to teach her how to prepare the formula and supplement.

2. Design a teaching tool for parents about the techniques and safeguards of feeding for breastfed and bottlefed babies.

CRITICAL EXPLORATION

1. Survey your community for agencies that promote infant nutrition and parental education. After compiling the list, inform your clients of these agencies before their discharge.

2. Review the nursing care plans in your clinical areas for a mother and infant scheduled for discharge planning at your hospital. Note the information pertinent to infant nutrition. Exercise your teaching skills by providing this information to a parent the day before discharge. On the day of discharge, assess the effectiveness of your teaching by interviewing your client. Create your own evaluation tool.

PRACTICING FOR NCLEX

MULTIPLE-CHOICE QUESTIONS

Circle the letter that corresponds to the best answer for each question.

1. Jane Albright is breastfeeding her baby girl, whom she delivered at 6 this morning, weighing 6 lb 7.5 oz. The labor and delivery for mother and infant were uneventful. During the first feeding, Mrs. Albright asked how long her baby should suck on each breast per feeding. The nurse's best response would be which of the following?
   a. The infant should start nursing about 15 minutes on each breast.
   b. Five minutes on each breast for each feeding will be sufficient for today.
   c. Nurse only on one breast today for 5 minutes per feeding and start alternating breasts with the first feeding tomorrow.
   d. Ten minutes at each breast will be sufficient and will also keep the infant from becoming fatigued.

2. When counseling a new mother on breastfeeding, the nurse would know that the most fundamental ingredient for success is to
   a. teach the client how to relax.
   b. place the infant correctly on the breast.
   c. teach the client about holding the newborn in the various feeding positions.
   d. wait until the newborn actively demands a feeding.

3. On the second postpartum day, the nurse observes that a new mother is washing her breast and hands with soap just before she is to receive her infant for the next feeding. The nurse's action, if any, would be governed by which of the following statements?
   a. Good breast hygiene is necessary to avoid the spread of pathogens from the mother's skin to the newborn.
   b. The client should not clean her breast and hands in preparation for feeding until the infant has arrived in the room.
   c. Cleansing the breast with soap may lead to nipple soreness and dryness.
   d. Washing the breasts increases milk production that may be wastefully expressed before the infant is to be fed.

4. On the third postpartum day, Mrs. Jacobs tells the nurse that she sometimes has difficulty getting the infant to suck. She describes the infant opening her mouth when the breast touches her face but turning her head in the opposite direction. The nurse would explain that this behavior is related to
   a. the infant's immaturity and unfamiliarity with the technique of feeding.
   b. the extrusion reflex, normal for newborns, and demonstrates the need for much assistance to ensure adequate nutrition.
   c. the rooting reflex, which suggests improper technique when placing the infant on the breast.
   d. turning neck reflex, which suggests that breastfed infants are most sensitive to tactile stimulation.

5. A new mother reports that her daughter often falls asleep at feedings before she has taken in enough nutrients. Which of the following statements would be a helpful suggestion?
   a. Wash the infant's face with cool water.
   b. Give the infant a bath before alternating breasts to complete the feeding.
   c. Rub the fontanel of the infant's head gently.
   d. Lightly tickle the bottom of the newborn's feet.

6. Which of the following preparations of commercial formulas would the nurse suggest as being the least expensive?
   a. Powder to be combined with water.
   b. Condensed liquid to be diluted with equal parts of water.
   c. "Ready to pour" type.
   d. Individually prepackaged.

7. Choose the correct statement to be used to calculate a nutrient needed for the newborn infant.
   a. Fluid needs are approximately 100 cc/kg body weight/day.
   b. Fat needs are approximately 20 g/kg body weight/day.
   c. Protein needs are 2.2 g/kg body weight/day.
   d. Caloric needs are 100 kcal/kg body weight/day.

ALTERNATE FORMAT QUESTIONS

Multiple-Answer Multiple-Choice Questions

Circle the letter(s) corresponding to the appropriate answer(s). Select all that apply.

1. Which of the following is true about newborn nutrition and nutritional needs?
   a. The caloric requirements in the neonatal period exceed those at any other age.
   b. An infant up to 2 months of age requires 50 to 60 cal/kg of body weight (22.7 to 27.3 kcal/lb) every 24 hours.
   c. The caloric requirement at 1 year of age is 100 kcal/kg or 45 kcal/lb/day
   d. The 6-month old has a caloric requirement similar to an adult requirement of 42 kcal/kg or 20 kcal/lb/day.
   e. The actual caloric requirement of an infant depends on an infant's individual activity level and growth rate.

2. Which of the following is an acceptable guideline for use and storage of canned formula?
   a. The nutrients in canned formula may be enhanced with whole milk.
   b. Spring water is found to be clean and more suitable in preparing infant formula.
   c. Store the unused portions of the infant's bottle at room temperature after feeding.
   d. Formula in an open can should be used or discarded in 24 hours.
   e. Avoid using a microwave to warm the formula

3. Which of the following is true for both breast milk and commercial formulas?
   a. They supply all the essential amino acids necessary.
   b. They contain linoleic acid, an essential fatty acid.
   c. Supplementation with iron is necessary since neither supply it.
   d. Vitamins A and C are found in both but vitamin D is lacking.
   e. Formulas and breast milk supply a similar amount of calories.

Nursing Care of a Family Experiencing a Pregnancy Complication From a Pre-existing or Newly Acquired Illness

CHAPTER OVERVIEW

Chapter 20 provides an overview of various systemic conditions that can result in a client assuming a high-risk pregnancy status. The effects of various physical illnesses on the woman and her fetus during pregnancy stages are discussed. The use of the nursing process to plan and provide care for the client, the fetus, and the family involved in a high-risk pregnancy is explored.

LEARNING OBJECTIVES

After mastering the content in this chapter, you should be able to do the following:

1. Define *high-risk pregnancy*, including pre-existing factors that contribute to its development.

2. Describe common illnesses such as cardiovascular disease, diabetes mellitus, or renal and blood disorders that can result in complications when they exist with pregnancy.

3. Identify National Health Goals related to complications of pregnancy that nurses can help the nation achieve.

4. Use critical thinking to analyze ways that nursing care can remain family centered when a pre-existing or newly acquired illness develops during pregnancy.

5. Assess a woman with an illness during pregnancy for changes occurring in the illness because of the pregnancy or the pregnancy because of the illness.

6. Formulate nursing diagnoses related to the effect of a pre-existing or newly acquired illness on pregnancy.

7. Identify expected outcomes that will contribute to a safe pregnancy outcome when illness occurs with pregnancy.

8. Plan nursing care for a woman with an illness during pregnancy, such as how a woman with heart disease could manage to get more rest.

9. Implement nursing care for a woman when illness complicates pregnancy.

10. Evaluate expected outcomes for achievement and effectiveness of care.

11. Identify areas related to illness and pregnancy that could benefit from additional nursing research or application of evidence-based practice.

12. Integrate knowledge of high-risk pregnancy and nursing process to achieve quality maternal and child health nursing care.

KEY TERMS

deep vein thrombosis
glucose tolerance test
glycosuria
glycosylated hemoglobin
high-risk pregnancy
hyperglycemia
hypoglycemia
megaloblastic anemia
orthopnea
paroxysmal nocturnal dyspnea
peripartal cardiomyopathy
proteinuria

MASTERING THE INFORMATION

FILL IN THE BLANKS

Supply the missing term or the information requested.

1. _____ _____ _____ could cause cardiac failure, anemia, and hypertensive vascular disease to result in fetal distress or low birth weight.

2. Three factors in pregnancy that can result in venous thromboembolic disease are _____ _____ , and _____ .

3. The organism most commonly responsible for UTIs is _____ _____ .

MATCHING

Match the terms in Column I with a definition, example, or related statement from Column II. Place the letter corresponding to the answer in the space provided.

Column I

1. ___ Functional heart murmur

2. ___ Paroxysmal nocturnal dyspnea

3. ___ Megaloblastic anemia

4. ___ Left heart failure

5. ___ Pyelonephritis

6. ___ Hiatal hernia

7. ___ Scoliosis

8. ___ Systemic lupus erythematosus

9. ___ Pseudoanemia

10. ___ Chlamydia trachomatis

Column II

a. Occurs when mitral valve stenosis, or insufficiency, or aortic coarctation causes a decrease in cardiac output and back pressure to the lungs.

b. A normal decrease in the red blood cell count due to the expanded blood volume of pregnancy.

c. An innocent, transient escape of fluid through heart valves due to increased blood flow past valves that can occur during pregnancy.

d. Low blood levels with enlarged red blood cells related to folic acid deficiency.

e. A multisystem connective tissue disease that may result in acute nephritis.

f. A portion of the stomach extended through the diaphragm that can result in inability to eat due to heartburn.

g. Lateral curvature of the spine that may cause pelvic distortion that can interfere with childbirth.

h. Suddenly waking during the night with sever shortness of breath.

i. Kidney infection that can result in premature labor or rupture of membranes.

j. The most common vaginal infection seen during pregnancy.

ADDITIONAL MATCHING EXERCISES

Match the terms in Column I with a definition, example, or related statement from Column II. Place the letter corresponding to the answer in the space provided.

Column I

1. ___ Viral hepatitis

2. ___ Human immunodeficiency virus

3. ___ Schizophrenia

4. ___ Tonic–clonic seizures

5. ___ Burns

Column II

a. Danger to mother and fetus due to carbon monoxide and fluid/electrolyte losses.

b. Jaundice occurs as a late symptom.

c. Maternal infection with this virus requires active interactions to reduce fetal exposure to maternal blood.

d. Treatment with teratogenic medication possibly necessary.

e. Possible anoxia occurring from spasm of chest muscles.

SHORT ANSWER

Supply the missing term or the information requested.

1. List one example each of psychological, social, and physical factors that can cause a pregnancy to be categorized as high risk during the prepregnancy, pregnancy, and labor and delivery periods.

   _____

   _____

2. Describe how pregnancy can cause a woman to develop a urinary tract infection.

   _____

   _____

3. Discuss the key issues that should be included in a teaching plan for a pregnant woman who is a diabetic or who develops diabetes during pregnancy. Address diet, exercise, insulin, and glucose monitoring.

   _____

   _____

APPLYING YOUR KNOWLEDGE

CASE STUDY

Melinda Jaffe is a 28-year-old mother of two, ages 5 and 3. Melinda is in for her second prenatal visit. She is 5 months pregnant and has a history of congestive heart failure secondary to valve disease from childhood rheumatic fever.

1. What is the most dangerous time in the pregnancy for a woman with heart disease and why?

   _____

   _____

   _____

2. How might the fact that Melinda has two young children affect her risk for complications from her heart disease? What nursing interventions would you plan?

   _____

   _____

   _____

CRITICAL INQUIRY EXERCISE

1. What would be the major points you would include in a teaching plan for adolescents that addresses the effects of sexually transmitted diseases on a fetus or on an infant after childbirth?

2. In what way, if any, would your teaching plan differ for an insulin-dependent diabetic who became pregnant, and for a pregnant woman who developed gestational diabetes?

CRITICAL EXPLORATION

While on a postpartal clinical unit, review the chart of a client with diabetes. Note the prenatal history, course of the pregnancy for glucose regulation, any complications experienced, postpartal glucose control, and status of the newborn.

PRACTICING FOR NCLEX

MULTIPLE-CHOICE QUESTIONS

Circle the letter that corresponds to the best answer for each question.

1. Melle, 12 years old, is 2 months pregnant and has a history of heart disease. Which of the following is true about her risk factors for high-risk pregnancy?

   a. Good nutrition and exercise will eliminate any added risk factors Melle may have for complications.

   b. Melle's heart condition will not affect her pregnancy, since she has not reached adolescence.

   c. Melle's youth will protect her from many problems experienced by older women with heart disease.

   d. Both Melle's age and heart condition will place her at risk for complications during pregnancy.

2. Which of the following could be included in the outcome for a client with the nursing diagnosis, "Ineffective tissue perfusion (fetal or maternal) related to maternal cardiovascular disease"?

   a. Bed rest is maintained at home after the 36th week of gestation.

   b. Fetal heart rate will remain between 120 and 160 beats per minute.

   c. Jugular vein distention is evident when lying at 45°.

   d. Maternal blood pressure is maintained above 150 mm Hg systolic.

3. When planning care for a pregnant woman with heart disease, the nurse should do which of the following?

   a. Assess complaints of fatigue and note any accompanying dyspnea or pulmonary congestion.

   b. Discourage the mother from taking any medications during pregnancy, since they will affect the baby.

   c. Instruct the client to eat as much food as desired to promote maximum fetal and maternal nutrition.

   d. Plan an exercise schedule to prevent thrombus formation during labor.

4. Which of the following interventions should be implemented with caution when caring for a postpartal woman who has heart disease or hypertensive vascular disease?

   a. Administering prenatal vitamins.

   b. Ensuring early ambulation with antiembolism stockings.

   c. Encouraging bulk and high fiber in the diet.

   d. Suggesting oral contraceptives as a birth control method.

5. Pregnant women with venous thromboembolic disease

   a. are at risk for death from a pulmonary embolism.

   b. must have oral fluids restricted throughout the pregnancy.

   c. receive heparin as soon as their labor begins.

   d. need teaching to keep their legs crossed at the knee when sitting.

6. Clients with megaloblastic anemia should be encouraged to do which of the following?

   a. Avoid pregnancy, since they cannot carry the baby to term.

   b. Avoid excessive fluid intake, which has caused this hemodilution.

   c. Take over-the-counter multivitamins.

   d. Take the prescribed folic acid supplements.

7. When planning care for a pregnant client with sickle-cell anemia, the nurse might establish which of the following as an outcome? The client

   a. lies on her back in a semi-Fowler's position when sleeping.

   b. rests with her legs elevated when sitting in a chair.

   c. reports intent to get a sickle-cell antigen shot after delivery.

   d. states understanding of need to limit fluid intake to 16 oz/day.

8. Clients with chronic renal disease or who have had kidney transplants may have difficulty in pregnancy for which of the following reasons?

   a. Fetal and maternal waste products must be excreted.

   b. Hormones released in pregnancy can cause rejection of transplant.

   c. Increased glomerular filtration rate causes decreased serum creatinine level.

   d. Steroids may cause excessive fetal growth stimulation.

9. Which of the following measures the nurse should implement for the pregnant client with rheumatoid arthritis?

   a. Discussing the woman's intent to breast-feed so that medications can be changed if necessary.

b. Instructing the woman to increase her intake of aspirin 2 weeks prior to term to offset the decrease in corticosteroids.

c. Encouraging the woman to contact her physician for a higher dosage, if methotrexate is prescribed.

d. Assessing the client each week to monitor for blood clots due to salicylate ingestion.

10. Teresa, who is at 20 weeks' gestation, has been diagnosed with acute appendicitis. She expresses concern that the doctor is going to perform surgery. The nurse could explain which of the following?

a. Delivery of the baby with a cesarean birth at this point would be safer than trying to complete the pregnancy.

b. Since the appendix cannot be removed at this stage of the pregnancy without disruption of the pregnancy, an abortion is necessary.

c. If she prefers, the doctor can delay removal of the appendix until later in the pregnancy.

d. Peritonitis could result from rupture of the appendix and would be dangerous for both mother and child.

11. Which of the following evaluation data would indicate that the nurse's teaching plan for the pregnant client with cholecystitis had been effective?

a. Aching occurs primarily in the right epigastrium after eating.

b. Jaundice and pain remain absent throughout the pregnancy.

c. The client prepares a menu that is fat-free.

d. The client reports ingestion of high-cholesterol foods.

12. A pregnant woman diagnosed with diabetes should be instructed to do which of the following to control her glucose level?

a. Discontinue insulin injections until pregnancy is completed, since hormones will regulate glucose levels.

b. Ingest a smaller amount of food prior to sleep to prevent nocturnal hyperglycemia.

c. Notify the physician if she is unable to eat because of nausea and vomiting.

d. Prepare foods with increased fat content to provide needed calories.

13. After delivery, a diabetic woman might need to do which of the following?

a. Change to oral hypoglycemia agents, which will control glucose levels more effectively than insulin.

b. Bottlefeed her infant, since insulin received through breastfeeding may cause hypoglycemia in the child.

c. Receive no insulin during the immediate postpartal period, since insulin resistance is gone.

d. Take medications to decrease uterine hypertonicity if hydramnios was present during pregnancy.

ALTERNATE FORMAT QUESTIONS

Multiple-Answer Multiple-Choice Questions

Circle the letter(s) corresponding to the appropriate answer(s). Select all that apply.

1. Which of the following is an appropriate as an outcome for the pregnant client who has seizures as a result of childhood meningitis? The client

a. demonstrates ability to recognize the Moro reflex as an early indication of fetal seizures.

b. requires no supplemental oxygen administration during convulsions.

c. states understanding that her child is not certain to have seizures just because she developed the condition.

d. refrains from taking anticonvulsant medications during the first trimester to prevent congenital defects.

e. understands chromosomal defects are not the etiology of her seizures.

2. When assessing a pregnant woman's risk for complications, which of the following would lead the nurse to suspect that the woman is considered high risk?

a. BMI between 18.5 and 30.

b. History of intimate partner abuse.

c. Previous pregnancy with twins.

d. Two previous miscarriages.

e. 30 years of age.

3. The nurse is reviewing the blood glucose levels of several pregnant women with diabetes. Which of the following results would demonstrate good control?

  a. Fasting level of 78 mg/dL.

  b. Fasting level of 110 mg/dL.

  c. Fasting level of 135 mg/dL.

  d. 2-hour postprandial level of 90 mg/dL.

  e. 2-hour postprandial level of 105 mg/dL.

  f. 2-hour postprandial level of 128 mg/dL.

Nursing Care of a Family Experiencing a Sudden Pregnancy Complication

CHAPTER OVERVIEW

Chapter 21 discusses the complications that can occur during pregnancy and the effects these complications may have on the woman and her family. The use of the nursing process to plan and provide care for the woman and her family under these circumstances is explored.

LEARNING OBJECTIVES

After mastering the content in this chapter, you should be able to do the following:

1. Describe complications of pregnancy that place a pregnant woman and her fetus at high risk.

2. Identify National Health Goals related to complications of pregnancy and specific measures nurses can take to help the nation achieve these goals.

3. Use critical thinking to analyze ways that nurses can help prevent complications of pregnancy while keeping care family centered.

4. Assess a woman who is experiencing a complication of pregnancy.

5. Formulate nursing diagnoses that address the needs of a woman and her family experiencing a complication of pregnancy.

6. Identify expected outcomes to minimize the risks to a pregnant woman and her fetus when a complication of pregnancy occurs.

7. Plan nursing interventions to meet the needs and promote optimal outcomes for a woman and her family during a complication of pregnancy.

8. Implement nursing care specific to a woman who has developed a complication of pregnancy such as teaching her how to recognize the symptoms of preterm labor.

9. Evaluate expected outcomes for effectiveness and achievement of care.

10. Identify areas of nursing care related to high-risk pregnancy that could benefit from additional nursing research or the application of evidence-based practice.

11. Integrate knowledge of complications of pregnancy with nursing process to achieve quality maternal and child health nursing care.

KEY TERMS

abortion
ankle clonus
cervical cerclage
chorioamnionitis
couvelaire uterus
early pregnancy failure
eclampsia
ectopic pregnancy
erythroblastosis fetalis
gestational trophoblastic
  disease
HELLP syndrome
hemolytic disease of
  the newborn
hydramnios
isoimmunization
miscarriage

oligohydramnios
placenta previa
postterm pregnancy
pre-eclampsia
premature cervical
  dilatation
premature separation
  of the placenta
preterm labor
preterm rupture of
  membranes
pseudocyesis
recurrent pregnancy
  loss
Rh incompatibility
tocolytic agent

MASTERING THE INFORMATION

FILL IN THE BLANKS

Supply the missing term or the information requested.

1. The two main causes of bleeding during the second trimester are _____ and _____.

2. Sudden placental separation from the uterus with bleeding is called _____.

3. Production of antibodies against Rh-positive blood results in _____.

MATCHING

Match the terms in Column I with a definition, example, or related statement from Column II. Place the letter corresponding to the answer in the space provided.

Column I

1. ____ Placenta previa

2. ____ Isoimmunization

3. ____ Cervical cerclage

4. ____ Imminent miscarriage

5. ____ Erythroblastosis

6. ____ Abruptio placentae

7. ____ Pseudocyesis

8. ____ Late spontaneous miscarriage

9. ____ Eclampsia

10. ____ Hydatiform mole

11. ____ Ectopic pregnancy

Column II

a. An interruption of pregnancy (natural causes) occurring between the 16th and 24th week.

b. Implantation occurring outside the uterine cavity.

c. Proliferation and degeneration of the trophoblast villi.

d. Low implantation of the placenta.

e. Pregnancy-induced hypertension, proteinuria, and cerebral edema with seizure.

f. Purse-string sutures applied to prevent recurrence of premature dilation and fetal expulsion (loss).

g. Event occurring when Rh-negative women are exposed to Rh-positive fetal blood.

h. Premature separation of the placenta.

i. Vaginal bleeding with uterine contractions and cervical dilation prior to fetal viability.

j. Hemolytic disease of the newborn.

k. Amenorrhea, nausea, and enlargement of the abdomen occurring in a nonpregnant woman.

IDENTIFICATION

For each of the pregnancy complications listed below, indicate when it usually occurs with the letter "A" for first trimester, "B" for second trimester, and "C" for the third trimester.

1. ____ Placenta previa

2. ____ Spontaneous miscarriage

3. ____ Hydatidiform mole

4. ____ Abruptio placentae

5. ____ Incompetent cervix

6. ____ Ectopic pregnancy

SHORT ANSWER

Supply the missing term or the information requested.

1. What term is used to denote an unplanned interruption of pregnancy before the fetus is viable?

   _____

   _____

2. Identify the condition in pregnancy in which implantation occurs outside the uterine cavity.

_____

_____

3. What condition involves hypertension of pregnancy with hemolysis, high liver enzymes, and low platelet levels?

_____

_____

4. What term is used to describe hypertension of pregnancy with blood pressure elevated 30 mm Hg systolic or 15 mm Hg diastolic above prepregnancy values?

_____

_____

5. Identify the condition described as excessive amniotic fluid formation.

_____

_____

6. Briefly explain why it is important to determine the week of pregnancy at which bleeding began to occur.

_____

_____

7. Contrast the symptoms noted by a woman with a normal pregnancy with those that may be noted by a woman with an ectopic pregnancy.

_____

_____

8. Describe the rationale for using heparin to treat disseminated intravascular coagulation.

_____

_____

9. Explain how a teaching plan for a client with multiple gestations would differ from a plan for a client with single gestation in the following areas: activity, nutrition, complications, and role changes.

_____

_____

APPLYING YOUR KNOWLEDGE

CASE STUDY

Danielle is a 38-year-old secretary who is pregnant with her first child. She is 5 ft 6 in and weighs 210 lb. When she arrived at the clinic for her seventh-month visit, the nurse notes her blood pressure is 148/92 mm Hg. She states she has had ankle edema for several months now but lately has noticed swelling in her face and hands.

1. What symptoms might signal the development of mild pre-eclampsia? How would you teach a client to monitor for them?

_____

_____

2. What nursing measures would you implement for a client with mild pre-eclampsia?

_____

_____

_____

CRITICAL INQUIRY EXERCISE

1. What would be the major points you would include in a teaching plan for adolescents that address the effects of sexually transmitted diseases on a fetus or on an infant after childbirth?

2. In what way, if any, would your teaching plan differ for an insulin-dependent diabetic who became pregnant, and for a pregnant woman who developed gestational diabetes?

CRITICAL EXPLORATION

Monitor the care of a client with pre-eclampsia or eclampsia. Note the nursing care provided and medications used.

PRACTICING FOR NCLEX

MULTIPLE-CHOICE QUESTIONS

Circle the letter that corresponds to the best answer for each question.

1. Mrs. Dean is 2 months pregnant and has a history of two spontaneous miscarriages. Which of the following assessments indicates a potential for a third miscarriage?

   a. Lab results revealing an elevation in protein-bound iodine.

   b. Dietary intake indicating 300 more calories than eaten by the nonpregnant female.

   c. Reports of exposure to a child with rubella over a period of time.

   d. Nervous, anxious behavior noted during the prenatal visits.

2. The nurse monitoring a client who is experiencing a miscarriage episode must consider which of the following facts?

   a. Miscarriages occurring before the sixth week of pregnancy often result in severe bleeding and hypovolemia.

   b. A D&C can be performed to prevent a threatened miscarriage from advancing to an imminent miscarriage.

   c. A missed miscarriage will result in no expulsion of blood or fetal material until the fetus actually dies.

   d. Incomplete miscarriages present a greater potential for hemorrhage than do complete miscarriages.

3. If an Rh-negative woman experiences a miscarriage during her first pregnancy, she should be instructed to do which of the following?

   a. Adopt children, since future pregnancies will result in future miscarriages.

   b. Avoid pregnancy for the next year to permit a decrease in Rh antigens.

   c. Consume high doses of vitamin D and vitamin K to prevent anemia.

   d. Receive Rh(D antigen) immune globulin (RhIG) to prevent isoimmunization.

4. When assessing a woman who is suspected of having an ectopic pregnancy, the nurse would report which of the following as a risk factor?

   a. A history of using intrauterine devices for birth control.

   b. Nausea and vomiting during early pregnancy.

   c. A soft, nontender abdomen with active bowel sounds.

   d. Absence of vaginal bleeding or menstrual flow.

5. Which of the following findings might be noted in a client with a hydatidiform mole?

   a. False-negative blood test results for pregnancy.

   b. Fetal heart tones that are louder and faster than normal.

   c. Marked (extreme) nausea and vomiting noted in early pregnancy.

   d. Uterine growth occurring more slowly than in normal pregnancy.

6. Which of the following nursing diagnoses may be indicated for a client diagnosed and treated for hydatidiform mole?

   a. Imbalanced nutrition, more than body requirements related to increased appetite.

   b. Fluid volume excess related to polycythemia resulting from drug therapy.

   c. Grieving related to feelings associated with the loss of a pregnancy.

   d. Ineffective family coping related to poor bonding with newborn.

7. Dee Ball is admitted with placenta previa with 75% coverage of the cervical os. The fetus is at 35 weeks' gestation. Which of the following nursing measures should be implemented?

   a. Encourage Ms. Ball to lie on her back as much as possible.

   b. Instruct Ms. Ball to use a tampon to halt the vaginal bleeding.

   c. Obtain oxygen equipment to keep on standby in case of fetal distress.

   d. Teach Ms. Ball the importance of limiting stair climbing.

8. Postterm pregnancy is dangerous to the fetus in which of the following ways?

   a. The fetus will suffer from decreased blood perfusion.

   b. Fetal inhalation results in aspiration of amniotic fluid.

c. Hydramnios leading to decreased fetal circulation will occur.

d. Microcephaly may result in increased biparietal diameter.

9. Which of the following is true about Rh incompatibility?

a. If the mother is Rh negative and the father is homozygous Rh positive, the child will have a 50% chance of being Rh negative.

b. If the mother is Rh negative and the father is heterozygous for the trait, 100% of the children can be expected to be Rh positive.

c. The Rh-positive fetus inside of an Rh-negative mother is perceived as a foreign agent and stimulates the formation of antibodies.

d. Women who are Rh negative and experience miscarriage of an Rh-positive fetus will not develop antibodies to foreign Rh antigen.

10. The client going through labor who knows her child will be stillborn will likely experience which of the following emotions?

a. Relief that the pregnancy will be terminated early so she can try again to have a baby.

b. Delight that she will not have to carry the heavy baby to term.

c. Grief at the loss of her infant and her inability to carry a pregnancy to term.

d. Confidence in her ability to conceive a child that will be viable.

ALTERNATE FORMAT QUESTIONS
Multiple-Answer Multiple-Choice Questions

Circle the letter(s) corresponding to the appropriate answer(s). Select all that apply.

1. Which of the following would be the cause for concern if it were noted during a prenatal assessment in the third trimester?

a. Frequent painless urination.

b. Fetal movement after eating.

c. Meconium appearing vaginal discharge.

d. Back pain and problems finding a comfortable sleeping position.

e. Additional, severe pain occurring with each contraction.

2. Which of the following findings would be most indicative of fetal death?

a. Failure of labor to begin before the 42nd week of gestation.

b. Reports that the fetus has been very lazy and has not moved or kicked.

c. Sonogram readings that reveal a rapid heart rate and rhythm.

d. Absence of fetal movement in the period of pregnancy after to quickening.

e. Dark green sticky substance noted when membranes ruptured.

3. Which of the following findings would lead the nurse to suspect hydramnios?

a. Rapid enlargement of the uterus.

b. Dark red vaginal bleeding.

c. Complaints of shortness of breath.

d. Decreased weight gain.

e. Lower extremity varicosities.

22

Nursing Care of a Pregnant Family With Special Needs

CHAPTER OVERVIEW

Chapter 22 discusses nursing care related to care of a pregnant family with special needs. The needs of an adolescent, a woman over age 40, a woman with a physical handicap, a woman with a drug dependency during pregnancy, and trauma during pregnancy are reviewed. The use of the nursing process to plan and provide appropriate teaching for a woman with special needs throughout pregnancy is explored.

LEARNING OBJECTIVES

After mastering the content in this chapter, you should be able to do the following:

1. Identify the characteristics and the risks of pregnancy of a pregnant woman who has special needs such as one who has been injured, an adolescent, a woman over age 40, someone who is physically or cognitively challenged, or a woman who is drug dependent.

2. Identify National Health Goals related to women with special needs that nurses can be instrumental in helping the nation achieve.

3. Use critical thinking to analyze ways that nursing care of a pregnant woman with a special need can be optimally family centered.

4. Assess a woman with special needs during pregnancy.

5. Formulate nursing diagnoses related to pregnancy for a woman with special needs.

6. Identify expected outcomes for a pregnant woman with special needs.

7. Plan nursing care to address the special needs of women at the extremes of the childbearing spectrum, have a physical or cognitive challenge who have been injured or who are substance dependent.

8. Implement nursing care for a woman with special needs, such as encouraging her to remain ambulatory during pregnancy.

9. Evaluate outcomes for effectiveness and achievement of care.

10. Identify areas related to care of a pregnant woman with special needs that would benefit from additional nursing research or application of evidence-based practice.

11. Integrate knowledge of the risks of pregnancy with women with special needs with the nursing process to achieve quality maternal and child health nursing care.

KEY TERMS

autonomic dysreflexia
emancipated minor
substance dependent

MASTERING THE INFORMATION

FILL IN THE BLANKS

Supply the missing term or the information requested.

1. A pregnant adolescent is regarded as an _____ _____ and can make her own health care decisions and sign permission for her own care.

2. In a pregnant adolescent, cephalopelvic disproportion is suggested by lack of _____ at the beginning of labor, a _____ first stage of labor and poor _____ _____.

3. In the woman over age 40, the uterus may not contract as readily in the postpartum period because of inelasticity placing her at higher risk for _____ _____.

MATCHING

Match the terms in Column I with a definition, example, or related statement from Column II. Place the letter corresponding to the answer in the space provided.

Column I

1. ___ Autonomic dysreflexia

2. ___ Substance dependent

3. ___ Cephalopelvic disproportion

4. ___ Trauma

5. ___ Day history

6. ___ Egocentric phenomenon

7. ___ Nest-building behavior

8. ___ Postpartal hemorrhage

9. ___ Striae

10. ___ Varicosities

Column II

a. Complication associated with pregnant adolescents and women over 40 due to overdistention of the uterus or decreased uterine contractility.

b. Pregnancy change that will probably fade from the adolescent's body following pregnancy.

c. Written account of nutritional practices, sleep and daily activity, use of drugs, and support/friendships of the pregnant adolescent.

d. A possible complication associated with a pregnant adolescent that may occur because of incomplete pelvic growth, necessitating a cesarean birth.

e. Symptoms include severe hypertension, throbbing headache, nausea, bradycardia, skin flushing, and profuse diaphoresis in a woman with a high spinal cord injury.

f. The development of withdrawal symptoms following discontinuation of a substance.

g. Common problem possibly prevented by resting daily with feet elevated and sleeping in Sims position to decrease venous congestion.

h. Evidence may not be noted in women over 40 until after aminocentesis results determine the baby is healthy.

i. An adolescent's belief that although she is sexually active she would not become pregnant.

j. Increased incidence during third trimester due to poor balance and fainting from orthostatic hypotension.

SHORT ANSWER

Supply the missing term or the information requested.

1. Identify three factors that have contributed to the inability to stop teenage pregnancies.

   _____

   _____

2. Name three physical conditions that a pregnant adolescent is at high risk for developing.

   _____

   _____

3. Explain how nurses can be instrumental in helping the nation achieve the goal of reducing pregnancy among girls aged 17 and younger.

   _____

   _____

4. Discuss nursing responsibilities relative to child safety for the pregnant woman who is experiencing moderate or severe cognitive challenges.

_____

_____

5. Discuss the reasons a pregnant woman with drug dependency might not comply with a prenatal visitation schedule or proper diet.

_____

_____

APPLYING YOUR KNOWLEDGE

CASE STUDY

Bertha, age 16, has a T1 spinal injury due to an automobile accident 2 years ago. She is 4 months pregnant and is in for her second prenatal visit.

1. What are some of the major areas you would assess to determine priorities in planning care for Bertha?

_____

_____

_____

2. In what ways will Bertha's age add to the complications normally present for a pregnant woman with a spinal cord injury?

_____

_____

_____

3. What issues might impact birth control measures that you suggest for Bertha during your postpartal teaching?

_____

_____

_____

CRITICAL INQUIRY EXERCISE

1. Prepare a teaching plan for a woman with cerebral palsy that addresses methods for maintaining an adequate rest and activity pattern.

2. Write a short essay about your feelings regarding adolescent pregnancy, women over age 40 who plan pregnancy, and women with drug addiction who become pregnant. What type of nursing care should they receive?

CRITICAL EXPLORATION

Visit a prenatal clinic for women who are mentally retarded. Observe the visit of a woman at each of the levels of retardation. Note the differences and similarities in instructions given regarding activities, rest, and nutritional needs.

PRACTICING FOR NCLEX

MULTIPLE-CHOICE QUESTIONS

Circle the letter that corresponds to the best answer for each question.

1. Bobby, age 14, is in her fourth month of pregnancy. To help prevent the development of anemia, the nurse would do which of the following?

a. Tell Bobby she needs to eat balanced meals and snacks to help her be well nourished.

b. Instruct Bobby to report black stools, which indicate that she is bleeding internally because of iron intake.

c. Instruct Bobby regarding the signs of labor before she completes her fifth month of pregnancy.

d. Tell Bobby if she takes an iron supplement each day she would not have to eat foods like liver.

2. When planning a teaching strategy for the pregnant adolescent, the nurse should do which of the following?

a. Inform the teen she should consider the needs of her baby first when eating or planning activity.

b. Omit information related to minor pains of pregnancy to prevent the adolescent from developing hypochondria.

c. Explain how healthy eating and exercise habits will help the teen look and feel better.

d. Emphasize the importance of frequent urine and blood testing to ensure that she is drug-free.

3. Bonnie, 16 years old and 7 months pregnant, has been diagnosed with early symptoms of pregnancy-induced hypertension (PIH). An outcome that would be appropriate for Bonnie would include which of the following? Bonnie

   a. regularly performs knee–chest exercises three times daily to strengthen her vascular system.

   b. verbalizes a plan for obtaining schoolwork while resting at home until her baby is born.

   c. states her intention to watch for pale mucous membranes and note any cravings, which are signs of PIH.

   d. verbalizes her understanding that she is ill and must remain in bed to get well.

4. Sheila, age 43, is pregnant and has been scheduled for a serum alpha-fetoprotein level. The nurse would explain which of the following to Sheila?

   a. One purpose of the test is to determine whether a chromosomal defect is present.

   b. An amniocentesis will not provide the fetal serum specimen needed for the test.

   c. Conditions like open spinal cord cannot be diagnosed through this test.

   d. The test must be performed before the 12th week of pregnancy to prevent fetal damage.

5. Your client has a T2 spinal cord injury and is 6 months pregnant. Which of the following information should be included in pregnancy counseling for her?

   a. Since she will not be able to feel uterine contractions, she needs to feel her abdomen often during the last months to detect the tightening of labor.

   b. She should adjust the footrests on her wheelchair so that she maintains her legs with a sharp bend at the knee to relieve the pressure on her abdomen.

   c. Pregnancy will decrease her risk for urinary tract infections since serum corticosteroid levels are increased in pregnancy.

   d. The enlarged uterus will assist her in urinating, so she will not need to use a catheter or perform the Credé method to be sure she empties her bladder.

6. Joan is in her fourth month of pregnancy and confides to the nurse that she is addicted to heroin and uses prostitution to afford her

habit. Which response by the nurse would be most appropriate?

   a. Plan to include tests for sexually transmitted diseases in Joan's future prenatal visits.

   b. Prepare Joan for the high possibility that her baby will be born dead because she has taken heroin.

   c. Record on Joan's chart the need to monitor her baby for hyperbilirubinemia, a complication of heroin abuse.

   d. Tell Joan her baby is in no danger because fetal exposure to narcotics actually strengthens the liver and the lungs.

7. During the postpartal period, the nurse would implement which of the following measures for the visually impaired woman to facilitate maternal–child well-being?

   a. Instruct the mother to secure a sighted assistant to help her care for her new infant after she is discharged home.

   b. Limit the time the mother has to care for her child during the first few days to prevent frustration and fatigue.

   c. Speak loudly when explaining self-care measures or infant care measures the mother must use with her baby.

   d. Stress the importance of the mother facing the infant when speaking, to establish eye-to-eye contact and develop trust.

8. Tina is a pregnant cocaine user. Which of the following, if undertaken by Tina, would indicate that a teaching plan for her had been effective?

   a. Tina plans to restrict her cocaine use to smoking a pipe during her last months of pregnancy.

   b. Tina decreases cocaine use once she has completed her pregnancy.

   c. Tina stated she will use crack instead of cocaine while she is pregnant.

   d. Tina voiced plans to seek assistance to help her stop using cocaine.

9. Which information would be most important to provide to a pregnant woman who is drug dependent?

   a. Her fetus may be born drug dependent and have withdrawal symptoms.

   b. Marijuana can be used to decrease withdrawal symptoms without fetal harm.

c. Pregnancy will temporarily take away her desire for drugs and alcohol.

d. Regular cocaine will not cross the placental barrier, but crack cocaine will.

ALTERNATE FORMAT QUESTIONS

Multiple-Answer Multiple-Choice Questions

Circle the letter(s) corresponding to the appropriate answer(s). Select all that apply.

1. When providing care to a 42-year-old pregnant woman, the nurse would be alert for signs and symptoms of which of the following?

   a. Hypertension of pregnancy.

   b. Preterm birth.

   c. Postterm birth.

   d. Rapid labor.

   e. Postpartum hemorrhage.

2. The nurse is teaching a community women's group about the effects of drug use on pregnancy. Which of the following would the nurse include as possible effects of heroin use?

   a. Fetal opiate dependence.

   b. Hyperbilirubinemia.

   c. Pregnancy-induced hypertension.

   d. Large-for-gestational age newborn.

   e. Hepatitis B.

   f. Subacute bacterial endocarditis.

3. A woman with a high thoracic spinal cord injury is in labor develops autonomic dysreflexia. Which of the following would the nurse expect to assess?

   a. Severe hypotension.

   b. Profuse diaphoresis.

   c. Throbbing headache.

   d. Flushing of the skin.

   e. Tachycardia.

Nursing Care of a Family Experiencing a Complication of Labor or Birth

CHAPTER OVERVIEW

Chapter 23 describes and summarizes the more common complications that occur during labor and birth. Women and their families who are most at risk are discussed. Nurses play a vital role in making labor safe. Common treatments are explained and illustrated. Nursing diagnoses and related intervention skills are emphasized to ensure protection of fetal and maternal health.

LEARNING OBJECTIVES

After mastering the content of this chapter, you should be able to do the following:

1. Define the terms *dystocia* and *dysfunctional labor* and how common deviations in the power (force of labor), the passage, or the passenger can cause dystocia or dysfunctional labor.

2. Identify National Health Goals related to complications of labor that nurses could help the nation achieve.

3. Use critical thinking to analyze ways to maintain family-centered nursing care when deviations from the normal in labor or birth occur.

4. Assess a woman in labor and during birth for deviations from the normal labor process.

5. Formulate nursing diagnoses related to deviations from normal in labor and birth.

6. Identify expected outcomes associated with deviations from normal labor and birth and resultant complications.

7. Plan nursing interventions to help the family meet expected outcomes when complications of labor occur.

8. Implement nursing care related to complications of labor or birth, such as preparing the family for a cesarean birth.

9. Evaluate expected outcomes for achievement and effectiveness of care.

10. Identify areas related to complications of labor that could benefit from additional nursing research or application of evidence-based practice.

11. Integrate the knowledge of deviations of normal in labor and birth with nursing process to achieve quality maternal and child health nursing care.

KEY TERMS

amnioinfusion
amniotic fluid embolism
augmentation of labor
battledore placenta
deceleration
dysfunctional labor
dystocia
external cephalic
    version
forceps birth
hypertonic uterine
    contractions
hypotonic uterine
    contractions

induction of labor
Leopold's maneuvers
oxytocin
pathologic retraction
    ring
placenta accreta
placenta circumvallata
placenta marginata
placenta succenturiata
precipitate labor
umbilical cord
    prolapse
uterine inversion
vacuum extraction

MASTERING THE INFORMATION

FILL IN THE BLANKS

Supply the missing term or the information requested.

1. _____ _____ causes a marked caput on the newborn's head when used.

2. Immediate management of umbilical cord prolapse is to place the patient in a _____- _____ position or _____ position.

3. _____ or _____ labor are terms used to describe sluggish contractions.

MATCHING

Match the terms in Column I with a definition, example, or related statement from Column II. Place the letter corresponding to the answer in the space provided.

Column I

1. ___ Cephalopelvic disproportion

2. ___ Cervical ripening

3. ___ Oxytocin

4. ___ Dystocia

5. ___ McRobert's maneuver

6. ___ Pathologic retraction ring

7. ___ Vacuum extraction

8. ___ Uterine inversion

9. ___ Piper forceps

10. ___ External cephalic version

Column II

a. Method that is advantageous over forceps births.

b. Method used to deliver the head in a breech presentation.

c. Ridge across abdomen that signals possible uterine rupture.

d. Turning of the uterus inside out.

e. Drug used to induce or augment labor.

f. Gentle external pressure used to rotate the position of the fetus.

g. Measure involving sharp flexion of woman's thighs onto the abdomen.

h. Fetal head too large for passage; small pelvis.

i. Change in consistency from firm to soft.

j. Sluggishness of contractions or force of labor.

DYSFUNCTION AND THE STAGES OF LABOR

Indicate whether the following dysfunctions occur in the first (A) or second (B) stage of labor by placing an "A" or "B" in the space provided.

1. ___ Protracted active phase

2. ___ Prolonged deceleration phase

3. ___ Arrest of descent

4. ___ Prolonged descent

5. ___ Secondary arrest of dilation

6. ___ Prolonged latent phase

SHORT ANSWER

Supply the missing term or the information requested.

1. A _____ _____ _____ is a warning sign of severe dysfunctional labor and may signal an impending _____ of the uterus.

2. Umbilical cords that have only two vessels are associated with congenital anomalies of the _____ and _____.

3. Management of a prolapsed cord is aimed toward relieving _____ _____ which will relieve fetal _____.

4. List and define the three main components of labor.

_____

_____

5. What is one of the major assessments used to detect deviations from normal labor and birth?

_____

_____

6. List three types of abnormal uterine contractions.

_____

_____

7. Name the dysfunctional labor patterns for the first stage of labor.

_____

_____

8. Name three common health problems associated with multiple gestation deliveries.

_____

_____

9. List two dangers of a breech delivery.

_____

_____

10. List four types of abnormal presentation.

_____

_____

11. Name three indications for a forceps delivery.

_____

_____

12. List the two types of breech presentation.

_____

_____

APPLYING YOUR KNOWLEDGE

CASE STUDY

Mrs. Price, age 36, is in premature labor, expecting twins. She is at 36 weeks' gestation, and one of the twins is a breech presentation. This is Mrs. Price's second multiple birth. Her previous delivery of twins resulted in the death of twin A; twin B survived and was later diagnosed with cerebral palsy.

1. How might Mr. and Mrs. Price be feeling about their current situation?

_____

_____

_____

2. What assessments would be critical for the nurse to make at this time?

_____

_____

_____

CRITICAL INQUIRY EXERCISE

1. Choose a potential health problem as a complication of labor and write a care plan for this high-risk patient.

2. Formulate a nursing care plan for a woman who is pregnant with her first child and is in prolonged labor.

CRITICAL EXPLORATION

Arrange to visit the labor and delivery care areas in your hospital. Seek assistance from the staff to accompany and monitor a patient who would need surgery after her labor has failed to progress.

PRACTICING FOR NCLEX

MULTIPLE-CHOICE QUESTIONS

Circle the letter that corresponds to the best answer for each question.

1. Labor may be induced in which of the following women? A woman with
   a. a fetus in transverse lie.
   b. presenting part engaged.
   c. a premature fetus.
   d. cephalopelvic disproportion.

2. A multiparous woman arrived 2 hours ago in active labor with 4 cm of cervical dilation. Now she states that she has a strong urge to push. Which answer most likely describes what is occurring?
   a. She may have cephalopelvic disproportion.
   b. She may need an analgesic or sedation.

c. She is having a precipitous delivery.

d. She is having a breech birth.

3. Which of the following would lead the nurse to suspect that a pregnant client has developed an amniotic fluid embolism?

a. Report of sudden severe chest pain and dyspnea.

b. Evidence of hypotonic contractions and poor force of labor.

c. Report of back pain when ambulating or lying in bed.

d. Rapid cervical dilation of 5 cm/hour.

4. To assess a laboring client for ineffective uterine force, the nurse would

a. check the electrolyte panel for the level of carbon dioxide.

b. assess for glucose in a specimen of amniotic fluid.

c. monitor contraction duration, strength, and resting tone.

d. watch the client for elevated respiratory rates during contractions.

5. A woman with a fetus in occipitoposterior position would commonly demonstrate which of the following?

a. Precipitate labor.

b. Acute chest pain.

c. Increased energy levels.

d. Intense back pressure.

ALTERNATE FORMAT QUESTIONS
Multiple-Answer Multiple-Choice Questions

Circle the letter(s) corresponding to the appropriate answer(s). Select all that apply.

1. Which conditions place a pregnant woman at high risk for a prolapsed cord? Select all that apply.

a. Premature rupture of membranes.

b. Cephalic fetal presentation.

c. Placenta previa.

d. Hydramnios.

e. A large fetus.

f. Cephalopelvic disproportion.

2. Conditions that may place the patient at high risk for uterine rupture during the birthing process include which of the following?

a. Premature labor.

b. Abnormal presentation.

c. Multiple gestation.

d. Previous episiotomy scar.

e. Obstructed labor.

f. Traumatic maneuvers of forceps or traction.

3. A woman is to undergo labor induction. Which of the following assessment findings should be present?

a. Breech fetal presentation.

b. Ripe cervix.

c. Engagement of presenting part.

d. Cephalopelvic disproportion.

e. Mature fetus.

f. Cervical dilation of 4 cm.

Nursing Care of a Family During Cesarean Birth

CHAPTER OVERVIEW

Interruptions in the predictable laboring process and the mechanics of delivery may require preparation of a woman and her family for delivery of the infant by cesarean birth. This chapter reviews both scheduled and emergency cesarean births and examines the preoperative and postoperative principles of nursing for the client experiencing a cesarean surgery. Reasons for cesarean birth, the surgical procedure, and physiologic and psychological responses of the woman and family are discussed.

LEARNING OBJECTIVES

After mastering the content in this chapter, you should be able to do the following:

1. Describe the usual indications for cesarean birth.

2. Identify National Health Goals related to cesarean birth that nurses can help the nation achieve.

3. Use critical thinking to analyze how to keep birth family centered when a cesarean birth is scheduled.

4. Assess a woman scheduled for cesarean birth for effective preoperative, intraoperative, and postoperative needs.

5. Formulate nursing diagnoses related to the family experiencing a cesarean birth.

6. Establish outcomes that meet the needs of a woman requiring a cesarean birth.

7. Plan appropriate nursing care for the family experiencing a cesarean birth.

8. Implement common preoperative and postoperative care measures for cesarean birth.

9. Evaluate expected outcomes for achievement and effectiveness of care.

10. Identify areas related to cesarean birth that could benefit from additional nursing research or application of evidence-based practice.

11. Integrate knowledge of cesarean birth with the nursing process to achieve quality maternal and child health nursing care

KEY TERMS

cesarean birth	dehiscence
classic cesarean incision	low segment incision

MASTERING THE INFORMATION

MATCHING

Match the terms in Column I with a definition, example, or related statement from Column II. Place the letter corresponding to the answer in the space provided.

Column I

1. ____ Transcutaneous electrical nerve stimulation (TENS)

2. ____ Patient-controlled analgesia (PCA)

3. ____ Stress response

4. ____ Epidural analgesia

Column II

a. May result in intense itching and nausea and vomiting.

b. Involves applying electrodes to the surface of the skin to effectively control pain by blocking the ability of the cerebral cortex to interpret the incoming sensation.

c. Requires self-administration of intravenous narcotic analgesia.

d. Results in the release of epinephrine and norepinephrine from the adrenal gland medulla.

TRUE OR FALSE

Indicate if the following statements are true or false by placing a "T" or "F" in the space provided.

1. ____ Obesity may predispose the skin line repair of a woman who had a cesarean birth to dehiscence.

2. ____ Unlike the cesarean birth client who has received general anesthesia, the cesarean birth client who has received an epidural is not at risk for intestinal paralysis.

3. ____ The woman who received epidural anesthesia for cesarean birth is limited to a supine position immediately after the procedure.

4. ____ Lochia should not be visible for assessment if the woman has a cesarean birth.

SHORT ANSWER

Supply the missing term or the information requested.

1. Why is it an effective nursing action to include the expectant woman's support person when giving anticipatory guidance?

_____

_____

2. Why is a sonogram useful to the physician before making the incision for a cesarean procedure?

_____

_____

3. Explain why it is of utmost importance that the surgical client be assessed for urinary output following surgery.

_____

_____

4. Identify and discuss three potential maladaptations that may occur in a woman following a cesarean birth procedure if her pain is not controlled.

_____

_____

5. Identify and discuss two supportive pain control methods that can be used to assist the postpartal surgical client. Explain the essential components of these devices.

_____

_____

6. Compare the amount of blood lost during a vaginal birth with that of a cesarean birth.

_____

_____

APPLYING YOUR KNOWLEDGE

CASE STUDY

Lorraine Murphy has undergone a cesarean birth of her first child with epidural anesthesia. The nurse is monitoring her closely for postpartal and postsurgical complications.

1. What position should Ms. Murphy be placed in when she is brought to the postanesthesia care unit?

   _____

   _____

   _____

2. What would be Ms. Murphy's immediate care needs?

   _____

   _____

   _____

3. Explain why Ms. Murphy would be in jeopardy for an imbalance of fluid and electrolytes.

   _____

   _____

   _____

CRITICAL INQUIRY EXERCISE

1. Formulate a nursing care plan that will focus on alleviating fears for the client and family awaiting a cesarean delivery.

2. Compare the preoperative and postoperative nursing care needed for the client who delivers vaginally with the client who has undergone a cesarean section delivery.

CRITICAL EXPLORATION

Formulate a teaching plan for a pregnant woman whom you will care for when assigned to the women's health unit. The plan should indicate that this patient has been scheduled for a preplanned surgical procedure. Identify those teaching advantages from your text that you propose will enable the nurse to prepare the patient more efficiently due to the nature of the birthing method. After you have been assigned to the patient on the floor, compare and contrast the teaching points that you selected from your text with those listed in the teaching care plan on the patient's chart.

PRACTICING FOR NCLEX

MULTIPLE-CHOICE QUESTIONS

Circle the letter that corresponds to the best answer for each question.

1. Mrs. Jordan has been admitted on the unit the day prior to a scheduled cesarean birth. Mrs. Jordan is unable to deliver vaginally due to cephalopelvic disproportion. The nurse instructs Mrs. Jordan on deep breathing exercises as part of the preoperative teaching plan. The rationale for this exercise is to

   a. promote involution on a traumatized uterus.

   b. prevent stasis of mucus in the lungs.

   c. prevent pulmonary edema.

   d. stimulate the diaphragm to contract.

2. Nurse administers ranitidine (Zantac) as ordered prior to a planned cesarean birth to

   a. neutralize urine acidity.

   b. promote uterine contractions.

   c. delay uterine contractions.

   d. decrease gastric secretions.

3. The surgeon plans to perform a low segment incision rather than a classic incision. This type of incision is more advantageous because

   a. it is made horizontally and high on the woman's abdomen.

   b. the procedure is faster with the incision being made simultaneously through the abdomen and uterus.

   c. the likelihood of a postpartal uterine infection is decreased.

   d. the procedure is made with a vertical incision to decrease the chances of reopening.

4. Which of the following would lead the nurse to suspect that a woman who has had a cesarean birth is developing peritonitis?

   a. Guarded abdomen.

   b. Elevated temperature.

c. Excessive lochia discharge.

d. Episode of painful involuntary contractions.

5. If oxytocin is ordered postoperatively for the client who has had a cesarean birth, the most important nursing intervention would be to

   a. monitor the woman's blood pressure.

   b. assess for increased lochia discharge.

   c. prevent infection at the incision site.

   d. implement measures to promote comfort.

ALTERNATE FORMAT QUESTIONS

Multiple-Answer Multiple-Choice Questions

Circle the letter(s) corresponding to the appropriate answer(s). Select all that apply.

1. A woman has undergone a cesarean birth is to be discharged. The nurse would instruct the woman to notify her health care provider is she develops which of the following?

   a. Burning on urination.

   b. Drainage at her incision line.

   c. Decrease in lochia.

d. Fever over 100.4°F (38°C).

e. No bowel movement for 2 days.

2. Which of the following would lead a nurse to suspect that woman who has had a cesarean birth is developing postpartum hemorrhage?

   a. Pulse rate of 140 beats per minute.

   b. Respiratory rate of 22 breaths per minute.

   c. Blood pressure of 110/60 mm Hg.

   d. Complaints of being thirsty.

   e. Restlessness.

3. Which of the following interventions would be most helpful to assist a woman to void after a cesarean birth?

   a. Withholding prescribed analgesic.

   b. Providing privacy for elimination.

   c. Assisting the woman to the bathroom every 2 hours.

   d. Pouring cold water over her perineal area.

   e. Running water from the tap within woman's hearing distance.

Nursing Care of a Family Experiencing a Postpartal Complication

CHAPTER OVERVIEW

A woman and her family who are experiencing a postpartal complication may have difficulty bonding with the child. If the illness responds poorly to treatment, the woman's potential to give birth to another child may be threatened. Many postpartal complications can be prevented with the support of a health team's assessment skills and the ability of each professional caring for the postpartal patient to evaluate findings and intervene appropriately.

LEARNING OBJECTIVES

After mastering the content in this chapter, you should be able to do the following:

1. Describe common deviations from the normal that can occur during the puerperium.

2. Identify National Health Goals related to postpartal complications that nurses can help the nation achieve.

3. Use critical thinking to analyze ways that promote family-centered nursing care when a postpartal complication occurs.

4. Assess a woman and her family for deviations from the normal during the puerperium.

5. Formulate nursing diagnoses related to deviations from the normal during the puerperium.

6. Identify expected outcomes for a postpartal woman experiencing a complication.

7. Plan interventions that meet the special needs of a family with a postpartal complication, such as planning for an extended hospitalization.

8. Implement nursing care when a postpartal complication such as hemorrhage, infection, pregnancy-induced hypertension, or postpartal psychosis develops.

9. Evaluate expected outcomes for achievement and effectiveness of care.

10. Identify areas related to care of women with postpartal complications that could benefit from additional nursing research or application of evidence-based practice.

11. Integrate knowledge of postpartal complications with the nursing process to achieve quality maternal and child health nursing care.

KEY TERMS

endometritis
mastitis
peritonitis
postpartal depression

postpartal psychosis
thrombophlebitis
uterine inversion

MASTERING THE INFORMATION

FILL IN THE BLANKS

Supply the missing term or the information requested.

1. When assessing lochia to detect a cervical tear that occurred during the birthing process, the nurse would note that blood from a cervical tear is _____ than normal lochia.

2. The nurse would weigh _____ _____ to get an accurate account of measuring blood loss from lochia.

3. _____ _____ refers to a prolapse of the fundus through the cervix so that the uterus turns inside out.

MATCHING

Match the terms in Column I with a definition, example, or related statement from Column II. Place the letter corresponding to the answer in the space provided.

Column I

1. ___ Thrombophlebitis

2. ___ Endometritis

3. ___ Perineal hematomas

4. ___ Postpartal depression

5. ___ Peritonitis

6. ___ Urinary retention

7. ___ Mastitis

Column II

a. A collection of blood in the subcutaneous layer of the perineum.

b. Infection of the breast.

c. Result of edema of the bladder from pressures during childbirth.

d. Overwhelming sadness extending beyond the immediate postpartum period.

e. Inflammation of the lining of a blood vessel with the formation of blood clots.

f. Infection of the peritoneal cavity.

g. Infection of the lining of the uterus.

TRUE OR FALSE

Indicate if the following statements are true or false by placing a "T" or "F" in the space provided.

___ 1. The majority of the complications occurring during the puerperium are preventable.

___ 2. Women who experience blood loss greater than 500 cc in 24 hours are traditionally considered to be hemorrhaging and may require blood replacement.

___ 3. An elevated level of human chorionic gonadotropin (hCG) is present if the postpartal woman has retained placental fragments after the birth of the placenta.

___ 4. Most postpartal infections are caused by staphylococcal organisms.

SHORT ANSWER

Supply the missing term or the information requested.

1. The four reasons that are most often found to be the precipitating causes of postpartal hemorrhage include _____, _____, _____, and _____.

2. Define disseminated intravascular coagulation (DIC).

   _____

   _____

3. What are the common causes of DIC during the postpartal period?

   _____

   _____

4. What is the rationale that supports teaching women to wipe the perineal area from front to back when cleansing or removing feces?

   _____

   _____

5. Endometritis is a preventable postpartal complication that may lead to a more serious illness. What are the important components of the nurse's assessment to determine the early signs of endometritis?

_____

_____

_____

6. Explain why it is important to inspect the placenta after an uncomplicated delivery?

_____

_____

_____

APPLYING YOUR KNOWLEDGE

CASE STUDY

Mrs. Lawson, age 36, gravida 3 para 3, is suffering from a puerperal infection during the postpartum period.

1. What factors might predispose Mrs. Lawson to the development of an infection?

_____

_____

_____

2. Review of Mrs. Lawson's medical record reveals endometritis. Which assessment findings would support this diagnosis?

_____

_____

_____

CRITICAL INQUIRY EXERCISE

1. Prepare a discharge-teaching packet for a client with thrombophlebitis.

2. Consider the risk of exposure to an infection during delivery. Develop a set of guidelines that can serve as protective measures against the development of endometritis.

CRITICAL EXPLORATION

Review the policy of the agency where you are doing your maternal health clinical rotation. Identify the ward's policy on the nurse's authority to order blood from the blood bank for a client who is experiencing a postpartal hemorrhage.

PRACTICING FOR NCLEX

MULTIPLE-CHOICE QUESTIONS

Circle the letter that corresponds to the best answer for each question.

1. Which assessment finding would lead the nurse to suspect a postpartal complication?
   a. Lochia rubra 12 hours after birth.
   b. Temperature of 100.4°F or less.
   c. Blood loss of more than 12 oz/24 hours.
   d. 20 to 24 sanitary pads saturated/24 hours.

2. Mrs. Jones is experiencing signs of shock about 3 hours after delivery. Which of the following would the nurse expect to find when assessing Mrs. Jones?
   a. Diastolic blood pressure increased more than 10 mm Hg.
   b. Decreased pulse rate.
   c. Rapid respirations.
   d. Flushed face.

3. Which medication would the nurse expect to administer as ordered for a client who is experiencing postpartum hemorrhage from uterine atony?
   a. Apresoline.
   b. Zaroxolyn.
   c. Methergine.
   d. Proventil.

4. Which of the following is viewed as a risk factor for a woman developing a postpartal infection?
   a. Thyroid toxicosis.
   b. Excessive blood loss.
   c. Pregnancy-induced hypertension.
   d. Negative Rh factor.

5. Which measure would be most appropriate when caring for the client who has experienced a fourth-degree perineal laceration?

   a. Encourage her to douche at least once a week to ensure cleanliness.

   b. Administer analgesic rectal suppositories to promote comfort.

   c. Encourage fluid intake and foods high in fiber.

   d. Administer an enema when necessary to prevent constipation.

ALTERNATE FORMAT QUESTIONS

Multiple-Answer Multiple-Choice Questions

Circle the letter(s) corresponding to the appropriate answer(s). Select all that apply.

1. Identify the cardinal signs of postpartal-induced hypertension. Select all that apply.

   a. Elevated blood pressure.

   b. Urinary frequency.

   c. Edema.

   d. Proteinuria.

   e. Perspiration.

2. Which of the following instructions would be most appropriate to teach a woman to prevent thrombophlebitis?

   a. Using the lithotomy position for birth.

   b. Drinking adequate amounts of fluid.

   c. Ambulating soon after birth as able.

   d. Sitting with the knees sharply bent.

   e. Wearing knee high stockings.

   f. Doing leg lifts while resting in bed.

3. Which of the following assessment findings would lead a nurse to suspect that a woman has developed postpartum depression?

   a. Six days since the birth of the newborn.

   b. Reports of feelings of loss.

   c. History of previous depression.

   d. Statements of wanting to harm self.

   e. Lack of support persons.

Nursing Care of a Family With a High-Risk Newborn

CHAPTER OVERVIEW

The family with a high-risk newborn will need care from a specialized skilled professional health team. The newborn may experience numerous problems that may be related to gestational age, physiologic complications, pregnancy complications, or unhealthy maternal lifestyle. The high-risk neonate may have difficulty establishing respirations at birth necessitating interventions such as resuscitation. After completion of this chapter, the student will be able to care for family with a high-risk newborn.

LEARNING OBJECTIVES

After mastering the content in this chapter, you should be able to do the following:

1. Define the following terms—small-for-gestational-age infant, term infant, large-for-gestational-age infant, preterm infant, and postterm infant—and describe common illnesses that occur in these and other high-risk newborns.

2. Identify National Health Goals related to high-risk newborns nurses can be instrumental in helping the nation achieve.

3. Use critical thinking to analyze the special crisis imposed on families when alterations of newborn development or neonatal illness occur to make nursing family centered.

4. Assess a high-risk newborn to determine whether safe transition to extrauterine life has occurred.

5. Formulate nursing diagnoses related to a high-risk newborn.

6. Identify expected outcomes for a high-risk newborn and family.

7. Plan nursing care focused on priorities to stabilize a high-risk newborn's body systems.

8. Implement nursing care for a high-risk newborn, such as monitoring body temperature.

9. Evaluate expected outcomes for achievement and effectiveness of care.

10. Identify areas related to the care of high-risk newborns that could benefit from additional nursing research or application of evidence-based practice.

11. Integrate knowledge of the needs of a high-risk newborn with nursing process to achieve quality maternal and child health nursing care.

KEY TERMS

apnea
apparent life-threatening
  event
appropriate for
  gestational age (AGA)
brown fat
caudal regression
  syndrome
developmental care
dysmature
extracorporeal membrane
  oxygenation (ECMO)
fetal alcohol syndrome
gestational age
hemorrhagic disease
  of the newborn
hydrops fetalis
hyperbilirubinemia
intrauterine growth
  restriction

large for gestational
  age (LGA)
low-birth-weight
  infant
macrosomia
ophthalmia neona-
  torum
periodic respirations
periventricular
  leukomalacia
postterm syndrome
preterm infants
retinopathy of
  prematurity
shoulder dystocia
small for gestational
  age (SGA)

MASTERING THE INFORMATION

FILL IN THE BLANKS

Supply the missing term or the information requested.

1. Retinopathy of prematurity (ROP) is an acquired ocular disease that leads to _____ and is caused by vasoconstriction of immature retinal blood vessels.

2. Kernicterus occurs as a result of the deposit of _____ in the brain.

3. The premature infant with hemolytic anemia might benefit from the administration of _____ to protect the red blood cell from oxidation.

4. To supply glucose to maintain increased metabolism, an infant begins anaerobic _____.

MATCHING

Match the terms in Column I with a definition, example, or related statement from Column II. Place the letter corresponding to the answer in the space provided.

Column I: Age/Weight Classification

1. ___ Term

2. ___ Low birthweight

3. ___ Postterm

4. ___ Small for gestational age

5. ___ Large for gestational age

Column II: Description of Infant

a. Infant whose weight falls below the 10th percentile of weight for gestational age.

b. Infant whose weight falls above the 90th percentile of weight for age.

c. Infant weighing less than 2500 g.

d. Infant born after the onset of week 43 of pregnancy.

e. Infant born after week 38 or before week 42 of pregnancy.

TRUE OR FALSE

Indicate if the following statements are true or false by placing a "T" or "F" in the space provided.

___ 1. A newborn's attempt to raise his or her body temperature increases his or her need for oxygen.

___ 2. A newborn's attempt to raise his or her body temperature increases his or her metabolic rate.

___ 3. Hypercalcemia is a common nutritional problem of the small-for-gestational-age infant.

___ 4. Infants of drug-dependent mothers become symptomatic approximately 48 hours after birth.

SHORT ANSWER

Supply the missing term or the information requested.

1. Describe the respiratory pattern of primary apnea.

_____

_____

2. Discuss two causes of intrauterine growth restriction and state one example of each.

_____

_____

3. Explain the concept of extracorporeal membrane oxygenation (ECMO).

_____

_____

4. Discuss how periodic respiration differs from true apnea and periodic apnea.

_____

_____

5. Why is the immediate administration of oxygen under pressure (bag and mask) contraindicated for infants who are born with meconium-stained amniotic fluid?

_____

_____

6. Discuss the physiology of transient tachypnea of the newborn (TTN).

_____

_____

APPLYING YOUR KNOWLEDGE

CASE STUDY

Mr. and Mrs. Boyd came to the hospital with Mrs. Boyd in active labor. She was 31 weeks pregnant and laboratory studies revealed an acute urinary tract infection. Fetal heart tones indicated fetal distress and Mrs. Boyd was prepared for a cesarean birth. The Boyds had decided that the name of a male child would be Roy. Roy was born with an Apgar score of 4 and 6, weighing 1980 g, and is preterm and small for gestational age. Six hours after birth, Baby Roy's assessment reveals severe acrocyanosis, progressive metabolic disturbances, hematocrit of 56, and specific gravity of 1.005. The infant is in severe respiratory distress and his urinary output is 1 mL/kg/hr.

1. What factors may have contributed or are contributing to Roy's respiratory distress?

_____

_____

_____

2. What interventions would be implemented to address Roy's respiratory distress?

_____

_____

_____

CRITICAL INQUIRY EXERCISE

1. Write a plan identifying the methods you would use to teach the mother how to implement a stimulation program at home for the preterm infant who has been deprived of environmental stimuli.

2. Identify all supporting devices and therapeutic procedures that might be used in direct support of an infant with respiratory distress syndrome. Synthesize how the devices and the procedures function to correct the pathologic processes demonstrated by assessment data and lab values.

CRITICAL EXPLORATION

1. Identify a preterm infant in the high-risk znursery. Examine the prenatal history and inpatient chart. Identify any existing factors that may have precipitated an early delivery.

2. Collaborate with two of your classmates to practice the sequential steps of external cardiac massage in the newborn using the cardiopulmonary resuscitation doll. Present your skill to the class and instructors with the assistance of your two partners.

PRACTICING FOR NCLEX

MULTIPLE-CHOICE QUESTIONS

Select the letter that corresponds to the best answer for each question.

1. Baby girl LaTrond is born with an Apgar score of 5 and 7. The infant is experiencing respiratory difficulty. The nurse's immediate goal for this infant would be to

   a. establish adequate circulatory pattern within 2 minutes.

   b. clear the airway and establish respirations in 2 minutes.

   c. prevent respiratory distress syndrome.

   d. obtain the oxygen concentration in the circulating blood volume.

2. After therapeutic interventions, a newborn demonstrates adequate lung expansion. The amount of pressure that would enable her to continue to reinflate the alveoli of her lungs would be

   a. 10 to 15 cm of water.

   b. 15 to 20 cm of water.

   c. 20 to 25 cm of water.

   d. 25 to 20 cm of water.

3. Which method would be most appropriate to stimulate initial respirations in the high-risk newborn?

   a. Spanking the buttocks.

   b. Slapping the face.

   c. Squeezing the thorax.

   d. Rubbing the back.

4. Baby Susan is about 21 hours old and has begun to exhibit signs and symptoms of respiratory compromise after an uneventful delivery and "normal" newborn assessment. The nurse's initial response would be to

   a. obtain blood gas levels and position the infant prone.

   b. increase the flow of oxygen and position the infant in Trendelenburg position.

   c. place the infant on her abdomen and lower the head of the bed.

   d. raising the head of the crib 15° and placing the infant on her back.

5. An infant whose temperature is being maintained by a radiant heat source should have the probe or disk placed

   a. over a scapula area near the midscapular line.

   b. on the abdomen between the umbilicus and the xiphoid process.

   c. over the rib cage between the costal structures.

   d. over the diaphragm below the lungs.

6. Baby girl Lathasa born vaginally was determined to be large for gestational age. The nurse would assess this newborn carefully for

   a. increased intracranial pressure.

   b. hypothermia.

   c. decreased red blood levels (anemia).

   d. hyperglycemia.

7. A newborn baby girl is diagnosed with Rh incompatibility. The nurses understand that this is most likely the result of which of the following?

   a. The exchange of fetal and maternal blood in utero.

   b. Rh-positive fetus and Rh-positive father.

   c. Rh-negative mother and Rh-positive father.

   d. Family history of a genetic disorder.

8. Which of the following newborn characteristics would suggest that there was nutritional deprivation during fetal growth?

   a. Widely separated sutures.

   b. Excessive lanugo.

   c. Excessive brown fat.

   d. Disproportionately small head to large body.

9. When administering intravenous fluids to a high-risk newborn, the nurse should be cautious to avoid which of the following?

   a. Heart failure.

   b. Polycythemia.

   c. Decreased intracranial hemorrhage.

   d. Increased tissue perfusion.

ALTERNATE FORMAT QUESTIONS
Multiple-Answer Multiple-Choice Questions

Circle the letter(s) corresponding to the appropriate answer(s). Select all that apply.

1. Which of the following would the nurse needs to incorporate in the plan of care for a newborn who is large for gestational age (LGA).

   a. Anticipate that the LGA newborn will have strong sucking ability.

   b. Be alert for respiratory problems due to increased intracranial pressure.

   c. Decrease feedings to reduce size and prevent obesity.

   d. Observe closely for signs of hyperbilirubinemia.

   e. Decrease stimulation, such as holding and talking to prevent seizures.

   f. Assess for possible impaired parenting due to newborn's high-risk status.

2. A nurse is assessing a newborn who was born at 32 weeks' gestation. Which of the following would the nurse most likely find?

   a. Copious vernix caseosa.

   b. Scant lanugo.

   c. Minimal acrocyanosis.

   d. High-pitched cry.

   e. Ruddy skin.

   f. Head small in proportion to chest.

3. A couple is concerned that their preterm infant will develop sudden infant death syndrome. Which of the following would the nurse suggest?

   a. Placing the infant on the back for sleeping.

   b. Avoiding the use of a pacifier when sleeping.

   c. Placing a fan in the room to keep air moving.

   d. Having the infant sleep with a bottle.

   e. Encoring the use of home apnea monitoring.

Nursing Care of the Child Born With a Physical or Developmental Challenge

CHAPTER OVERVIEW

Chapter 27 reviews common physical or developmental challenges that appear at birth or soon after. When a child is born with an apparent physical or developmental challenge, nurses must play a major role in supporting and educating the parents to help them move forward from this point. Some concerns require surgery but the prognosis is good, so this is only a temporary concern. Other challenges, however, represent serious, even life-threatening concerns for infants and financially draining long-term responsibilities for parents. This chapter also assists students in synthesizing the knowledge needed to formulate appropriate plans of care and evaluate the outcomes for children with physical or developmental challenges.

LEARNING OBJECTIVES

After mastering the content in this chapter, you should be able to do the following:

1. Describe common physical and developmental birth disorders.

2. Identify National Health Goals related to children born physically or developmentally challenged that nurses can help the nation achieve.

3. Use critical thinking to analyze the effect of a physically or developmentally challenged child on a family and propose ways to make care more family centered.

4. Assess a child who is born physically or developmentally challenged.

5. Formulate nursing diagnoses for children born with a physical or developmental challenge.

6. Establish expected outcomes to meet the needs of a child with a physical or developmental challenge.

7. Plan nursing care to meet the needs of a child born with a physical or developmental challenge, such as encouraging mobility.

8. Implement nursing interventions for care of children born with physical or developmental challenges, such as preventing infection in a child with a neural tube disorder.

9. Evaluate expected outcomes to determine achievement and effectiveness of care.

10. Identify areas related to physically or developmentally challenged infants that could benefit by additional nursing research or application of evidence-based practice.

11. Integrate knowledge of congenital physical or developmental challenges with the nursing process to achieve quality maternal and child health nursing care.

KEY TERMS

ankyloglossia	meconium plug
atresia	omphalocele
cleft lip	polydactyly
cleft palate	spina bifida
developmental hip dysplasia	stenosis
fistula	syndactyly
frenulum	transillumination
hydrocephalus	volvulus

MASTERING THE INFORMATION

FILL IN THE BLANKS

Supply the missing term or the information requested.

1. _____ is the absence of the cerebral hemisphere of the brain.

2. _____ is the audible noise heard when the femoral head dislocates from the acetabulum.

3. _____ _____ deformity refers to an elongation of the lower brain stem and displacement of the fourth ventricle into the upper cervical canal.

4. A _____ _____ is a hard portion of meconium completely obstructing the intestinal lumen.

5. Developmental hip dysplasia may involve _____ or _____.

MATCHING

Match the terms in Column I with a definition, example, or related statement from Column II. Place the letter corresponding to the answer in the space provided.

Column I

1. ___ Ankyloglossia
2. ___ Pierre Robin syndrome
3. ___ Diaphragmatic hernia
4. ___ Torticollis
5. ___ Meconium ileus
6. ___ Hydrocephalus
7. ___ Craniosynostosis
8. ___ Thyroglossal cyst
9. ___ Polydactyly
10. ___ Umbilical hernia
11. ___ Talipes
12. ___ Achondroplasia
13. ___ Microcephaly
14. ___ Atresia
15. ___ Gastroschisis
16. ___ Fistula
17. ___ Frenulum
18. ___ Pectus excavatum

Column II

a. Slow brain growth resulting in mental retardation.

b. Occurrence almost exclusively in newborns who are later diagnosed with cystic fibrosis due to absent enzyme.

c. Defect arising from an embryogenic fault leaving a growth at the base of the tongue which drains through a fistula.

d. Protrusion of abdominal organs into the chest cavity through a defect in the diaphragm.

e. Restriction of the tongue caused by an abnormally tight frenulum.

f. Birth defect identified as a trait anomaly small mandible, cleft palate, and glossoptosis.

g. Defect in cartilage production resulting stunted growth of arms and legs.

h. Protrusion of a portion of the intestine through umbilical ring, muscle, fascia.

i. One or more additional fingers.

j. Ankle–foot deformity.

k. Injury to sternocleidomastoid muscle during birth, resulting in infant holding head tilted to the side.

l. Premature closure of sutures of the skull.

m. Indentation of the lower portion of the sternum decreasing lung volume and displacing the heart to the left.

n. Opening in the esophagus leading to the trachea.

o. Membrane attached to lower anterior tip of tongue.

p. Complete closure occurring such as due to absence of canalization in the bowel.

q. An excess of cerebrospinal fluid in the ventricles and subarachnoid spaces of the brain.

r. Herniation of abdominal contents without peritoneal membrane to contain it.

APPLYING YOUR KNOWLEDGE

CASE STUDY

Patrick is approximately 24 hours old. The doctors are implementing tests and procedures to determine if his congenital neural tube defect is a meningocele or a myelomeningocele.

1. What are the physical characteristics that Patrick would exhibit if diagnosed with a myelomeningocele?

   _____

   _____

   _____

2. Preoperatively, what would be the priority for Patrick and how would the nurse intervene?

   _____

   _____

   _____

CRITICAL INQUIRY EXERCISE

1. Create a teaching plan for parents to perform a neurologic assessment on a child discharged from the hospital in a spica cast.

2. Identify the major components of the assessment when examining an infant for a diaphragmatic hernia. What are the physiologic explanations for the positive findings that you might find on assessment?

CRITICAL EXPLORATION

1. Visit the physical therapy department at your clinical facility. Identify the equipment used for motor development by the patients in the hospital and by the patients who visit for outpatient therapy.

2. Visit a community agency that sponsors the annual Special Olympics in your area. Speak with an appropriate staff member to learn some basic psychosocial skills on how to communicate with and motivate the child who has a chronic physical developmental defect.

PRACTICING FOR NCLEX

MULTIPLE-CHOICE QUESTIONS

Circle the letter that corresponds to the best answer for each question.

1. Leonard, age 8 months, is visiting the health clinic for a well-baby checkup. He is diagnosed with developmental hip dysplasia. The physician describes the defect as no communication between the femoral head and the acetabulum. This dysplasia is called

   a. preluxation.

   b. subluxation.

   c. dislocation.

   d. acetabular subluxation.

2. A nurse performing the assessment on an infant with hip dysplasia would find that the affected extremity

   a. appears slightly shorter than the normal one.

   b. is resistant to extension.

   c. will not allow the child to lie supine with feet flexed.

   d. is obviously malformed.

3. Dayle is 3 months old admitted to the hospital with a diagnosis of hydrocephalus. Which of the following findings would the nurse interpret as least indicative of increased intracranial pressure?

   a. Overriding sutures.

   b. Shrill cry.

   c. Hyperactive reflexes.

   d. Prominent scalp veins.

4. After a shunt to relieve intracranial pressure, which of the following would lead the nurse to suspect an infection?

   a. Subnormal temperature.

   b. Decreased pulse.

   c. Marked irritability.

   d. Flexible neck.

5. Crying is to be avoided in a child who has had a cleft lip repair because it

   a. sustains a traumatic experience.

   b. places tension on the suture line.

   c. threatens maternal–infant bonding.

   d. predisposes to respiratory difficulties.

6. After repair of a tracheoesophageal fistula, the nurse would watch the infant carefully at postoperative days 7 to 10 for which of the following that would indicate a leak at sites of anastomosis?

   a. Serous drainage.

   b. Acute indigestion.

   c. Profuse diarrhea.

   d. Respiratory distress.

ALTERNATE FORMAT QUESTIONS

Multiple-Answer Musltiple-Choice Questions

Circle the letter(s) corresponding to the appropriate answer(s). Select all that apply.

1. When caring for an infant with a meningocele preoperatively, the nurse should

   a. irrigate the back of the head with saline every 2 hours.

   b. place a rolled towel under the abdomen to flex the hips.

   c. position the infant supine with the head of bed at 45°.

   d. place a piece of plastic on the child's back below the meningocele.

   e. replace the wet compress every 4 hours with a fresh saline compress.

2. Desmond is admitted to the surgical floor of the pediatric hospital several hours after birth for a tracheoesophageal fistula. Which of the following would the nurse expect to assess?

   a. Constantly blowing mucus bubbles from the mouth.

   b. Absence of stools.

   c. Absence of rooting reflex.

   d. Inability to swallow.

   e. Respiratory distress.

3. Which of the following assessment findings would suggest that a newborn has a diaphragmatic hernia?

   a. Protuberant abdomen.

   b. Vomiting.

   c. Respiratory distress immediately after birth.

   d. Absent breath sounds on one side of the chest.

   e. Intercostal retractions.

28

Principles of Growth and Development

CHAPTER OVERVIEW

Chapter 28 examines and summarizes the basic concepts of hereditary and environmental factors that influence a child's growth and development. The theories of development according to Freud, Erikson, Piaget, and Kohlberg are discussed. The chapter also explores the developmental tasks of parenting as the child progresses through various growth stages. The implications of growth and development for the nursing care of children from various age groups are explored, and interviewing and therapeutic communication skills needed by the nurse when caring for children in various stages of growth and development are also discussed. A case study presents a contrasting view of the developmental characteristics for each stage.

LEARNING OBJECTIVES

After mastering the content in this chapter, you should be able to do the following:

1. Describe principles of growth and development and developmental stages according to major theorists.

2. Identify National Health Goals related to growth and development that nurses can help the nation achieve.

3. Use critical thinking to analyze ways that paths to achieving a new developmental stage remain family centered.

4. Assess a child to determine the stage of development that has been achieved.

5. Formulate nursing diagnoses that address wellness as well as both a potential for and an actual delay in growth and development.

6. Identify expected outcomes for nursing goals for a growing child.

7. Plan nursing interventions to assist a child in achieving and maintaining normal growth and development such as encouraging a parent to read to a child.

8. Implement nursing care such as suggesting age-appropriate play materials to support normal growth and development.

9. Evaluate outcome criteria for achievement and effectiveness of care.

10. Identify areas of nursing care related to growth and development that could benefit from additional nursing research or application of evidence-based practice.

11. Integrate knowledge of growth and development with nursing process to achieve quality maternal and child health nursing care.

KEY TERMS

abstract thought	industry versus
accommodation	inferiority
assimilation	initiative versus guilt

autonomy versus
   shame or doubt
centering
cognitive development
conservation
development
developmental milestones
developmental task
egocentrism
growth
identity versus role
   confusion

integrity versus
   despair
maturation
permanence
reversibility
role fantasy
schemas
sensorimotor stage
temperament
trust versus mistrust

Column II

a. A time in which a child's libido is diverted into concrete thinking.

b. Possible factor interfering with parents' ability to provide adequate health care and nutrition.

c. A child's inherited background.

d. A stage of cognitive development displayed by adolescents as they begin to have abstract thoughts about standards of conduct.

e. An individual child's particular manner of thinking, behaving, or reacting to environmental stimuli.

f. Loss of this crucial environmental influence can interfere with a child's growth and development.

MASTERING THE INFORMATION

FILL IN THE BLANKS

Supply the missing term or the information requested.

1. _____ and _____ are essential physical data when making an assessment and should be accurately plotted on a growth chart.

2. _____ _____ includes provision of information regarding further expectation of a child's ability to function in his/her environment.

3. _____ is a synonym for development.

4. _____ is a term used to express an increase in physical size or a quantitative change.

5. _____ denotes an increase in skill or the ability to function.

MATCHING

Match the terms in Column I with a definition, example, or related statement from Column II. Place the letter corresponding to the answer in the space provided.

Column I

1. ____ Genetic makeup

2. ____ Temperament

3. ____ Parent-child relationship

4. ____ Latent phase

5. ____ Socioeconomic level

6. ____ Postconventional development

ADDITIONAL MATCHING EXERCISES

Match the terms in Column I with the description from Column II. Place the letter corresponding to the answer in the space provided.

Column I: Piaget's Stages of Development

1. ____ Sensorimotor

2. ____ Preoperational thought

3. ____ Intuitive thought

4. ____ Concrete operational thought

5. ____ Formal operational thought

Column II

a. Thinking in terms of what could be rather than what currently exists.

b. Inductive reasoning, from specific to general.

c. Development of the concept of permanence and goal directed behavior.

d. Object viewed as having only one characteristic.

e. Symbolic thought, egocentric and static thinking.

SHORT ANSWER

Supply the missing term or the information requested.

1. Complete the chart by naming the five psychoanalytic stages of development as defined by Sigmund Freud. Assign the

appropriate childhood division and age range to these stages (see example).

	Stage	Childhood Division	Age Range
a.	Oral stage	Infant	1 month to 1 year
b.			
c.			
d.			
e.			

2. Identify the psychosocial stage of development identified by Erikson that is described by each of the following statements.

   a. _____ Strives to obtain a sense of independence, taking pride in new accomplishments, and wanting to do everything for himself/herself.

   b. _____ Expends effort to gain a sense of identity, bringing together experiences previously learned.

   c. _____ Concentrates on perfecting learned skills while seeking to enlarge his or her environment with school and community.

   d. _____ Recognizes that needs are met as they arise, with discomfort being quickly removed.

   e. _____ Learns how to do things, and the need for freedom and opportunity to initiate motor skills increases.

STAGES OF MORAL DEVELOPMENT

State the appropriate stage of moral development described in the sentences below.

1. _____ Imitates behavior and practices doing gestures only for gestures in return.

2. _____ Internalizes standards of conduct, doing what he or she thinks is right regardless of an existing social rule.

3. _____ Learns that certain actions may elicit positive or negative behaviors from parents.

4. _____ Punishment–obedience orientation, governed easily by parental authority.

5. _____ Behaviors are influenced more by what is "nice" than by what may be right or wrong.

APPLYING YOUR KNOWLEDGE

CASE STUDY

You are providing care to a 3.5-year-old girl who is hospitalized for a recurrent infection necessitating intravenous antibiotic therapy.

1. Summarize the characteristics that you would expect to find related to the child's cognitive development.

   _____

   _____

   _____

2. Describe the typical characteristics that you would expect to see with this child's psychosocial development.

   _____

   _____

   _____

3. Where would this child be at in his moral development?

   _____

   _____

   _____

CRITICAL INQUIRY EXERCISE

1. Write a teaching plan that could be used to prepare the parent of a 13-month-old for the next stage of the child's development.

2. Compile a list of potentially dangerous areas in the average household environment that would be accessible to a toddler. Write to the nearest pediatric hospital's education department to obtain information that they provide to their clients and families on safety and anticipatory guidance.

CRITICAL EXPLORATION

Choose a stage of childhood and interview a parenst with a child in that age range. Attempt to identify the type of temperament reactivity pattern manifested by the child in each of the nine categories and evidence that the parent has, or has not, met the developmental tasks of parenting for the child's developmental stage.

PRACTICING FOR NCLEX

MULTIPLE-CHOICE QUESTIONS

Circle the letter that corresponds to the best answer for each question.

1. Mrs. Peters complains that her daughter Millie, age 1 month, is very fussy and will not sit in her car seat. She states that Millie never responds well to new people or toys. The nurse should explain which of the following to Mrs. Peters?

   a. When children are ill they are often fussy and respond poorly to new stimuli; these children often need to be hospitalized.

   b. Children have different approaches to life, and some children naturally demonstrate withdrawal when faced with new stimuli.

   c. The behavior she described is a sign of Millie's rhythmicity and activity level, which are inborn reactivity patterns.

   d. Infants are seldom adaptable to new stimuli; as time passes Millie will probably have a less intense reaction to stimuli.

2. Jason is 2 months old. His mother reports that he wiggles and squirms constantly in his crib and wakes up at different times every day. The nurse recognizes these behaviors as examples of which of the following reaction patterns?

   a. Adaptability and attention span.

   b. Distractibility and approach.

   c. Mood and reaction intensity.

   d. Activity and rhythmicity.

3. When discussing temperament reactivity patterns of children with parents, which of the following would the nurse include?

   a. Early training and instruction can correct a child's apprehensive approach to new stimuli.

   b. Even children with poor adaptability can be expected to become accustomed to a new environment by the third exposure to the area.

   c. While some children will accept a substitute toy when crying for their favorite toy, others may refuse to accept anything else.

   d. Children who spend only 1 to 2 minutes with a toy before wanting a new one are usually mentally ill and sociopathic to a small degree.

4. When discussing care for Winston, who is 15 months old, with his mother, the nurse should consider the developmental tasks of parenting for which of the following divisions of childhood?

   a. Toddler.

   b. Neonate.

   c. Infant.

   d. Preschooler.

5. The nurse might discuss which of the following with the parents of Ida, a 2-year-old, during a parenting workshop?

   a. Ida can be expected to be cooperative and easily controlled at this stage of development.

   b. Ida may prefer finger foods and clothing she can put on without assistance at this age.

   c. Expect Ida to want to be held and cuddled a great deal at this stage of her development.

   d. At this age, Ida will take the initiative in activities and will question everything.

6. A key developmental task of parenting is learning to determine if their child is crying from hunger, discomfort, or some other reason. This task is most important for parents of a(n)

   a. preschooler.

   b. infant.

   c. toddler.

   d. school-aged child.

7. When planning the care of a 4-month-old child hospitalized with a respiratory tract infection and placed on strict bed rest, the nurse would include interventions to promote growth and development due to the child's

   a. decreased exposure to appropriate stimulation.

   b. reduced opportunities for initiative development.

   c. overexposure to varied stimuli.

   d. limited opportunities for independence.

8. An appropriate goal when caring for a 4-year-old hospitalized child might be that

   a. the child will demonstrate initiative, within limits, evidenced by asking for paper and crayons to draw a picture.

b. the parents will demonstrate appropriate parenting task achievement by dressing and feeding the child each day.

c. the child will demonstrate formal operational thought by discussing the importance of being in the hospital.

d. the parents will demonstrate the ability to interpret the child's behavioral cues.

ALTERNATE FORMAT QUESTIONS
Multiple-Answer Multiple-Choice Questions

Circle the letter(s) corresponding to the appropriate answer(s). Select all that apply.

1. Which of the following would be most accurate about the parents of an adolescent?

   a. They must set strict limits on activities to prevent the child from becoming independent and taking initiative.

   b. They often experience difficulty in becoming independent of their child's life and in developing their own interests again.

   c. They should not offer support or help to the child during this stage, so a sense of independence can be developed by the child.

   d. They must take an active authoritarian role in planning the child's daily activities and future experiences.

   e. They should educate their child about the long-term consequences of alcohol use.

2. The nurse would determine that the parents of a preschooler had achieved their developmental tasks if which of the following behaviors were noted?

   a. The mother and father alternately attending kindergarten with the child each day.

   b. The child is allowed to play without limits in the home to encourage free expression and growth.

   c. The mother or father sits with the child and sips imaginary tea from a toy teacup.

   d. The child is punished for talking too much and asking too many questions.

   e. The parents refrain from punishing or disciplining the child when masturbation is exhibited.

3. Freud's stages of childhood are listed below. Place them in the proper sequence from infancy through adolescence.

   a. Phallic.

   b. Oral.

   c. Genital.

   d. Anal.

   e. Latent.

CHAPTER 29

Nursing Care of a Family With an Infant

CHAPTER OVERVIEW

This chapter discusses the growth and development patterns of the infant and family. Emphasis is placed on specific growth and development parameters and common health deviations that should be assessed during routine child health visits. Nursing interventions aimed at family support, anticipatory guidance, and alleviating common health problems are highlighted. The case study explores appropriate interventions and rationales during a well-child visit in a health facility.

LEARNING OBJECTIVES

After mastering the contents of this chapter, you should be able to do the following:

1. Describe normal infant growth and development and associated parental concerns.

2. Identify National Health Goals related to infant growth and development that nurses can help the nation achieve.

3. Use critical thinking to analyze methods of care for an infant to be certain care is family centered.

4. Assess an infant for normal growth and development milestones.

5. Formulate nursing diagnoses related to infant growth and development and associated parental concerns.

6. Identify expected outcomes to promote optimal infant growth and development needs.

7. Plan nursing care to meet an infant's growth and development needs, such as teaching parents to childproof their home.

8. Implement nursing care related to normal growth and development of an infant, such as encouraging eye/hand coordination.

9. Evaluate expected outcomes for achievement and effectiveness of care.

10. Identify areas related to nursing care of an infant that could benefit from additional nursing research or application of evidenced-based practice.

11. Integrate knowledge of infant growth and development with nursing process to achieve quality maternal and child health nursing care.

KEY TERMS

baby-bottle syndrome	neck-righting reflex
binocular vision	seborrhea
deciduous teeth	social smile
eighth-month anxiety	neonatal teeth
extrusion reflex	object permanence
hand regard	pincer grasp
natal teeth	thumb opposition

MASTERING THE INFORMATION

FILL IN THE BLANKS

Supply the missing term or the information requested.

1. An infant's immune system becomes functional at age _____ months.

2. The first tooth eruption is expected at age _____ months.

3. Thumb opposition is beginning around the age of _____ months.

4. Tracey, a 6-month-old, is undergoing a hearing assessment. The nurse would expect Tracey to be able to locate sounds made _____ the head.

5. A 6-week-old infant smiles in return to an interested person's nodding and smiling. This is called a _____ smile.

MATCHING

Match the terms in Column I with a definition, example, or related statement from Column II. Place the letter corresponding to the answer in the space provided.

Column I

1. ____ Laughs out loud

2. ____ Uses palmar grasp

3. ____ Says first word, "da-da"

4. ____ Pulls self to a standing position

5. ____ Shows beginning stranger anxiety

6. ____ Brings hands together and pulls at clothes

7. ____ Sits securely without support

8. ____ Can draw a semi-straight line with a crayon.

Column II

a. 3 months

b. 4 months

c. 6 months

d. 7 months

e. 8 months

f. 9 months

g. 10 months

h. 12 months

SHORT ANSWER

Supply the missing term or the information requested.

1. State four benefits derived from well-child follow-up visits.

   _____

   _____

2. What is the most serious complication for infants with supernumerary teeth?

   _____

   _____

3. Identify the four body positions from which to assess gross motor development in an infant.

   _____

   _____

4. List three ways parents can childproof their homes.

   _____

   _____

5. Identify two benefits to the growth and development of infants that may be promoted when bathing the infant.

   _____

   _____

6. How can parents provide tooth and oral care for their infants?

   _____

   _____

7. State three ways to prevent diaper dermatitis.

   _____

   _____

8. What are three factors that should be assessed when an infant is experiencing diarrhea?

   _____

   _____

APPLYING YOUR KNOWLEDGE

CASE STUDY

Stephen is a 5-month-old infant visiting the well-child clinic for his second series of immunizations.

1. Stephen weighed 7 lb and was 20 in long at birth. On the basis of normal growth and development parameters, what should his weight be at this visit?

_____

_____

_____

2. List a normal set of vital signs that may be assessed from Stephen.

_____

_____

_____

3. On what physiologic principle might the physician prescribe a vitamin with iron?

_____

_____

_____

4. Stephen's mother is eager to feed him solid foods and asks the nurse if it would be recommended. What response would the nurse give? Why?

_____

_____

_____

CRITICAL INQUIRY EXERCISE

1. Formulate a nursing care plan for the following case scenario: David, a 7-month-old infant, is experiencing diarrhea. His weight was 18 lb before the diarrhea; now it is 16 lb. His anterior fontanel is slightly sunken, mucous membranes are dry, urine output is diminished, and the specific gravity is 1.035.

2. Contrast the developmental milestones occurring during infancy relating to fine and gross motor skills and physiologic and cognitive development.

CRITICAL EXPLORATION

Assess two infants of the same chronologic age, but one born at term and one born 2 to 3 months prematurely. Make an assessment of the developmental behaviors that are seen in the adjusted chronologic age groups for these infants. Comparatively evaluate the infants' performances. What principles of growth and development should be researched for this exercise?

PRACTICING FOR NCLEX

MULTIPLE-CHOICE QUESTIONS

Circle the letter that corresponds to the best answer for each question.

1. During a routine well-child visit, the nurse should educate the parents regarding
   a. the infant's need for meat by 4 months of age.
   b. expected growth and development patterns.
   c. specific yearly milestones the child must meet.
   d. the signs and symptoms of failure to thrive.

2. According to Erikson's theory of emotional development, infants will develop a sense of trust when
   a. they can identify and distinguish their mother and father.
   b. they feel a sense of belonging and be accepted as part of the family.
   c. they can predict what is coming and needs are consistently met.
   d. nutritional and hygiene needs are provided on a daily basis.

3. Keeping in mind the leading cause of accidents in infants, the nurse should advise parents to
   a. buy clothes for the infant with buttons rather than snaps.
   b. check all toys for small removable parts.
   c. provide round, cylinder-type toys.
   d. avoid finger foods before the age of 15 months.

4. Since falls are a common cause of injury to infants, parents should be advised to
   a. avoid using pillows around the infant placed on a bed.
   b. use an infant seat when placing the infant on a table top.
   c. use blankets around the infant on a couch.
   d. place protective gates at the top and bottom of stairs.

5. Palliative measures aimed at relieving colic should include
   a. placing a warm heating pad on the abdomen.
   b. diluting the formula to a weaker strength.
   c. administering simethicone at 30-minute intervals.
   d. sitting the infant upright for a half-hour after feedings.

6. Alice is 4 months of age. Her mother is singing to her. Why type of response should be expected of Alice?
   a. Imitating the sounds.
   b. Smiling, cooing, and babbling.
   c. Saying "da-da."
   d. Watching her mother's face without making a sound.

7. At what age should an infant begin to locate an object hidden under a blanket?
   a. 6 months.
   b. 8 months.
   c. 10 months.
   d. 12 months.

8. When assessing the visual ability of a 7-month-old boy, the nurse should
   a. attempt to place a familiar object in the infant's hand and observe his response.
   b. use a brightly colored object and check the infant's ability to follow the object.
   c. use a mirror to observe the infant's response to his image.
   d. observe the infant's ability to follow hand motions.

9. When teaching parents about their infant's need for sleep, the nurse would be correct in stating that most infants usually sleep
   a. 10 to 12 hours per night, with one or more naps.
   b. 14 to 16 hours per night, with one nap.
   c. an average of 18 to 20 hours each day.
   d. at 4-hour intervals and throughout the night.

10. What type of device would enhance the development of an 8-month-old infant through play activity?
   a. Stroller.
   b. Floor mat.
   c. Crib.
   d. Play pen.

11. A major developmental task for the family of an infant girl should be
   a. interpreting her cues to decipher her needs.
   b. allowing her to gain her autonomy and freedom to express herself.
   c. providing an environment for learning new skills.
   d. allowing her to take initiative and respond to her environment.

12. An 8-month-old infant who loves to suck her thumb visits the clinic. Her mother is very worried that this habit will cause permanent dental problems. What should the nurse suggest to the mother?
   a. Wrap the infant's thumb with adhesive tape.
   b. Distract the infant with toys.
   c. Ignore this behavior.
   d. Remove the infant's thumb from her mouth as often as possible.

ALTERNATE FORMAT QUESTIONS
Multiple-Answer Multiple-Choice Questions

Circle the letter(s) corresponding to the appropriate answer(s). Select all that apply.

1. Parents report their infant frequently wakes up from a sound sleep. What should the nurse advise the parents to do to help the child sleep through the night?
   a. When the infant awakens, wait a while and let her fall back to sleep.
   b. Go to the child immediately when she awakens and comfort her back to sleep.

c. Provide soft music or toys to allow her to play quietly alone.

d. Pick her up and rock her back to sleep.

e. Place pillows around the infant to cushion the crib.

2. Patrick is 10 months old. What type of play activity is appropriate for his expected level of development?

a. Rolling a ball.

b. Shaking a rattle.

c. Winding up a toy.

d. Playing patty-cake.

e. Peek-a-boo.

f. Playing marbles.

3. A nurse is assessing a 6-month-old infant. Which of the following would the nurse expect to find?

a. Ability to creep.

b. Use of palmar grasp.

c. Ability to hold a cup.

d. Ability to turn both ways.

e. Strong stepping reflex.

f. Fading Moro reflex.

CHAPTER 30

Nursing Care of a Family With a Toddler

CHAPTER OVERVIEW

This chapter explores the patterns of normal growth and development of the toddler. The developmental accomplishments related to fine and gross motor skills and language skills are presented. Anticipatory guidance with a reference to making the toddler's environment safe is also addressed. The case study provides the student with the opportunity to provide teaching for the parents of a toddler through a teaching plan for health promotion.

LEARNING OBJECTIVES

After mastering the contents of this chapter, you should be able to do the following:

1. Describe normal growth and development of a toddler as well as common parental concerns.

2. Identify National Health Goals related to the toddler age group that nurses can help the nation achieve.

3. Use critical thinking to analyze methods of care for toddlers to be certain care is family centered.

4. Assess a toddler for normal growth and development milestones.

5. Formulate nursing diagnoses related to toddler growth and development or parental concerns regarding growth and development.

6. Identify expected outcomes for nursing care of a toddler.

7. Plan nursing care to meet a toddler's growth and development needs, such as anticipatory guidance to prevent problems such as sleep disturbances.

8. Implement nursing care to promote normal growth and development of a toddler, such as discussing toddler developmental milestones with parents.

9. Evaluate expected outcomes for achievement and effectiveness of care.

10. Identify areas related to care of a toddler that could benefit from additional nursing research or application of evidence-based practice.

11. Integrate knowledge of toddler growth and development with nursing process to achieve quality maternal and child health nursing care.

KEY TERMS

assimilation	parallel play
autonomy	preoperational thought
deferred imitation	punishment
discipline	tertiary circular reaction
lordosis	stage

MASTERING THE INFORMATION

FILL IN THE BLANKS

Supply the missing term or the information requested.

1. The toddler has the developmental task of achieving _____ versus shame or doubt.

2. _____ is the type of accident that occurs most frequently in toddlers.

3. Allowing self-feeding is a major way to strengthen _____ in a toddler.

MATCHING

Match the terms in Column I with a definition, example, or related statement from Column II. Place the letter corresponding to the answer in the space provided.

Column I

1. ___ Deferred imitation

2. ___ Negativism

3. ___ Separation anxiety

4. ___ Lordosis

5. ___ Discipline

6. ___ Preoperational thought

Column II

a. Universal fear that begins at about 6 months of age and persists throughout the preschool period.

b. Remembering an action to mimic at a later time.

c. A forward curve of the spine at the sacral area.

d. A positive stage in toddler development; the toddler sees himself or herself as a separate individual with separate needs.

e. Major period of cognitive development that usually occurs at the end of the toddler period.

f. Setting rules to teach children what is expected of them.

SHORT ANSWER

Supply the missing term or the information requested.

1. Describe the gross motor, language, and play developmental milestones that

are accomplished at ages 15, 24, and 30 months.

2. How does head circumference change in the second year of life when compared with that which occurs during the first year?

3. A toddler engages in which type of play?

APPLYING YOUR KNOWLEDGE

CASE STUDY

Mr. and Mrs. Stargell and their 18-month-old son, Cody, are being seen today in the pediatrician's office where you are a nurse for a follow-up visit. The night before, Mr. Stargell discovered that Cody had tumbled down the stairs. The Stargells called the emergency room (ER) at a local children's hospital; they were instructed to bring Cody to the ER immediately. Cody was given a thorough examination and was treated for a small laceration to the head and a severely sprained arm. He was discharged in stable condition from the ER with instructions to see the pediatrician the following morning.

1. What information regarding toddler safety should you include in your plan to teach health promotion to Cody's parents?

2. You begin your assessment of Cody with a careful health history. What is the rationale for taking this health history?

3. Explain how information from a health history will help you develop a teaching plan for Cody's parents.

_____

_____

_____

CRITICAL INQUIRY EXERCISE

1. Formulate a nursing care plan that will focus on setting safety guidelines for an 18-month-old child in the home environment.

2. List outcome criteria that might be established before the parents leave the pediatrician's office.

CRITICAL EXPLORATION

1. Visit a day-care setting and observe a group of toddlers during a free play period for 30 minutes or more. Select one toddler from the group and describe how he or she plays among the group members.

2. Visit the Red Cross center in your community and obtain the name and address of an agency that will furnish literature to institutions or families on poison prevention and child safety. Write for the literature and ask your instructor for assistance to distribute the materials to the parents of the children at your pediatric clinical site.

PRACTICING FOR NCLEX

MULTIPLE-CHOICE QUESTIONS

Circle the letter that corresponds to the best answer for each question.

1. The child's universal language is
   a. behavior.
   b. crying.
   c. touching.
   d. play.

2. Which of the following describes the type of play observed with toddlers?
   a. Solitary.
   b. Parallel.
   c. Competitive.
   d. Fantasy.

3. When developing a plan of care to reduce the incidence of lead poisoning, which of the following would be most important for the nurse to include?
   a. Parent education.
   b. Early detection.
   c. Family planning.
   d. Chelating therapy.

4. Which of the following would the nurse be least likely to assess in a child with lead poisoning?
   a. Irritability.
   b. Cardiomegaly.
   c. Headaches.
   d. Abdominal pain.

5. When planning the care for a toddler who is to be hospitalized, the nurse plans interventions based on minimizing the toddler's emotional stress related to which of the following?
   a. Loss of control.
   b. Fear of bodily injury.
   c. Fear of death.
   d. Separation anxiety.

6. Which of the following would the nurse suggest as appropriate for promoting adequate nutrition in an active toddler?
   a. Use of skim milk after age 2.
   b. Unrestricted fat intake until age 3.
   c. Daily calorie intake of 1400 kcal.
   d. Limit exposure to finger foods.

ALTERNATE FORMAT QUESTIONS

Multiple-Answer Multiple-Choice Questions

Circle the letter(s) corresponding to the appropriate answer(s). Select all that apply.

1. Which interventions would be most appropriate for a toddler?
   a. _____ Leaving toddlers alone in the tub for a brief moment while bathing them.
   b. _____ Offering high-protein snacks rather than high-carbohydrate snacks.
   c. _____ Placing a gate on the door to a toddler's room.
   d. _____ Informing parents that sleep times will be shorter for toddlers than for infants.

e. _____ Offering a toddler something pleasurable in the middle of a temper tantrum to stop the tantrum.

f. _____ Assisting the child in putting his clothes on correctly to develop neatness.

2. The nurse is assessing a 2-year-old at a health maintenance visit. Which of the following would the nurse expect to find?

   a. Sunken abdomen.

   b. Chest circumference greater than head circumference.

   c. 20 deciduous teeth.

   d. Speaking in two-word sentences.

   e. Walking with a narrow stance gait.

   f. Pretending to drive a car.

3. When developing a teaching plan for the parents of a toddler in preparation for toilet training, which of the following suggestions would be most helpful?

   a. "Wait until the child is at least 3 years old."

   b. "Use training pants that have snaps to secure them snugly."

   c. "Follow a regular schedule for using the potty."

   d. "Praise the child if he urinates or defecates."

   e. "Flush the toilet while the child is still sitting there."

   f. Have the child sit on the potty until he urinates or defecates."

31

Nursing Care of a Family With a Preschool Child

CHAPTER OVERVIEW

Preschool-age children demonstrate the desire to care for themselves through daily activities. They insist on dressing themselves and often resist assistance from parents. The nurse should include the need for parent education related to these behaviors when planning nursing care. This chapter discusses the developmental tasks and anticipatory guidance for children in this age group. The case study provides a learning opportunity for educating about growth and development during the preschool years.

LEARNING OBJECTIVES

After mastering the contents of this chapter, you should be able to do the following:

1. Describe normal growth and development as well as common parental concerns of the preschool period.

2. Identify National Health Goals related to the preschool period that nurses can help the nation achieve.

3. Use critical thinking to analyze methods of care for preschoolers to be certain care is family centered.

4. Assess a preschooler for normal growth and developmental milestones.

5. Formulate nursing diagnoses related to preschool growth and development and common parental concerns.

6. Identify expected outcomes for nursing care of a preschooler.

7. Plan nursing care to meet a preschooler's growth and development needs, such as planning age-appropriate play activities.

8. Implement nursing care related to normal growth and development of a preschooler, such as preparing a preschooler for an invasive procedure.

9. Evaluate expected outcomes for achievement and effectiveness of care.

10. Identify areas related to care of the preschool-age child that could benefit from additional nursing research or application of evidence-based practice.

11. Integrate knowledge of preschool growth and development with nursing process to achieve quality maternal and child health nursing care.

KEY TERMS

broken fluency	genu valgus
bruxism	intuitional thought
conservation	Oedipus complex
ectomorphic body build	endomorphic body build
Electra complex	secondary stuttering

MASTERING THE INFORMATION

FILL IN THE BLANKS

Supply the missing term or the information requested.

1. The developmental task for the preschool-age child is to achieve a sense of _____.

2. _____ _____ refers to the strong emotional attachment of a preschool boy to his mother.

3. Grinding the teeth at night is called _____.

MATCHING

Match the terms in Column I with a definition, example, or related statement from Column II. Place the letter corresponding to the answer in the space provided

Column I

1. ____ Initiative

2. ____ Play

3. ____ Regression

4. ____ Broken fluency

5. ____ Intuitional thought

Column II

a. Reverting to behaviors practiced in earlier years.

b. Repetition and prolongation of sounds.

c. Method by which preschoolers use imaginations.

d. Lacking insight to view themselves as others see them and think of themselves as always right.

e. Achievement leading to knowledge that learning new things is fun.

SHORT ANSWER

Supply the missing term or the information requested.

1. Define the following terms.

   a. Endomorphic.

   b. Ectomorphic.

   c. Genu valgus.

2. Describe the Oedipus and Electra complexes.

3. Explain how the preschooler's inability to understand the law of conservation may affect your ability to care for him or her.

4. What are some therapeutic methods that can be practiced by the nurse and family to alleviate the preschooler's fear of the dark?

5. Identify four basic rules recommended to resolve secondary stuttering.

APPLYING YOUR KNOWLEDGE

CASE STUDY

Mrs. Bell and her two children, Amy (age 8) and Bryan (age 4), are visiting the health center today for a well-child appointment. Mrs. Bell is 6 months pregnant. After the physician's visit, Mrs. Bell asks if she could speak with you for a few moments about Bryan. She explains that she is very concerned about Bryan's fixation on his genitals. Mrs. Bell began to notice this behavior about 2 weeks after she enrolled him in a day-care center. She says that he masturbates often and seems to have forgotten what the family has taught him about his "private parts."

1. What guidelines would you use to advise Mrs. Bell regarding Bryan's masturbating in public?

2. What basic rule concerning sex education should you be sure to mention to help protect Bryan from sexual abuse?

_____

_____

_____

3. Outline a teaching plan to help the mother explain pregnancy and the arrival of a new baby.

_____

_____

_____

CRITICAL INQUIRY EXERCISE

1. Contrast the developmental milestones across the life span of the 3, 4, and 5 years old.

2. Prepare a teaching plan for the parent and preschooler about developing safety measures in the home.

CRITICAL EXPLORATION

1. Visit a kindergarten and talk with a preschool child near the end of the day. Ask the child to tell you what happened during the day. Assess the child's language development, understand how the term "egocentrism" applies to the preschooler, and identify if the child is accomplishing the developmental tasks of that age group.

2. Visit a preschool child who is hospitalized for an elective surgery. Talk to the child before the surgery. Obtain three or four pictures depicting a pediatric hospital area, including the patient's room and the operating room. Do not include any pictures suggestive of invasive procedures or treatment. Show these pictures to the preschooler and ask him or her to make up a story about the pictures. Record the story as the preschooler talks to you. Identify the statements indicating fear and stress. Notice in the story how the child's ability to fantasize allows him or her to stretch the imagination to include even mutilation, although the pictures do not suggest aggressive or invasive subjects.

PRACTICING FOR NCLEX

MULTIPLE-CHOICE QUESTIONS

Circle the letter that corresponds to the best answer for each question.

1. Which of the following types of play is primarily demonstrated by preschoolers?
   a. Parallel.
   b. Imaginary.
   c. Solitary.
   d. Cooperative.

2. When preparing a preschooler for an invasive procedure, the nurse would plan interventions to address which fear?
   a. Fear of the dark.
   b. Fear of abandonment.
   c. Fear of losing control.
   d. Fear of multilation.

3. Which action would be most appropriate to help lessen the feelings of rivalry among siblings?
   a. Punish for unacceptable behavior.
   b. Separate siblings and give individual attention separately.
   c. Interact with younger and older siblings together.
   d. Allow the older sibling to practice adult roles to comfort him or her.

4. A preschooler appropriately explores his body by
   a. dressing up in parents' clothing.
   b. masturbating.
   c. inflicting harm.
   d. comparing his body parts with playmates.

5. Which of the following is an appropriate activity for the preschooler?
   a. Cutting paper dolls.
   b. Playing house.
   c. Stacking blocks.
   d. Dart board game.

ALTERNATE FORMAT QUESTIONS

Multiple-Answer Multiple Choice Questions

Circle the letter(s) corresponding to the appropriate answer(s). Select all that apply.

1. Which of the following are appropriate nursing interventions for a preschooler?
   a. Encourage the preschooler to speak during the health examination.
   b. Assess weight and height or standard growth chart at each health visit.
   c. Include head circumference on each physical examination.
   d. Encourage constructive play.
   e. Provide a helmet for bicycle riding.
   f. Avoid parental use of medications while child is watching.

2. Which of the following would a nurse identify as a common fear of the preschool period?
   a. Fear of the dark.
   b. Fear of attending school.
   c. Fear of mutilation.
   d. Fear of separation.
   e. Fear of abandonment.

3. Which of the following would a nurse expect a 4-year-old child be able to accomplish?
   a. Draw a six-part man.
   b. Lace his shoes.
   c. Undress himself.
   d. Do simple buttons.
   e. Throw a ball overhand.
   f. Enjoy playing a game with numbers.

Nursing Care of a Family With a School-Age Child

CHAPTER OVERVIEW

The school-age years (ages 6 to 12) represent a time of slow physical growth, but cognitive and developmental growth is rapid. When caring for this age group, it is important to stress the physical growth and accomplishment of emotional, cognitive, and moral developmental tasks. The school-age period is the time the child becomes independent and begins to separate from the family for long periods of time. The nurse should know the principles of development related to this age group to promote developmental needs and safety. This chapter contains exercises that help the student in learning developmental tasks and in assisting the family of a school-age child by providing anticipatory guidance. The case study emphasizes the principles of school-age growth and development.

LEARNING OBJECTIVES

After mastering the contents of this chapter, you should be able to do the following:

1. Describe the normal growth and development pattern and common parental concerns of the school-age period.

2. Identify National Health Goals related to school-age children that nurses can help the nation achieve.

3. Use critical thinking to analyze ways in which the care of school-age children can be more family centered.

4. Assess a school-age child for normal growth and development milestones.

5. Formulate nursing diagnoses that speak to both school-age children and their families.

6. Identify expected outcomes for nursing care of a school-age child.

7. Plan anticipatory guidance to prevent problems of growth and development in a school-age child, such as teaching about normal puberty.

8. Implement nursing care to help achieve normal growth and development of a school-age child, such as counseling parents about helping their child adjust to a new school.

9. Evaluate expected outcomes for achievement and effectiveness of care.

10. Identify areas related to care of school-age children that could benefit from additional nursing research or application of evidence-based practice.

11. Integrate knowledge of school-age growth and development with nursing process to achieve quality maternal and child health nursing care.

KEY TERMS

accommodation
caries
class inclusion
conservation
decentering

inclusion
latchkey child
malocclusion
nocturnal emissions

MASTERING THE INFORMATION

FILL IN THE BLANKS

Supply the missing term or the information requested.

1. Talent for music or art becomes evident and children respond well by age _____.

2. For the first 1 to 2 years after menarche, most girls experience menstrual irregularity primarily because the cycle is _____.
Cycles become more regular with the onset of _____.

3. As seminal fluid is produced, boys begin to notice ejaculation during sleep, called _____ _____.

MATCHING

Match the terms in Column I with a definition, example, or related statement from Column II. Place the letter corresponding to the answer in the space provided.

Column I: Chronologic School Age

1. ____ Age 6

2. ____ Age 7

3. ____ Age 8

4. ____ Age 9

5. ____ Age 10

6. ____ Age 11

7. ____ Age 12

Column II: Physical or Psychosocial Development

a. Best friends important; whispering and giggling.

b. Teacher as the authority figure.

c. Social and cooperative.

d. Conservation learned.

e. Ready for competitive games.

f. Clubs are formed, all boys or all girls.

g. Insecure with members of opposite sex.

SHORT ANSWER

Supply the missing term or the information.

1. Compare and contrast the accomplishment or failure of the developmental task industry versus inferiority.

_____

_____

2. Describe the characteristics of the following forms of cognitive development:

a. Decentering.

_____

_____

b. Accommodation.

_____

_____

c. Conservation.

_____

_____

d. Class inclusion.

_____

_____

3. What advice would you give parents to improve or increase their child's interest in reading?

_____

_____

4. Define school phobia. Discuss why this occurs and give ways to help the family cope with and resolve these fears.

_____

_____

5. Describe measures that can be taken to avoid the following accidents with the school-age child:

a. Drowning.

_____

_____

b. Motor vehicle accidents.

_____

_____

c. Sports injuries.

_____

_____

d. Firearms.

_____

_____

APPLYING YOUR KNOWLEDGE

CASE STUDY

Mrs. Elway brings her daughter Clois, age 11, to the well-child care center for an annual checkup. The nurse obtains the history and begins the assessment. Clois's vital signs are within normal limits: temperature 98.6°F, pulse 75, respirations 26, blood pressure 110/58. Mrs. Elway tells the nurse she is concerned about Clois's sudden outbreaks of perspiration; although the episodes are not frequent, they do not seem to correlate with environmental temperatures.

1. What anticipatory guidance should the nurse give to Mrs. Elway regarding breast development and vaginal secretion?

_____

_____

_____

2. Clois wants to play soccer at school; Mrs. Elway asks the nurse if she thinks this would be a good idea. What principles regarding structured activities should the nurse call upon to formulate a response?

_____

_____

_____

CRITICAL INQUIRY EXERCISE

1. Develop a teaching plan for parents to explain the physical growth related to sexuality occurring during the school-age years.

2. Create a set of key points to discuss when providing anticipatory guidance for parents on detection of recreational drug use.

CRITICAL EXPLORATION

1. Observe students in an elementary school classroom. Record the behaviors of the teacher that may be considered positive and valuable to the children's transition to the school environment.

2. Observe several students for gross and fine motor development. Compare the findings to the expected motor development for that chronologic age group.

3. Visit a school during a recess period and observe the behaviors of children that are active with the following types of play: (a) group, (b) cooperative, (c) grouping, (d) same gender, and (e) consisting of rules.

PRACTICING FOR NCLEX

MULTIPLE-CHOICE QUESTIONS

Circle the letter that corresponds to the best answer for each question.

1. Sex education should be introduced at
   a. high school.
   b. junior high school.
   c. middle school.
   d. grade/elementary school.

2. Peer relationships are important to the school-age child. Which of the following is a characteristic of the 9-year-old child?
   a. Boys and girls love to play together.
   b. Activities are very complete.
   c. Boys and girls begin to have social interactions.
   d. Loyalty and affiliation are directed to a same-sex peer groups.

3. Which of the following permanent teeth would the nurse expect to be present when assessing a 7-year-old child?
   a. Lower cuspids.
   b. Upper central incisor.
   c. First bicuspid.
   d. Second molar.

4. Which of the following is correct regarding physical maturation before puberty?

   a. Boys are usually taller than girls.

   b. Girls are usually taller than boys.

   c. Boys and girls are usually the same height.

   d. There is no pattern of height based on gender.

ALTERNATE FORMAT QUESTIONS

Multiple-Answer Multiple-Choice Questions

Circle the letter(s) corresponding to the appropriate answer(s). Select all that apply.

1. Gross motor development will allow a 6-year-old child to do which of the following?

   a. Jump.

   b. Tumble.

   c. Skip rope easily.

   d. Play hopscotch.

   e. Ride a bicycle.

2. Which of the following would be most helpful in promoting a sense of industry in a school-age child?

   a. Having the child read a book with many short chapters.

   b. Assembling a complicated model car kit.

   c. Receiving a reward for completing a task.

   d. Reassuring the child that he is doing something correctly.

   e. Allowing the child to learn through frustration.

3. When describing the typical socialization activities of 9-year-old children, which of the following would most likely apply?

   a. Peer groups are extremely important.

   b. Clubs consisting of boys and girls.

   c. Readiness for away from home camps.

   d. Increased episodes of homesickness.

   e. Intense need for privacy.

Nursing Care of a Family With an Adolescent

CHAPTER OVERVIEW

Chapter 33 provides an overview of adolescent growth and development, nursing care related to health promotion, and the management of illness in the adolescent. The physiologic and psychological needs of the adolescent and common health concerns encountered during adolescence are reviewed. The use of the nursing process to plan and provide appropriate health care for the adolescent and his or her family is explored.

LEARNING OBJECTIVES

After mastering the contents of this chapter, you should be able to do the following:

1. Describe normal growth and development and common parental concerns of the adolescent period.

2. Identify National Health Goals related to adolescents that nurses could help the nation achieve.

3. Use critical thinking to analyze ways in which care of an adolescent could be more family centered.

4. Assess an adolescent for normal growth and development milestones.

5. Formulate nursing diagnoses for the family of an adolescent.

6. Identify expected outcomes for nursing care of an adolescent.

7. Plan nursing care related to growth and development concerns of an adolescent, such as planning health teaching necessary to accept pubertal changes.

8. Implement nursing care related to growth and development or special needs of an adolescent, such as organizing a discussion group on ways to prevent drug abuse.

9. Evaluate expected outcomes for achievement and effectiveness of care.

10. Identify areas related to care of adolescents that could benefit from additional nursing research or application of evidence-based practice.

11. Integrate knowledge of adolescent growth and development with nursing process to achieve quality maternal and child health nursing care.

KEY TERMS

adolescence	puberty
comedones	role confusion
formal operational thought	stalking
glycogen loading	substance abuse
identity	

MASTERING THE INFORMATION

FILL IN THE BLANKS

Supply the missing term or the information requested.

1. Females generally stop growing within _____ years from menarche.

2. Adolescents will experience a slight _____ in pulse rate as they move toward adulthood.

3. Adolescents will experience a slight _____ in blood pressure as they move toward adulthood.

4. One major dilemma encountered by adolescents that leads to many growth and development concerns is that they are _____ in some respects but still _____ in others.

5. Early adolescence generally occurs between the ages of _____ and _____ years; middle adolescence occurs between _____ and _____ years; and late adolescence occurs between _____ and _____ years.

6. Cognitive development over the adolescent years involves the stage of _____ _____ , which begins at age _____ or _____.

7. The goal of therapy for acne treatment is to decrease the formation of _____ , prevent _____ , and control _____ proliferation.

8. As many as 90% of high school seniors report having used _____.

MATCHING

Match the terms in Column I with a definition, example, or related statement from Column II. Place the letter corresponding to the answer in the space provided.

Column I

1. ____ Adolescence

2. ____ Formal operational thought

3. ____ Empathy

4. ____ Intimacy

5. ____ Substance abuse

6. ____ Puberty

7. ____ Pustular acne

8. ____ Runaway

9. ____ Suicide

10. ____ Secondary sex characteristics

Column II

a. The physiologic period between the beginning of puberty and the cessation of bodily growth.

b. Use of chemicals to improve the mental state.

c. Deliberate self-injury with the intent to end one's life.

d. Body hair configuration and breast growth distinguishing males from females.

e. Feeling for another by projecting one's self into the other person's situation.

f. Development of a sense of compassion or concern for others of both sexes.

g. The stage at which the individual first becomes capable of sexual reproduction.

h. A 10- to 17-year-old absent from home at least overnight without permission of parent or guardian.

i. Condition often treated with systemic antibiotics.

j. Ability to think in abstract terms and use the scientific method.

SHORT ANSWER

Supply the missing term or the information requested.

1. Discuss two reasons the nurse should obtain an adolescent's health history in private, separately from his or her parents.

   _____

   _____

2. List three common factors (primary assessment areas) that explain why adolescents may suffer fatigue.

   _____

   _____

3. What major task must the adolescent achieve in each of the following developmental areas: sense of intimacy, emancipation from parents, and value system?

   _____

   _____

4. State two ways nurses can be instrumental in helping to achieve National Health Goals related to adolescent health.

_____

_____

5. Describe the common social behaviors manifested by adolescents at ages 13, 14, 15, 16, and 17.

_____

_____

6. Identify 7 of the 14 danger signs for adolescent suicide.

_____

_____

APPLYING YOUR KNOWLEDGE

CASE STUDY

Angelique Rodriguez, age 14, was referred to you, the school nurse, by her guidance counselor. Angelique's grades have dropped from A's to low C's over the past two semesters, and she has become aggressive and refuses to talk to the teachers or counselors. The counselor suspects drugs, pregnancy, or depression but does not know how to help Angelique.

1. What would three of your first actions be when approaching Angelique?

_____

_____

_____

2. If Angelique admitted depression and drug abuse, what initial steps would you take to get help for her?

_____

_____

_____

CRITICAL INQUIRY EXERCISE

1. Prepare a teaching plan for an adolescent group that addresses methods for maintaining adequate nutrition, rest, and exercise.

2. How could the usual social behaviors noted in adolescents ages 13 through 17 contribute to problems or concerns that may be experienced by the adolescent and his or her family?

CRITICAL EXPLORATION

Attend a group session at an adolescent drug rehabilitation center (either in person or via two-way mirror). Note common themes related to why adolescents use drugs.

PRACTICING FOR NCLEX

MULTIPLE-CHOICE QUESTIONS

Circle the letter that corresponds to the best answer for each question.

1. Because of changes occurring in the sebaceous glands and sweat glands of adolescents, the nurse would include which of the following in health care teaching?
   a. Increased hygiene requirements to reduce body odor and acne.
   b. Information regarding the need for increased fat-soluble vitamins.
   c. Instructions regarding medications for inadequate sweat production.
   d. Exercises that will minimize the production of sweat.

2. When planning a teaching strategy for an adolescent, the nurse should do which of the following?
   a. Give information about how the teen can manage the specific problems he or she identifies.
   b. Maintain an air of authority by providing explanations for care procedures to parents only.
   c. Provide information related to long-term health needs, since adolescents respond best to long-range planning.
   d. Teach the parents first, since they will be better able to teach the teen.

3. At his physical, Bob, 14 years old, tells the nurse he is "a short, clumsy klutz." The nurse should respond in which of the following ways?

   a. Discuss with Bob the fact that his clumsiness is probably a sign of an easily curable disease.

   b. Instruct Bob in methods of relieving clumsiness through muscle exercises and improving nutrition.

   c. Explain to Bob that adolescent boys are usually taller than adolescent girls, so he should be examined.

   d. Inform Bob that what he is experiencing will lessen becoming more co-ordinated as he grows taller over the next 4 to 6 years.

4. The mother of Sheila, age 13, reports that Sheila "talks for hours to her girlfriends, and spends most of her waking hours with girls." The nurse could reassure Sheila's mother by explaining which of the following?

   a. If Sheila spends less time on the phone during the next 2 years, she will mature normally.

   b. Sheila is probably talking to boys when her parents are not around.

   c. Talking on the phone and spending time with girlfriends is normal for a girl of Sheila's age.

   d. There is no current threat of homosexuality due to Sheila's young age.

5. Marla is 15 years old. Marla's mother tells the nurse that she fears that her daughter will get into serious trouble soon because she is always "going for a walk or sitting outside somewhere." The nurse should respond in which of the following ways to this information?

   a. Encourage Marla's mother to follow her to determine why Marla is being so distant.

   b. Inform the mother that Marla is probably all right and is seeking the privacy she needs.

   c. Schedule Marla for a blood and urine drug screening immediately.

   d. Tell Marla's mother to call a psychologist to help her deal with the stress of adolescence.

6. Which of the following would be a positive sign of identity formation in a client in late adolescence?

   a. Obtaining a job to save money.

   b. Continuous dieting.

   c. Getting pregnant and having a baby.

   d. Living with parents.

7. Daryl, age 17, states he should not have sex and get girls pregnant "mostly because my parents would be really mad." Daryl's response may indicate a lack of development in which of the following areas?

   a. Cognitive development.

   b. Moral development.

   c. Physiologic development.

   d. Religious development.

8. Which of the following would be a realistic outcome related to an adolescent with a history of experimentation with marijuana? The adolescent will

   a. stop using drugs immediately without assistance.

   b. discuss ways to enjoy life without drugs.

   c. use only marijuana, with no additional drug use.

   d. smoke marijuana in moderation.

9. Which of the following would be a realistic outcome related to an adolescent with a medical condition requiring a special diet?

   a. The adolescent with diabetes will eat no sweet, sugary foods.

   b. The adolescent with hypertension will not eat potato chips.

   c. The adolescent with fatigue will choose preferred foods high in vitamins and minerals.

   d. The adolescent with acne will discuss the need for foods high in lipids to replace the deficient body supply.

10. Anna, age 17, has been identified as a suicide risk. The nurse should watch her carefully and during discharge teaching discuss the need for the family to watch her particularly closely

    a. before the beginning of the school year.

    b. between noon and 3 pm.

    c. during her menstrual period.

    d. During the evening hours.

ALTERNATE FORMAT QUESTIONS

Multiple-Answer Multiple-Choice Questions

Circle the letter(s) corresponding to the appropriate answer(s). Select all that apply.

1. Which of the following would be appropriate nursing interventions for an adolescent who is abusing the specific drug?

   a. *Alcohol*: Investigate the presence of alcohol abuse by parents or other close family members.

   b. *Amphetamines*: Monitor for symptoms such as aggressive and demanding behavior and paranoia.

   c. *Anabolic steroids*: Instruct athletes that these drugs cause fatigue and depression, which will lead to weight gain.

   d. *Barbiturates*: Allow the suicide-prone adolescent the control of managing oral administration alone, since these are generally harmless drugs.

   e. *Cigarettes*: Have a nurse who smokes discuss with the teen the evils and problems caused by smoking as one who knows the problems personally.

   f. *Cocaine/crack*: Educate adolescents on the potential for immediate death even with the first use.

2. When developing a plan of care for an adolescent runaway who will be returning home to the family, which of the following would be appropriate?

   a. Enlisting the aid of a mediator.

   b. Establishing a contract for behavior.

   c. Setting up ground rules for communication.

   d. Allowing the adolescent to do come and go as desired.

   e. Ensuring that the adolescent has limited privacy.

3. Which of the following medications would be appropriate for treating acne in an adolescent?

   a. Prednisone.

   b. Isotretinoin.

   c. Cefoxitin.

   d. Penicillin.

   e. Tetracycline.

Child Health Assessment

CHAPTER OVERVIEW

Chapter 34 offers an in-depth discussion of the nursing techniques used in child health assessment. Interviewing skills and procedures for performing physical and developmental assessments are described. Nursing interventions aimed at reducing the child's anxiety during assessment procedures are given. Normal growth and development parameters and health deviations are explained for each component of the health assessment. A case study is presented to help the student apply the principles used in conducting an abdominal assessment.

LEARNING OBJECTIVES

After mastering the contents of this chapter, you should be able to do the following:

1. State the purposes of health assessment in children of all ages.

2. Identify National Health Goals related to health assessment of children nurses can help the nation achieve.

3. Use critical thinking to analyze ways health assessment skills can be incorporated into nursing care procedures to maintain family-centered care.

4. Assess a child and family by health interview, physical examination, and development screening.

5. Formulate nursing diagnoses based on health assessment findings.

6. Identify expected outcomes based on health assessment findings.

7. Plan nursing care based on health assessment findings such as informing parents of health deviations.

8. Implement nursing care such as conducting an age-appropriate health interview or physical examination by modifying techniques based on the child's age.

9. Evaluate expected outcomes for achievement and effectiveness of care.

10. Identify areas related to health assessment of children that could benefit from additional nursing research or application of evidence-based practice.

11. Integrate nursing process with knowledge of health assessment to achieve quality maternal and child health nursing care.

KEY TERMS

antitoxins	geographic tongue
audiogram	hordeolum
auscultation	hydrocele
bruit	hypospadias
chief concern	inspection
conjunctivitis	intelligence
deep tendon reflexes	intercostal spaces
diaphragmatic	kwashiorkor
excursion	palpation
epispadias	percussion
esotropia	physiologic splitting
exotropia	point of maximum
gamma globulin	impulse

ptosis
retractions
review of systems
sinus arrhythmia
strabismus

temperament
toxoid
turgor
varicocele

MASTERING THE INFORMATION

FILL IN THE BLANKS

Supply the missing term or information requested.

1. The mobility of the eardrum (tympanic membrane) can be tested by injecting _____ into the ear canal.

2. _____ _____ is a rough-appearing tongue surface that accompanies general symptoms of illness such as fever.

3. Sinus arrhythmias are considered a normal phenomenon in children of _____ age. They are characterized by a marked heart rate increase on _____ and a marked heart rate decrease on _____.

MATCHING

Match the terms in Column I with a definition, example, or related statement from Column II. Place the letter corresponding to the answer in the space provided.

Column I: Body Mass Index Interpretation

1. ___ Underweight

2. ___ Normal

3. ___ Overweight

4. ___ Obese

Column II: Body Mass Index Finding

a. 32
b. 27
c. 20
d. 17.5

ADDITIONAL MATCHING QUESTIONS

Match the terms in Column I with a definition, example, or related statement from Column II. Place the letter corresponding to the answer in the space provided.

Column I: Child Health Problems

1. ___ Iron deficiency anemia

2. ___ Cyanosis

3. ___ Endocarditis

4. ___ Chromosomal abnormalities

Column II: Signs and Symptoms That May Be Noted on the Extremities

a. Simian crease
b. Concave nails
c. Clubbed fingers
d. Linear hemorrhages under the nails

SHORT ANSWER

Supply the missing term or the information requested.

1. List and explain the nine categories for data gathering in performing the initial health assessment for the child and family.

2. What are the height and weight deviations that indicate failing to thrive in a child?

3. Name two tests used to detect strabismus.

4. Describe the assessment technique used to detect choanal atresia.

5. Name three prominent features of chronic serous otitis media.

APPLYING YOUR KNOWLEDGE

CASE STUDY

Jennifer, age 14, is visiting the primary care center for a routine "return to school" physical checkup. She will be examined by the physician to determine her diagnosis and the immediate care necessary.

1. What is an important consideration related to the examination and privacy that the nurse should be aware of regarding Jennifer?

2. On examination, how would the nurse divide the abdomen for inspection?

3. What would be the appearance of the abdomen if the contour and structure are normal?

4. Describe the sounds to be heard when auscultating the abdomen.

CRITICAL INQUIRY EXERCISE

1. Pair off with another nursing student and practice performing an initial assessment using the eight categories for data gathering.

2. There is a significant change in the growth and development of the child moving from a toddler to a preschooler stage of development. Contrast the physical differences that you may find between the two groups of children.

CRITICAL EXPLORATION

1. Visit a well-child clinic or pediatrician's office and observe the performance of health assessments on children in various age groups. Focus on communication styles and techniques used by the parent, child, and health care provider.

2. Select a parent group, and explain to them why the Denver Developmental Screening Tool is used and how it is scored and interpreted.

PRACTICING FOR NCLEX

MULTIPLE-CHOICE QUESTIONS

Circle the letter that corresponds to the best answer for each question.

1. When obtaining information regarding the day history of a child, the nurse should ask
   a. "How much food does your child normally eat?"
   b. "Does your child socialize well with others?"
   c. "Describe your child's normal sleep patterns."
   d. "What types of stools does your child normally have?"

2. Which of the following is a priority when performing a physical assessment on a newborn?
   a. Preventing the newborn from squirming.
   b. Maintaining body temperature.
   c. Examining ears and throat before the eyes and nose.
   d. Assessing the newborn's brachial pulse.

3. When performing an assessment of the throat, depressing the tongue of a child who has acute epiglottitis is contraindicated because this
   a. may precipitate upper airway obstruction.
   b. overstimulates the cough and gag reflex.
   c. may be a source of bacterial infections.
   d. may rupture the epiglottis.

4. The most effective way to assess a toddler's gait is to
   a. observe play activity.
   b. perform a specific motor test.
   c. ask the child to walk toward the parent.
   d. ask the child to hop on one foot.

5. To assess hearing in a 1-month-old infant the nurse should
   a. play a musical toy 4 ft from the infant's ear and observe for eye movement.
   b. repeat the infant's name in a soft tone and observe facial expressions.
   c. perform the Rinne test and observe for head turning.
   d. make a loud noise and observe for the startle reflex.

6. When assessing a child's abdomen, which technique would the nurse perform first?
   a. Percussion.
   b. Palpation.
   c. Inspection.
   d. Auscultation.

7. Which of the following would the nurse interpret as possibly indicating a bowel obstruction in a toddler?
   a. Increased peristalsis with absence of stools for 2 or more days.
   b. Abdominal distention with absence of peristalsis.
   c. Severe abdominal pain with a loud bruit on auscultation.
   d. Presence of an abdominal hernia with dry, foul-smelling stools.

8. Which assessments would be a priority for a child who complains of a sore throat and dizziness?
   a. Otoscopic and throat exam.
   b. Nasal and ophthalmic exam.
   c. Mental status evaluation and complete neurologic exam.
   d. Respiratory and cardiovascular system assessments.

9. When performing an assessment for the presence of an inguinal hernia, which of the following should be considered a positive test result?
   a. Palpable femoral lymph nodes.
   b. Extreme pain and discomfort in rectal and perineal area.
   c. Bulging of the intestine while coughing.
   d. Pelvic pain on palpation.

10. To assess the school-age child for scoliosis the nurse should
    a. ask the child to stand straight with feet together.
    b. measure the leg lengths and pelvic girth.
    c. have the child bend over, inspecting for a dimpling.
    d. ask the child to walk to observe posture.

11. Tina is a preschooler who is brought to the clinic by her mother for a checkup? Which of the following statements made by Tina's mother would most likely indicate that Tina has a vision problem?
    a. "Tina is always rubbing her eyes, blinking, and squinting."
    b. "Tina sits so close to the television when she's watching it."
    c. "Tina still doesn't know her colors."
    d. "Tina doesn't seem to like to pay attention to what's in front of her."

12. To conduct the Denver Articulation Screening Examination (DASE), the nurse would ask the child to
    a. repeat some familiar words or phrases.
    b. read a favorite short story.
    c. recite a poem with age-appropriate words.
    d. read a phrase and interpret it.

ALTERNATE FORMAT QUESTIONS

Fill in the blanks

Multiple-Answer Multiple-Choice Questions

Circle the letter(s) corresponding to the appropriate answer(s). Select all that apply.

1. Assessment revealing which of the following would lead the nurse to suspect that a child is at increased risk for hearing impairment?
   a. Perinatal infections.
   b. High birth weight.
   c. Hyperbilirubinemia.
   d. Bacterial meningitis.
   e. Anatomical malformation.

2. Which of the following statement(s) is correct regarding the assessment findings of the female genitalia?
   a. Hair growth in the pubic area typically appears triangular in shape.
   b. A vaginal discharge in a young child may be a sign of sexual abuse.
   c. An enlarged clitoris in an adolescent girl is a sign of sexual activity.
   d. Vaginal warts are common findings in most children under the age of 13.
   e. Pelvic examination is usually performed when the girl reaches 16 years of age.

3. A nurse is performing an abdominal assessment of a school-aged child. Place the actions below in the proper sequence reflecting how the nurse would proceed.
   a. Percuss the liver.
   b. Inspect abdominal contour.
   c. Ausculate for bowel sounds.
   d. Palpate for tenderness.
   e. Palpate for rebound tenderness.

35

Communication and Teaching With Children and Families

CHAPTER OVERVIEW

Chapter 35 discusses communication and health-teaching techniques as related to children, beginning with an overview of nursing process specific to communication with children. Types of learning, the influence of age on learning, and techniques for developing and implementing a teaching plan are included. A case study is presented to help the students apply health teaching to a child requiring special communication skills.

LEARNING OBJECTIVES

After mastering the contents of this chapter, you should be able to do the following:

1. Describe principles of effective communication and teaching and learning as they relate to health teaching with children.

2. Identify National Health Goals related to communication and teaching with children that nurses could help the nation achieve.

3. Use critical thinking to analyze ways therapeutic communication and health teaching can be further incorporated into the nursing care of children and families to make it more family centered.

4. Assess children for their ability to communicate and readiness to learn.

5. State nursing diagnoses related to communication and health teaching with children.

6. Identify expected outcomes for a specific child based on the child's age, developmental maturity, emotional needs, and communication or learning style.

7. Plan nursing care based on the use of communication and health-teaching priorities.

8. Implement health teaching such as devising a puppet show using principles of effective communication and teaching–learning.

9. Evaluate expected outcomes for achievement and effectiveness of care.

10. Identify areas of care related to effective communication or health teaching of children that could benefit from additional nursing research or application of evidence-based practice.

11. Integrate knowledge of effective communication and teaching–learning with the nursing process to achieve quality maternal and child health nursing care.

KEY TERMS

affective learning
behavior therapy
clarifying
cognitive learning
communication
demonstration
empathy
feedback
focusing
nontherapeutic
  communication

paraphrasing
perception checking
positive reinforcement
psychomotor learning
redemonstration
reflecting
teaching plan
therapeutic
  communication

MASTERING THE INFORMATION

FILL IN THE BLANKS

Supply the missing term or the information requested.

1. _____ _____ is a method that examines statements, thoughts, and responses to determine effectiveness with therapeutic communication.

2. Teaching in the home gives the nurse an opportunity to assess the child's _____ , interactions with _____ _____, and overall _____ _____.

3. Provide the term for the type of learning described.

   a. _____ depends on muscle and neurologic coordination.

   b. _____ requires adequate development, intelligence, and attention span.

   c. _____ is gained best through role-modeling, role-playing, or shared experience discussion.

4. _____ is exact imitation of a demonstrated procedure.

5. Outcomes for learning should reflect the _____ of learning desired and should establish _____ and _____ guidelines.

6. When teaching a psychomotor skill, always assess the child's _____ _____ to perform the procedure.

7. Teaching strategies are most effective when they are _____.

8. The use of flash cards or board games may assist a child in _____ certain information.

9. Since children often absorb one piece of information at a time, preparation for surgery should be taught in _____.

10. Children learn best those things that hold a particular _____ for them.

11. Learning occurs best with _____ reinforcement.

MATCHING

Match the terms in Column I with a definition, example, or related statement from Column II. Place the letter corresponding to the answer in the space provided.

Column I

1. ___ Nontherapeutic communication
2. ___ Therapeutic communication
3. ___ Feedback
4. ___ Reflecting
5. ___ Clarifying
6. ___ Perception checking
7. ___ Focusing
8. ___ Paraphrasing

Column II

a. Helping someone center on a subject that you suspect is causing anxiety because he or she comments about it indirectly or completely avoids it.

b. Interaction that is planned, has structure, and is helpful and constructive.

c. Repeating statements someone has made so that you both can be certain you understood.

d. Restating the last word or phrase someone has said when there is a pause in the communication.

e. Documenting a feeling or emotion that someone has expressed to you.

f. Restating what someone has said not only to indicate that you have heard correctly but also to help explain what the person is trying to say.

g. Interaction that lacks structure, planning, and deliberate purpose.

h. A response acknowledging a message has been received and understood.

Column I

1. ____ Behavior modification

2. ____ Cognitive learning

3. ____ Informal teaching

4. ____ Learning

5. ____ Lifestyle

6. ____ Psychomotor learning

7. ____ Puppetry

8. ____ Resource people

9. ____ Role modeling

10. ____ Teaching

11. ____ Affective learning

Column II

a. A two-step process involving the acquisition of knowledge resulting in a measurable change in behavior.

b. Process that involves a change in an individual's ability to perform a skill.

c. Process that involves a change in the individual's level of understanding or knowledge.

d. Individuals specializing in teaching particular information or skills.

e. A system aimed at erasing some form of activity that interferes with health functioning.

f. Presentation of information so as to increase someone's knowledge or insight.

g. The common pattern of a child's life.

h. A helpful method for teaching preschool children about the hospital and health care staff.

i. Process occurring when a nurse spontaneously answers a child's or parent's question about a care measure.

j. Demonstration of a certain attitude that you want a child to learn.

k. Process that involves a change in a person's attitude.

SHORT ANSWER

Supply the missing term or the information requested.

1. Discuss three benefits of group teaching.

_____

_____

2. Describe the first step in developing a teaching plan.

_____

_____

3. Discuss the benefit of using visual aids when teaching children.

_____

_____

4. Explain the concept of learning ability plateaus.

_____

_____

5. Discuss nursing measures that will help the nation achieve health goals related to communication and health teaching as an important mechanism of preventive health care.

_____

_____

APPLYING YOUR KNOWLEDGE

CASE STUDY

Six-year-old Raoul Mendelez has been newly diagnosed with diabetes. He understands both English and Spanish, although his parents communicate with him and each other almost exclusively in Spanish.

1. As the nurse caring for Raoul, what communication and teaching techniques will you use to maximize his and his parents' comprehension of the disease and the lifestyle changes it will necessitate?

_____

_____

2. During your first teaching session, you notice the parents are constantly interrupting and questioning Raoul, and they appear anxious. You realize you must modify your teaching plan to improve effectiveness. What adjustments would you make?

_____

_____

3. How might your teaching plan change if Raoul were 16 years old?

_____

_____

_____

4. What effects might Raoul's Hispanic culture have on your communication and teaching plan?

_____

_____

_____

CRITICAL INQUIRY EXERCISE

1. Prepare and execute a teaching plan for an adolescent and a school-age child on some aspect of health maintenance or health promotion. Evaluate the effectiveness of your communication and teaching and note the differences in approach and content needed for each group.

2. Prepare a teaching plan for a toddler related to nutrition. Use a creative approach and evaluate its effectiveness in helping the child learn the content presented.

CRITICAL EXPLORATION

Examine the discharge-teaching forms or documentation at a local health care facility. Evaluate the clarity of instructions for children of various age groups.

PRACTICING FOR NCLEX

MULTIPLE-CHOICE QUESTIONS

Circle the letter that corresponds to the best answer for each question.

1. Which of the following indicates appropriate use of teaching-learning principles?

    a. Explaining to a school-age child that the kidney transplant is being done because it will be good for him.

    b. Providing a booklet that encourages a preschool child to eat extra meat because it will help to repair his incision.

    c. Having the mother of an infant use a game to teach the infant a desired activity.

    d. Using a firm tone to tell a toddler not to touch her bandage.

2. A child may have the greatest difficulty learning which of the following?

    a. Dietary adjustments.

    b. Insulin administration.

    c. Colostomy irrigation.

    d. Range of motion exercises.

3. Which of the following is true about children relative to learning?

    a. One child's learning style may differ from another's.

    b. Admitting your discomfort with teaching a subject will negatively affect learning.

    c. Chronologic age is more indicative of learning capability than mental age.

    d. The older the child, the shorter the attention span.

4. Sally has to teach a group of preschoolers to dial 911. The most effective strategy for this teaching would be

    a. pamphlets.

    b. lecture.

    c. discussion.

    d. demonstration.

5. Which of the following should be included in the teaching-learning process with a young child?

    a. Focusing information solely to the child, since parents cannot change the child's behavior.

    b. Evaluating if the child is performing the desired behavior when indicated.

    c. Letting the child decide the depth of information to be taught.

    d. Teaching the child special ways to prepare the food on a restricted diet.

ALTERNATE FORMAT QUESTIONS

Multiple-Answer Multiple-Choice Questions

Circle the letter(s) corresponding to the appropriate answer(s). Select all that apply.

1. Which of the following interventions would be most appropriate when teaching a child and family?

   a. _____ Provide a long, clear explanation about procedures to preschool clients to facilitate understanding.

   b. _____ Have parents present each time health teaching is performed with adolescents.

   c. _____ Offer an immediate, concrete reward to school-aged children to encourage learning.

   d. _____ Assess the child's family patterns before planning the timing for exercise or medication activities after discharge.

   e. _____ Avoid using puppets for teaching preschool children.

   f. _____ Correct a wrong action by first acknowledging a positive aspect of what the child did or how the child performed the action.

2. A nurse is describing the five levels of communication. Place the levels listed below in their proper sequence from lowest to highest depth.

   a. Fact reporting.

   b. Shared feelings.

   c. Cliché conversation.

   d. Shared personal ideas and judgments.

   e. Peak communication.

3. Which of the following would be most appropriate to use facilitate affective learning?

   a. Role-playing.

   b. Demonstration.

   c. Lecture.

   d. Shared value discussion.

   e. Pamphlet reading.

Nursing Care of a Family With an Ill Child

CHAPTER OVERVIEW

Chapter 36 provides an overview of the experience of hospitalization and its effect on children from infancy through adolescence and their families. The meaning of the hospital experience to children is discussed. The role of play therapy in the preparation and care of the hospitalized child is reviewed. The use of the nursing process to plan and provide care for the hospitalized child and the family is described.

LEARNING OBJECTIVES

After mastering the contents of this chapter, you should be able to do the following:

1. Describe illness and illness experiences, as they must appear to children.

2. Identify National Health Goals related to care of ill children nurses can help the nation achieve.

3. Use critical thinking to analyze ways in which illness care can be made more family centered and less traumatic for children.

4. Assess the impact of an illness, especially one requiring a hospital stay, on a child.

5. Formulate nursing diagnoses related to the stress of illness in children.

6. Establish expected outcomes for an ill child.

7. Plan nursing care to reduce the stress of illness, such as helping parents plan for ambulatory care or hospitalization.

8. Implement measures such as orientation, education, and therapeutic play to reduce the stress of illness.

9. Evaluate expected outcomes for achievement and effectiveness of care.

10. Identify areas related to illness in children that could benefit from additional nursing research or application of evidence-based practice.

11. Integrate knowledge about a child's response to illness with the nursing process to achieve quality maternal and child health nursing care.

KEY TERMS

calorie counting
case management nursing
nonrapid eye movement (NREM) sleep
play therapy
primary nursing
rapid eye movement (REM) sleep
sensory deprivation
sensory overload
sleep deprivation
therapeutic play

MASTERING THE INFORMATION

FILL IN THE BLANKS

Supply the missing term or the information requested.

1. The way children deal with hospitalization is based on the following factors: _____ of the event, _____ _____ available, and effectiveness of past _____.

2. The response of children to illness depends on their ____ _____, past _____, and level of _____.

3. Nurses can help the nation meet health care goals related to mental health of children by helping with assessment of children's _____level and reducing the _____of the hospitalization.

4. Parents of infants who will be hospitalized should bring the child's _____ ____ with the child to the hospital.

5. The three chief fears of the hospitalized toddler or preschooler are fear of the _____, _____, and _____.

6. The school-aged child and adolescent should have _____ explanations of what will happen in the hospital.

MATCHING

Match the terms in Column I with a definition, example, or related statement from Column II. Place the letter corresponding to the answer in the space provided.

Column I

1. ___ Observation play

2. ___ Cooperative play

3. ___ Creative play

4. ___ Dramatic play

5. ___ Parallel play

6. ___ Play

7. ___ Play therapy

8. ___ Therapeutic play

Column II

a. A psychoanalytic technique used by psychiatrists to help children understand their feelings, thoughts, and motives.

b. A play technique that is divided into three parts: energy release, dramatic play, and creative play.

c. The "work" of children: a means by which children develop increasing cognitive, psychomotor, and social capabilities.

d. Acting out an anxiety situation; most effective with preschoolers.

e. Type of play in which children watch play intently but are not actively engaged in it.

f. Two children playing side by side but seldom attempting to interact with each other.

g. Children playing with an organized structure or competing for a desired goal or outcome.

h. The child's drawing a picture or making a list to express emotions or knowledge level.

TRUE OR FALSE

Indicate if the following statements are true or false by placing a "T" or "F" in the space provided.

___ 1. Children are not just small adults.

___ 2. Children should be told that the doctor will be "taking their tonsils out."

___ 3. New foods should be introduced to the hospitalized infant to promote growth and development.

___ 4. School-aged children cannot describe symptoms with accuracy.

___ 5. Children can be reliable for monitoring their own care and speaking up about incorrect procedures and medications.

___ 6. Children need more nutrients than adults, and thus may require hospitalization for vomiting or diarrhea when adults would not.

___ 7. Children tend to respond to disease locally rather than systemically.

___ 8. Assess patient needs relative to cultural differences by using textbook descriptions of the needs of persons of that culture.

___ 9. Separation is most damaging to a child between ages 2 and 3 months.

___10. Children older than age 7 should be told of a pending hospitalization as soon as the parents are aware of it.

SHORT ANSWER

1. List five hazards common to all hospitalization regardless of the reason or length of stay.

   _____

   _____

2. Describe why explanations of procedures to young children are not always successful in relieving stress of illness and hospitalization.

   _____

   _____

3. Determine the appropriate age group for the following childhood play activities. Indicate the answer in the space provided.

   a. _____ Need toys in their cribs, such as mobiles.

   b. _____ Would enjoy watching a soap opera and then discussing the people and their problems.

   c. _____ Need put-in and take-out toys, such as blocks that can be stacked.

   d. _____ Need quiet toys such as crayons, markers, or books.

APPLYING YOUR KNOWLEDGE

CASE STUDY

Devon, a 3-year-old who had emergency surgery while on vacation, has been separated from her single mother, who had to return home because of her job, and 14-year-old sister. Devon has been without her family for 4 days.

1. What behaviors would you expect Devon to display to nursing staff over the next days?

   _____

   _____

2. What effect might Devon's hospitalization and absence have on her mother and older sister?

   _____

   _____

   _____

3. What interventions might you plan for Devon and her family?

   _____

   _____

   _____

CRITICAL INQUIRY EXERCISE

1. What measures would you take to prepare a 4-month-old infant and family members for open heart surgery? How would this preparation differ if the surgery were minor?

2. Design a teaching plan for parents whose 2-year-old child will be admitted to the hospital for surgery.

CRITICAL EXPLORATION

1. While on a pediatric clinical unit, assess children in varying age groups. Determine if separation anxiety is present, and note the age levels of the children experiencing the highest levels of anxiety.

2. Interview the parent of a hospitalized child. Determine the type of preparation the parent used before bringing the child to the hospital.

PRACTICING FOR NCLEX

MULTIPLE-CHOICE QUESTIONS

Circle the letter that corresponds to the best answer for each question.

1. A 6-year-old child is to be admitted to the hospital for an elective surgery. The nurse should advise the parents to tell the child about the surgery how many days before admission to prevent unnecessary worry?

   a. 1.

   b. 2.

   c. 4.

   d. 6.

2. The nurse might initiate which of the following interventions when caring for a hospitalized child with a disability or chronic illness?

   a. Avoid using information from previous hospitalizations when planning to prepare the child for the current hospitalization.

   b. Help the child avoid contact with peers while hospitalized to decrease self-consciousness and the sense of being different.

   c. Limit visiting hours of family and friends to prevent overtiring the child.

   d. Suggest the child write letters to friends or call family members.

3. Alice, age 2 years, is in the intensive care unit with multiple tubes and bandages. Her parents are present frequently but appear reluctant to handle Alice's tubes and bandages, although they asked to feed her at meals. The nurse should do which of the following?

   a. Inform the parents that it is important that they learn to change Alice's dressings and perform this procedure often.

   b. Encourage the parents to irrigate Alice's tubing to make them feel more involved in her plan of care.

   c. Allow the parents to feed Alice and do other care measures as they express interest and comfort.

   d. Limit the parents from performing any care for Alice so they will understand that nurses are capable of fully caring for her.

4. When preparing a child for procedures or surgery, the nurse might do which of the following?

   a. Instruct the child to place the thermometer into his or her arm and hold it there.

   b. Prepare the child for surgery by providing the child with a doll and a small scalpel.

   c. Provide a doll and syringe, alcohol wipes, and a tourniquet to prepare the child for a blood-drawing procedure.

   d. To help a child cope with a dressing change, allow the child to hand the sterile gauze to the nurse during the procedure.

5. Which of the following would be an appropriate method for influencing a child to assist with a care measure?

   a. Encourage fluid intake by explaining to the child that fluid will keep him from drying up.

   b. Have the child lift hand weights every 2 hours to strengthen muscles.

   c. Originate board games and crossword puzzles to help the child learn about health teaching.

   d. Place an incentive spirometry machine in front of the child and instruct him or her in deep breathing.

ALTERNATE FORMAT QUESTIONS
Multiple-Answer Multiple-Choice Questions

Circle the letter(s) corresponding to the appropriate answer(s). Select all that apply.

1. Which of the following nursing interventions would be appropriate when providing care for an ill child?

   a. _____ Saying grace before administering a tubefeeding if the child commonly says grace before meals.

   b. _____ Standing close to the child, at full adult height, during admission to establish a rapport with the child.

   c. _____ Calling the child "sugar" or "sweetie" when addressing him or her to create a warm environment and close relationship.

   d. _____ Determining the child's routines and attempt to adapt the hospital routine as much as possible.

   e. _____ Letting the child wear his or her own clothes if possible rather than change to a hospital gown.

   f. _____ Limiting the number of readmissions and length of stay by teaching parents how to safely monitor their child after a procedure.

2. Which of the following activities would be most appropriate for a nurse to do to provide play opportunities for a preschooler?

   a. Making a mobile from roller gauze to hang over the child's bed.

b. Making puzzle pieces from a picture from a magazine.

c. Singing nursery rhymes with the child.

d. Making a puppet out of a paper bag.

e. Getting paper and markers for coloring.

f. Making a deck of cards to play "go fish."

3. Which of the following would the nurse expect to include when conducting therapeutic play?

a. Choosing the articles that the child will use.

b. Allowing the play to be unstructured.

c. Not criticizing the child's play.

d. Using real equipment.

e. Telling the child how to use the equipment.

Nursing Care of a Family When a Child Needs Diagnostic or Therapeutic Modalities

CHAPTER OVERVIEW

Chapter 37 provides an overview of the nursing care required for the ill child and family during diagnostic and therapeutic procedures. Adaptations required for children when undergoing diagnostic procedures and various therapeutic techniques are discussed. The use of the nursing process to plan and provide care for the hospitalized child and the family is explored.

LEARNING OBJECTIVES

After mastering the contents of this chapter, you should be able to do the following:

1. Describe common nursing interventions used in the health care of children to aid diagnosis and therapy.

2. Identify National Health Goals related to diagnostic and therapeutic procedures for children that nurses could help the nation achieve.

3. Use critical thinking to analyze ways diagnostic and therapeutic procedures can be modified to be more family centered.

4. Assess children about developmental stage and knowledge level before beginning diagnostic or therapeutic procedures.

5. Formulate nursing diagnoses related to common diagnostic or therapeutic procedures used with children.

6. Identify expected outcomes for a child who needs a diagnostic or therapeutic procedure.

7. Plan nursing interventions to aid in diagnosis or therapy for children.

8. Implement nursing interventions relevant to diagnostic or therapeutic procedures, such as preparing a child for magnetic resonance imaging.

9. Evaluate expected outcomes for achievement and effectiveness of care.

10. Identify areas related to nursing procedures with children that could benefit from additional nursing research or application of evidence-based practice.

11. Integrate knowledge of common diagnostic and therapeutic procedures with nursing process to achieve quality maternal and child health nursinkg.

KEY TERMS

aspiration studies
barium contrast
   studies
bronchoscopy
clean-catch urine
   specimen
colonoscopy
computed
   tomography (CT)
electrical impulse
   studies
endoscopy

gavage feedings
magnetic resonance
   imaging (MRI)
positron emission
   tomography (PET)
radiopharmaceuticals
single-photon emission
   computerized tomog-
   raphy (SPECT)
total parenteral
   nutrition (TPN)
ultrasound

MASTERING THE INFORMATION

FILL IN THE BLANKS

Supply the missing term or the information requested.

1. Restraints should be checked every _____ minutes to ensure that circulation is intact.

2. When securing a dressing on infants and young children, use _____, _____ tape to protect it.

3. A _____-_____ specimen involves collecting urine after usual voiding after the external meatus has been cleaned.

MATCHING

Match the terms in Column I with a definition, example, or related statement from Column II. Place the letter corresponding to the answer in the space provided.

Column I

1. ___ Barium contrast studies

2. ___ Gavage feedings

3. ___ Total parenteral nutrition (TPN)

4. ___ Bronchoscopy

5. ___ Radiopharmaceutical

Column II

a. Infusion of a concentrated hypertonic solution into a central or peripheral intravenous site.

b. Radioactive-combined substances that when given orally or by injection flow to designated body organs for a diagnostic picture.

c. Direct visualization of the larynx, trachea, and bronchi through a fiberoptic tube.

d. Use of radiopaque dye to outline the gastrointestinal tract.

e. Provision of adequate nutrition through a nasogastric tube.

SHORT ANSWER

Supply the missing term or the information requested.

1. Name two problems associated with the use of an ostomy appliance for an infant.

   _____

   _____

2. Discuss the psychological and physical preparation needed for a child undergoing surgery.

   _____

   _____

3. List four common types of restraints used with children.

   _____

   _____

4. Describe two ways in which nurses can help the nation achieve goals related to reducing the length of hospital stay for children.

   _____

   _____

APPLYING YOUR KNOWLEDGE

CASE STUDY

Iesha Jackson, age 2, is admitted to your care after stabilization of a sickle cell crisis. She is screaming for her mother and trying to get out of bed. Her mother, age 18, is in the waiting room making a call. She says Iesha's father is the custodial parent and this crisis happened on "her weekend" with Iesha. She does not want to call Iesha's father for fear he will blame her.

1. Iesha will require several invasive procedures during her stay. What teaching responsibilities do you have in this situation?

   _____

   _____

   _____

2. How will the fact that Iesha's parents are separated affect your discharge-teaching plan?

   _____

   _____

   _____

CRITICAL INQUIRY EXERCISE

1. Review five skills listed in a fundamentals text that were not discussed in this chapter, and note ways in which those skills might need to be adjusted for an infant or child.

2. Plan a schedule for a 4-year-old child who must have blood drawn for lab work, an abdominal radiograph, a CT scan, and an endoscopy during her 2-day hospital stay.

CRITICAL EXPLORATION

Tour a pediatric unit and observe the procedures being performed. Compare the techniques used with those noted on an adult floor, and note any variations.

PRACTICING FOR NCLEX

MULTIPLE-CHOICE QUESTIONS

Circle the letter that corresponds to the best answer for each question.

1. When a procedure is being performed that requires a consent form, which of the following is true?

   a. A consent form can be omitted if the procedure involves only a minimal risk.

   b. The nurse must explain the procedure and obtain signed consent if the physician does not.

   c. Emancipated minors must have parental permission to sign a consent form.

   d. In single-parent families, the custodial parent must sign the consent form.

2. The nurse's role in assisting with diagnostic procedures includes which of the following?

   a. Helping the child to forget the experience of the procedure as quickly as possible.

   b. Using complex medical terms to explain procedures to children and parents to demonstrate knowledge and competence.

   c. Explaining the preparation and actual procedure before beginning either.

   d. Sending mature children to different test departments without supervision to increase independence.

3. Which of the following is appropriate when modifying procedures for children?

   a. Parents should be asked to restrain infants when indicated.

   b. Toddlers should be given procedures quickly and without warning to decrease resistance.

   c. Adolescents should be expected to tolerate procedures maturely and without fear.

   d. School-aged children should be given an explanation about reasons for the procedures.

4. When performing contrast dye studies with children, the nurse should

   a. tell the child the flavored barium will taste like a milkshake to increase cooperation.

   b. isolate the child after the test until the radioactivity resolves.

   c. explain to the child that a warm feeling may be experienced with IV dye.

   d. restrict all activity for the duration of the procedure to prevent distracting the child.

5. When teaching parents about temperature reduction in children, the nurse should include which of the following interventions?

   a. Administering acetylsalicylic acid every 4 hours until the child's temperature is less than 101°F.

   b. Dressing the child in warm flannel night clothes to prevent chilling.

   c. Giving the age-appropriate dose of ibuprofen (Motrin) to reduce temperature.

   d. Place an ice cloth on the child's forehead and refresh it every hour.

ALTERNATE FORMAT QUESTIONS

Multiple-Answer Multiple-Choice Questions

Circle the letter(s) corresponding to the appropriate answer(s). Select all that apply.

1. Which of the following intervention(s) are appropriate?

   a. _____ Allowing the child to look at the incision during a dressing change.

   b. _____ Taking a radial pulse for children under 1 year of age.

   c. _____ Ensuring that an infant is calm before assessing respiratory rate.

   d. _____ Sponging children with cold water to lower the temperature.

   e. _____ Assessing blood pressure in routine assessment of children over 3 years of age.

   f. _____ Instructing adolescents on the cleaning procedure for clean-catch specimens.

2. After an upper gastrointestinal endoscopy study, which of the following interventions would be most important?

   a. Check for gag reflex before giving any oral fluids.

   b. Monitoring airway and respiratory function for the first 4 hours.

   c. Applying a warm compress to the neck to reduce spasm.

   d. Administering atropine to reduce pulmonary secretions.

   e. Verifying allergy to iodine or shellfish.

3. Which of the following instructions would the nurse include when teaching the parents about their child's ostomy care?

   a. Check the appliance for stool at least every 4 hours.

   b. Remove a self-adhering bag if it becomes full.

   c. Rinse the bag with clear water after flushing it with warm water and soap solution.

   d. Use a solvent to remove sealant from the old appliance when applying a new appliance.

   e. Irrigate the ostomy with 100 mL of tap water daily.

Nursing Care of the Family When a Child Needs Medication Administration or Intravenous Therapy

CHAPTER OVERVIEW

Chapter 38 provides an overview of the nursing care required for the ill child and family regarding medication administration and intravenous therapy. Adaptations required for children during the preparation and administration of medications and when planning and implementing intravenous therapy are discussed. The use of the nursing process to plan and provide care for the child and the family involved in medication administration and intravenous therapy is explored.

LEARNING OBJECTIVES

After mastering the contents of this chapter, you should be able to do the following:

1. Describe common methods of medication and intravenous therapy used in the health care of children.

2. Identify National Health Goals related to medication or intravenous therapy that nurses could help the nation achieve.

3. Use critical thinking to analyze ways that medicine or intravenous therapy can be modified to be more family centered.

4. Assess the developmental stage and knowledge level of children and adolescents before beginning medication or intravenous therapy.

5. Formulate nursing diagnoses related to medication or intravenous therapy with children.

6. Identify expected outcomes for children receiving medication or intravenous therapy.

7. Plan nursing interventions to aid in making medicine and intravenous therapy maximally effective.

8. Implement nursing interventions concerned with medication and intravenous therapy and children, such as introducing patient-controlled analgesia.

9. Evaluate expected outcomes for achievement and effectiveness of care.

10. Identify areas related to medication or intravenous therapy with children that could benefit from additional nursing research or application of evidence-based practice.

11. Integrate knowledge of medication and intravenous therapy with nursing process to achieve quality maternal and child health nursing.

KEY TERMS

absorption
distribution
excretion
intermittent
  infusion devices

Intracath
metabolism
pharmacokinetics
vascular access port

MASTERING THE INFORMATION

FILL IN THE BLANKS

Supply the missing term or the information requested.

1. When administering nose drops, place the child on his or her _____.

2. The mandatory site for intramuscular injections in infants is the _____ _____. muscle.

3. _____ therapy is the quickest and most effective means of administering fluid or medicine to the ill infant or child.

4. The _____ of body systems in infants and children plays a major role in drug action.

5. To administer ear drops to a child under 2 years, straighten the ear canal by pulling the pinna _____ and _____.

MATCHING

Match the terms in Column I with a definition, example, or related statement from Column II. Place the letter corresponding to the answer in the space provided.

Column I

1. ____ Absorption

2. ____ Distribution

3. ____ Excretion

4. ____ Metabolism

Column II

a. Removal of the drug or metabolites from the body to prevent drug toxicity.

b. Conversion of the drug into an active form or an inactive form.

c. Movement of the drug through the bloodstream to a specific site of action.

d. Transfer of the drug from its point of entry into the bloodstream.

SHORT ANSWER

Supply the missing term or the information requested.

1. Identify four routes by which medications are given to children.

_____

_____

2. State what is used for determining the correct dosage of drugs for most children.

_____

_____

3. What can be used to obtain frequent venous blood samples?

_____

_____

4. List three fluid infusion safety measures to be used with children.

_____

_____

5. Identify the critical rights to follow when administering drugs safely to children.

_____

_____

APPLYING YOUR KNOWLEDGE

CASE STUDY

India Jeilhal is admitted to your care after a playground accident. The 5-year-old is sitting up in bed holding her mother's hand. The doctor has ordered an intravenous antibiotics and oral pain medication. India's mother is asking you to give India something for pain.

1. What would you need to do when responding to India's mother's request?

_____

_____

_____

2. How will you prepare for the initiation of intravenous therapy?

_____

_____

_____

3. What measures will you take to prepare India and her mother for the procedure?

_____

_____

_____

CRITICAL INQUIRY EXERCISE

1. Discuss ways in which you might need to alter your approach when administering an intramuscular injection to a 1-month-old, a 1-year-old, a 5-year-old, a 10-year-old, or a 16-year-old child.

2. Plan instructions for the parents of a 4-year-old child who must administer an oral medication that comes in tablet form only.

CRITICAL EXPLORATION

Tour a neonatal unit and pediatric unit and observe intravenous therapy in place with children of various ages. Compare the techniques and equipment used with the different age groups.

PRACTICING FOR NCLEX

MULTIPLE-CHOICE QUESTIONS

Circle the letter that corresponds to the best answer for each question.

1. Sites frequently used for intravenous insertion in young children or infants include which of the following?
   a. Veins in the antecubital space and on the extensor surface of the wrist.
   b. Jugular vein and veins on the ventral surface of the hand.
   c. Veins located in the leg or on the surface of the foot.
   d. Radial or ulnar surface veins or the subclavian vein.

2. The nurse preparing to initiate intravenous therapy with a newborn infant would obtain which of the following size catheters?
   a. 16 gauge.
   b. 18 gauge.
   c. 22 gauge.
   d. 25 gauge.

3. A child weighing 20 kg is to begin fluid therapy. On the basis of caloric expenditure per 24 hours, the child should receive how many milliliters of maintenance intravenous solution?
   a. 1500 mL.
   b. 1725 mL.
   c. 2000 mL.
   d. 2300 mL.

4. The nurse can be instrumental in helping the nation achieve national health goals related to children and drug or medication administration by
   a. stressing the importance of using medications to treat every discomfort.
   b. educating parents regarding the importance of steroid use to treat acne in adolescents.
   c. teaching stress management techniques to children and parents for use to address anxiety.
   d. instructing parents to keep medication at the bedside for ease of access.

5. A 3-year-old child may receive a medication dosage consistent with the dosage usually given to a 1-year-old child if the 3-year-old child
   a. was developmentally delayed.
   b. was tall for his or her age.
   c. had a body surface area of a 1-year-old child.
   d. weighed more than a 1-year-old child.

6. When assessing a child before medication administration, it is important to determine which of the following?

  a. The child's dosage preference.

  b. Past medication-taking experiences.

  c. Parental developmental status.

  d. Whether the medication is having the desired effect.

ALTERNATE FORMAT QUESTIONS

Multiple-Answer Multiple-Choice Questions

Circle the letter(s) corresponding to the appropriate answer(s). Select all that apply.

1. Which of the following would be appropriate for a child who is receiving oral medication therapy?

  a. Instructing parents to store drugs in locked, elevated cabinets.

  b. Asking a child, "Will you drink this for me?" to help the child feel respected.

  c. Telling the child it is time to take the medicine.

  d. Asking the child's preference of fluid to take the medicine with.

  e. Mixing bitter medicine with a full glass of juice to dilute the taste.

  f. Crushing a tablet and mixing it with applesauce for better taste when appropriate.

2. A child is receiving deferoxamin via hyperdermoclysis. Which of the following sites would the nurse expect to use?

  a. Pectoral region.

  b. Back.

  c. Anterolateral thigh.

  d. Dorsal hand surface.

  e. Scalp vein.

3. When administering nose drops to a preschooler, which of the following would the nurse expect to do?

  a. Have the child extend his head over the side of the bed prior to administration.

  b. Turn the child's head to the same side as the nostril used after administration.

  c. Ask the child to "sniff" the medicine once it has been instilled.

  d. Allow the child to get up immediately after the drops have been given.

  e. Praise the child for how he acted when the drops were being administered.

Pain Management in Children

CHAPTER OVERVIEW

Chapter 39 discusses the management of pain in children. The causes of pain as well as the assessment and measurement of pain are discussed, with emphasis on developmental considerations. Varied pain management strategies are reviewed, including pharmacologic and nonpharmacologic measures. The use of the nursing process to plan and provide appropriate care and teaching to promote appropriate pain management in children is discussed.

LEARNING OBJECTIVES

After mastering the contents of this chapter, you should be able to do the following:

1. Describe the major methods and techniques of pain management in children.

2. Identify National Health Goals related to pain management in children that nurses can help the nation achieve.

3. Use critical thinking to analyze ways nursing care for a child in pain could be more family centered.

4. Assess a child as to whether pain management is needed or adequate.

5. Formulate nursing diagnoses for a child in pain.

6. Identify expected outcomes for a child in pain.

7. Plan nursing care for a child in pain.

8. Implement nursing care related to a child in pain, such as suggesting an alternative therapy.

9. Evaluate outcomes for achievement and effectiveness of care of a child in pain.

10. Identify areas related to care of children in pain that could benefit from additional nursing research or application of evidence-based practice.

11. Integrate knowledge of pain in children with nursing process to achieve quality maternal and child health nursing care.

KEY TERMS

acute pain
conscious sedation
chronic pain
cutaneous pain
distraction
epidural analgesia
gate control theory
nociceptors
pain
pain threshold

pain tolerance
patient-controlled
   analgesia
referred pain
somatic pain
substitution of meaning
thought stopping
transcutaneous electrical
   nerve stimulation
visceral pain

MASTERING THE INFORMATION

FILL IN THE BLANKS

Supply the missing term or the information requested.

1. The technique that allows the child to be both pain-free and sedated for a procedure and leaves protective reflexes intact is called _____ _____.

2. A numerical or _____ _____ scale uses a straight line with endpoints marked 0 for no pain on the left and 10 for worst pain on the right.

3. _____ __ _____ or guided imagery is a distraction technique that helps a child place another, nonpainful meaning on a painful procedure.

4. To reduce the pain of procedures such as venipuncture or lumbar puncture, a _____ _____ cream may be applied.

MATCHING

Match the terms in Column I with a definition, example, or related statement from Column II. Place the letter corresponding to the answer in the space provided.

Column I

1. ____ Distraction
2. ____ Gate control theory
3. ____ Patient-controlled analgesia
4. ____ Thought stopping
5. ____ Transcutaneous electrical nerve stimulation

Column II

a. A technique whereby children are taught to substitute a positive or relaxing thought for anxious thoughts.

b. Use of current to interfere with the transmission of the pain impulse across small nerve fibers

c. Explanation of pain impulses travelling between a site of injury and the brain, where the impulse is actually registered as pain.

d. Cells of the brainstem that register an impulse as pain becoming preoccupied with other stimuli so the pain impulse cannot register.

e. Self-administering of intravenous opiate boluses with a medication pump to control pain.

SHORT ANSWER

Supply the missing term or the information requested.

1. Discuss two of three reasons that nurses do not provide adequate pain relief to children.

2. Explain why pain assessment might be difficult with children.

3. Briefly discuss the gate control theory.

APPLYING YOUR KNOWLEDGE

CASE STUDY

Patricia Walters, age 4, is admitted onto your unit after having abdominal surgery. Her mother is concerned that Patricia might have pain but says she is afraid of injections.

1. Patricia's mother asks if you will need to hold Patricia down because she hates needles but needs something for pain. What are some responses you might give?

2. What are some methods you might use to assess Patricia's pain? Which pain assessment tools would be inappropriate?

CRITICAL INQUIRY EXERCISE

1. What key points would you address in a teaching plan for a school-aged child and parents when the child is discharged home after a painful day surgery? In addition to pain

medication, what other pain relief measures might you include in this teaching plan?

2. What should you do if a school-aged child or adolescent who is 1 day postsurgery and has had no pain medication since surgery denies pain but shows signs of discomfort?

CRITICAL EXPLORATION

Visit a pediatric cancer unit and a postoperative inpatient care unit at a pediatric hospital. Compare the pain control methods used on each unit. Note the route of administration and the types of analgesics used.

PRACTICING FOR NCLEX

MULTIPLE-CHOICE QUESTIONS

Circle the letter that corresponds to the best answer for each question.

1. When assessing the pain of an infant, the nurse should consider which of the following?
   a. Infants are preverbal, so cues such as tears or guarding a body part can be helpful.
   b. Infants will be comforted completely solely by a parent if the pain is very intense.
   c. An infant can indicate if he or she has pain and exactly where the pain is located.
   d. Since infants think concretely, they may associate words like "sharp" with knives.

2. Which of the following is true about pain assessment for the school-aged child and adolescent?
   a. A scale of 1 to 10 should be used for younger children to provide the child with maximum choices.
   b. Some children may require preassessment work to evaluate if they understand incremental measurements.
   c. School-aged children use mechanisms for controlling pain that are unique and different from adult mechanisms.
   d. Preadolescents think very concretely, so they can describe pain with little difficulty.

3. Which of the following tools allows the health care provider to rate pain without the need of self-report input by the child and evaluates behaviors usually seen with pain?
   a. Logs and diaries of pain episodes.
   b. Oucher pain-rating scale.
   c. FLACC pain assessment tool.
   d. Poker chip tool.

4. Analgesia instilled in the space just outside the spinal canal is called
   a. local anesthesia.
   b. epidural analgesia.
   c. intranasal analgesia.
   d. intravenous analgesia.

ALTERNATE FORMAT QUESTIONS

Multiple-Answer Multiple-Choice Questions

Circle the letter(s) corresponding to the appropriate answer(s). Select all that apply.

1. When preparing a teaching plan about the physiology of pain, the nurse includes the following events. Place these events in the proper sequence from first to last.
   a. Pain impulse perceived as pain.
   b. Pain stimulus occurs.
   c. Activation of nociceptors.
   d. Interpretation of the sensation by the brain.
   e. Sensation is routed to the spinal cord.

2. A child is using distraction to assist with pain relief. Which of the following would be appropriate?
   a. Blowing soap bubbles.
   b. Using the fingers to count down from 5 to 1.
   c. Applying EMLA cream to the site.
   d. Playing a hand-held computer game.
   e. Reciting a list of positive things.

3. A nurse is using the COMFORT behavior scale to assess pain in young infant. Which of the following would the nurse evaluate?
   a. Alertness.
   b. Physical movement.
   c. Facial expression.
   d. Leg movement.
   e. Consolability.
   f. Need for oxygen administration.

CHAPTER 40

Nursing Care of a Family When a Child has a Respiratory Disorder

CHAPTER OVERVIEW

Respiratory diseases are serious in children because the lumens of respiratory structures are small in children and likely to become obstructed in disease. Nurses need good assessment skills to assess clinical status. This chapter presents the most common disorders of the upper and lower respiratory tract, along with their therapeutic management. Care that incorporates the maintenance of airway patency and promotion of oxygenation via therapeutic techniques such as administration of aerosols and bronchodilators, chest physiotherapy, and position changes, and antibiotics for infection is also addressed.

LEARNING OBJECTIVES

After mastering the contents of this chapter, you should be able to do the following:

1. Describe common respiratory disorders in children.

2. Identify National Health Goals related to children with respiratory disorders that nurses could help the nation achieve.

3. Use critical thinking to analyze ways nursing care for a child with a respiratory disorder could be more family centered.

4. Assess a child with a respiratory disorder.

5. Formulate nursing diagnoses related to respiratory disorders in children.

6. Identify expected outcomes that address the priority needs of a child with a respiratory disorder.

7. Plan nursing care for a child with a respiratory disorder.

8. Implement nursing care for a child with a respiratory disorder such as administering oxygen to a child.

9. Evaluate expected outcomes for achievement and effectiveness of care.

10. Identify areas related to care of children with respiratory disorders that could benefit from additional nursing research or application of evidence-based practice.

11. Integrate knowledge of respiratory disorders in children with nursing process to achieve quality maternal and child health nursing care.

KEY TERMS

adventitious sounds
anoxia
arterial blood gases
aspiration
atelectasis
clubbing
cyanosis
expiration
hypoxemia
hypoxia
inspiration
paroxysmal coughing

percussion
pneumothorax
rales
retraction
steatorrhea
stridor
tachypnea
tracheostomy
tracheotomy
vibration
wheezing

MASTERING THE INFORMATION

FILL IN THE BLANKS

Supply the missing term or the information requested.

1. The upper respiratory tract functions to
_____, _____, and _____
air.

2. Identify the normal values for each of these
blood gas components: (a) Po_2 _____; (b)
Pco_2 _____; (c) O_2 saturation _____; (d)
pH _____; (e) HCO_3._____.

3. The most dangerous periods following a
tonsillectomy are the _____, and days
_____ to _____.

4. If a child has no complications following a
tonsillectomy, he or she is discharged the
same day or the following morning. Three
danger signs you would tell the parents to
watch for are _____,
_____, and
_____.

5. Children with symptoms of epiglottitis should
never be examined with a tongue blade
because the gagging might cause _____
_____ _____.

6. Three symptoms of epiglottitis are _____,
_____, and _____.

7. The first indicator of airway obstruction in
children is _____.

8. The respiratory centers are located in the
_____ and the _____.

MATCHING

*Match the terms in Column I with a definition,
example, or related statement from Column II.
Place the letter corresponding to the answer in
the space provided.*

Column I

1. ___ Hypoxia
2. ___ Cyanosis
3. ___ Hypoventilation
4. ___ Apnea
5. ___ Hyperventilation
6. ___ Anoxia
7. ___ Tachypnea
8. ___ Hypoxemia
9. ___ Bronchopulmonary dysplasia
10. ___ Stridor
11. ___ Rales
12. ___ Wheezing

Column II

a. Lack of respiration.
b. Rapid deep breathing.
c. Bluish tint to the skin.
d. Decreased oxygen in body cells.
e. Reduction below adequate levels of oxygen in
tissue.
f. Rapid respiration.
g. Deficit oxygen content in the blood.
h. Shallow breathing.
i. Fine crackling sounds.
j. Harsh high-pitched sound heard on
inspiration.
k. A chronic lung condition seen in infants with
acute respiratory distress at birth.
l. Expiratory whistling sound due to obstruction
of lower trachea or bronchioles.

APPLYING YOUR KNOWLEDGE

CASE STUDY

Rebecca O'Shea is a 2-year-old girl with cystic
fibrosis. Her mother is a working single parent.

Rebecca was admitted to your unit with a diagnosis of pneumonia. Her mother expresses concern that Rebecca will die because working makes it difficult for her to perform the respiratory care Rebecca requires.

1. What are the major problems you would address for Rebecca during her hospital stay?

_____

_____

_____

2. Your discharge plan would need to address what family needs?

_____

_____

_____

3. How might community agencies be beneficial in assisting Rebecca and her mother?

_____

_____

_____

CRITICAL INQUIRY EXERCISE

1. In what way, if any, would you need to alter your approach and process when practicing respiratory assessment on a child compared with an adult?

2. Develop a discharge-teaching plan for parents of infants or children with an upper respiratory infection.

CRITICAL EXPLORATION

1. Spend a day at the cystic fibrosis clinic at a local hospital to observe follow-up care and treatment.

2. Spend a day with a respiratory therapist on a pediatric unit to observe various treatments and modalities.

PRACTICING FOR NCLEX

MULTIPLE-CHOICE QUESTIONS

Circle the letter that corresponds to the best answer for each question.

1. Which of the following actions would be most appropriate when assessing a newborn for choanal atresia?

 a. Make the newborn cry, then gently compress one nostril, then the second.

 b. Compress both nostrils at the same time and open the newborn's mouth.

 c. Hold the newborn's mouth closed, then compress one nostril, then the other.

 d. Have the newborn suck on a bottle as you compress the nostrils.

2. Baby Jane was diagnosed with acute nasopharyngitis (common cold). Her mother is being taught how to use a bulb syringe and a vaporizer to clear the congestion. Which of the following would the nurse include in the teaching plan?

 a. The bulb should be compressed before inserting the syringe into the child's nostril.

 b. The vaporizer should be kept at the bedside so the mist will be close to the child's face.

 c. The vaporizer will not require cleaning since the steam is very hot and sterile.

 d. The bulb syringe filled with saline nose drops should be squeezed into the nostril.

3. Baby John was admitted with streptococcal pharyngitis. When he was discharged, his mother was told to return to the doctor's office in 2 weeks with a urine specimen. The nurse understands that the rationale for this instruction is that the urine would be examined most likely

 a. for fat and lipids to see if the kidneys are working.

 b. for protein to determine if acute glomerulonephritis is developing.

 c. to determine if the child is developing otitis media.

 d. to determine whether to increase the child's diet from liquid to soft.

4. Which of the following would be inappropriate to include in the plan of care for a child who has had a tonsillectomy?

 a. Observing for signs of bleeding.

 b. Encouraging the child to eat ice cream hourly to soothe the child's throat.

c. Placing the child on his or her abdomen with a pillow under the chest.

d. Observing for excessive swallowing and throat clearing.

5. If bleeding occurs in a child following a tonsillectomy, the nursing action would be to

a. elevate the child's head and turn him or her on his or her side.

b. place the child in a prone position.

c. place the child in a Trendelenburg position.

d. elevate the child's feet and turn him or her in a prone position.

6. Which of the following would be most appropriate to give to a child following a tonsillectomy?

a. Sips of clear liquid.

b. Milkshakes.

c. French fries.

d. Popcorn.

7. Elisa, a 14-month-old child, is admitted to the hospital with laryngotracheobronchitis (croup). On assessment, the nurse would expect to find

a. cyanosis and dyspnea.

b. productive coughing and a high fever.

c. pale laryngeal tissue and dyspnea.

d. barking cough and inspiratory stridor.

8. Which of the following would the nurse include in the plan of care for a child with bronchitis?

a. Ensuring bed rest with minimal oral fluid intake.

b. Keeping room air cool and dry.

c. Encouraging shallow inspiration to decrease chest pain.

d. Using expectorants and coughing to clear secretions.

9. A 5-month-old child is admitted to your unit with bronchiolitis. Assessment reveals the following: temperature 102°F, apical pulse 154 beats per minute, respirations 68, and irritability. Oxygen therapy is ordered. The nurse understands that the rationale for this therapy is to

a. liquefy secretions.

b. promote rest.

c. relieve hypoxemia.

d. decrease coughing.

10. When developing a teaching plan for a group of parents about cystic fibrosis, the nurse would be least likely to include which statement?

a. It is inherited as an autosomal recessive trait.

b. It occurs in about 1 in 2000 births, mostly among whites.

c. Symptoms include patchy consolidations and tumors throughout the lungs.

d. It has an improved mortality with 50% of children now living to the age of 21.

ALTERNATE FORMAT QUESTIONS
Multiple-Answer Multiple-Choice Questions
Circle the letter(s) corresponding to the appropriate answer(s). Select all that apply.

1. Which of the following test results would the nurse expect to find in a child with cystic fibrosis?

a. Decreased levels of pancreatic enzymes in duodenal secretions.

b. Elevated plasma cholesterol.

c. Elevated chloride in sweat.

d. Increase fat content of the stool.

e. Decreased chloride in sweat.

2. It is very important that the nurse prevent aspiration following bronchoscopy. Which of the following interventions would be appropriate?

a. Feed the client slowly for the first hour.

b. Keep NPO until the gag reflex has returned.

c. Provide postural drainage for the first postoperative day.

d. Keep head elevated at 90° for the first postoperative day.

e. Maintain the bed flat and the client prone for the first hour.

3. Which of the following medications would the nurse expect the physician to order for a child with asthma?

a. Cough suppressant.

b. Long-acting bronchodilator.

c. Inhaled corticosteroid.

d. Mast cell stabilizer.

e. Leukotriene receptor antagonist.

41

Nursing Care of a Family When a Child has a Cardiovascular Disorder

CHAPTER OVERVIEW

Chapter 41 provides an overview of various cardiovascular conditions found in children. The potential effects of these conditions on the physical and psychological growth and development of the child are discussed. The use of the nursing process to plan and provide care for the client and for the family coping with a cardiovascular disorder is explored. The case study provides the student with an exercise involving preparation and management of a client undergoing a cardiac catheterization.

LEARNING OBJECTIVES

After mastering the contents of this chapter, you should be able to do the following:

1. Describe the common cardiovascular disorders of childhood.

2. Identify National Health Goals related to children with cardiovascular disorders that nurses could help the nation achieve.

3. Use critical thinking to analyze ways that nursing care of children with cardiovascular disorders could be more family centered.

4. Assess a child with a cardiovascular dysfunction.

5. Formulate nursing diagnoses for a child with a cardiovascular disorder.

6. Identify appropriate outcomes based on the priority needs of a child with a cardiovascular disorder.

7. Plan nursing care for a child with a cardiovascular disorder.

8. Implement nursing care for a child with a cardiovascular disorder such as teaching about the importance of taking prescribed medication.

9. Evaluate expected outcomes for achievement and effectiveness of care.

10. Identify areas related to the care of children with cardiovascular disorders that could benefit from additional nursing research or application of evidence-based practice.

11. Integrate knowledge of cardiovascular disorders with nursing process to achieve quality maternal and child health nursing care.

KEY TERMS

acyanotic heart disease
afterload
balloon angioplasty
cardiac catheterization
congestive heart failure
contractility
cyanosis
cyanotic heart disease
diastole
innocent heart murmur
left-to-right shunt

organic heart murmur
polycythemia
postcardiac surgery
  syndrome
postperfusion
  syndrome
preload
right-to-left shunt
systole
vasculitis

MASTERING THE INFORMATION

FILL IN THE BLANKS

Supply the missing term or the information requested.

1. In heart defects in which a connection exists between the right and left heart, the blood through the connective structure flows from _____ to _____.

2. Newborns and infants with heart disease are commonly brought to the health care facility by parents because the child is having

   _____ _____.

3. Chest tubes inserted in a child during open heart surgery will include an upper tube draining _____ and a lower one draining

   _____.

4. Rejection after cardiac transplant can occur as _____, _____, or _____ forms.

5. _____ refers to a structural or functional abnormality of the ventricular myocardium that occurs after an infection and results in severe dilation of the left or both ventricles.

6. _____ _____ is the most frequent cause of cardiac arrest in children.

7. Identify the name of the congenital heart disorder described.

   a. Includes pulmonary artery stenosis, ventricular septal defect, dextroposition of the aorta and right ventricular hypertrophy.

   _____

   b. The aorta rises from the right ventricle instead of the left ventricle; usually

accompanied by atrial and septal defects.

   _____

   c. The tricuspid valve is closed and the foramen ovale and ductus arteriosus remain patent.

   _____

8. One of the first signs of congestive heart failure in children is _____.

MATCHING

Match the terms in Column I with a definition, example, or related statement from Column II. Place the letter corresponding to the answer in the space provided.

Column I

1. ____ Endocarditis

2. ____ Dyslipidemia

3. ____ Patent ductus arteriosus

4. ____ Polycythemia

5. ____ Postperfusion syndrome

6. ____ Chest radiography

7. ____ Atrial septal defect

8. ____ Phonocardiography

9. ____ Echocardiography

10. ____ Pulmonic stenosis

11. ____ Truncus arteriosus

12. ____ Heart failure

13. ____ Kawasaki disease

14. ____ Calcium chloride

15. ____ Rheumatic fever

Column II

a. Agent used to increased heart contractility, possibly in place of epinephrine; contraindication for patients with digitalis toxicity.

b. An extreme increase in red blood cells in an attempt to increase tissue oxygenation.

c. Fever, splenomegaly, general malaise, and a maculopapular rash that occurs after open heart surgery.

d. Condition involving increased fatty acid level in the blood.

e. Infection of the valves of the heart, generally caused by streptococci.

f. Abnormal communication between the two atria where blood flows from left to right.

g. Left-to-right shunting of blood due to connection of the pulmonary artery to the aorta.

h. Autoimmune condition that typically results manifested a wide pulse pressure and systolic–diastolic murmur.

i. Condition that involves a narrowing of the pulmonary valve.

j. One major artery arises from the left and right ventricles instead of separate vessels.

k. Condition resulting when the myocardium of the heart cannot circulate and pump enough blood to supply the tissues of the body.

l. Mucocutaneous lymph node syndrome occurring almost exclusively in children before puberty.

m. A diagram of heart sounds translated into electrical energy by a microphone placed on the child's chest.

n. An ultrasound produced by high-frequency sound waves used to locate and study the movements and dimensions of cardiac structures.

o. Study that furnishes an accurate picture of the heart size and contour and size of the heart chambers.

SHORT ANSWER

Supply the missing term or the information requested.

1. In addition to fever, name three other criteria for the diagnosis of Kawasaki disease.

_____

_____

2. List the prenatal and birth information that should be discussed while obtaining a nursing history for a child with a cardiovascular disorder.

_____

_____

3. Relate two major areas of information to be discussed with parents when they are taking home their child who has a heart disorder.

_____

_____

4. Discuss the preparatory teaching necessary for a child and family before open heart surgery.

_____

_____

5. Describe how innocent and organic murmurs differ relative to duration, quality, and intensity.

_____

_____

APPLYING YOUR KNOWLEDGE

CASE STUDY

Harriette Borders, age 5, has been complaining of headaches and fatigue. She also experienced syncope at school. She was seen at the pediatrician's office and referred to the children's hospital for a cardiac catheterization. Mr. and Mrs. Borders bring Harriette to the hospital and you are assigned to care for her during the procedure.

1. Mrs. Borders was instructed not to allow Harriette to eat or drink fluids after midnight the morning before the procedure. What was the reasoning for these instructions?

_____

_____

_____

2. What is the purpose of the cardiac catheter?

_____

_____

_____

3. The child undergoing this procedure receives conscious sedation. It is likely that she would be anxious, afraid, and uncooperative if not prepared appropriately. What are some measures you can use to reduce Harriette's anxiety?

_____

_____

_____

4. You inform Mr. Borders that Harriette must lie flat in bed for 3 hours after returning to her

room. Explain the physiologic rationale for this statement.

_____

_____

_____

CRITICAL INQUIRY EXERCISE

1. Prepare a plan to teach cardiopulmonary resuscitation to family members of a child with a cardiac anomaly.

2. Prepare a teaching plan to instruct the family on how exercising and modifying nutritional intake can improve cardiovascular health. Include the National Health Goals in your plan.

3. Prepare for a class presentation an outline contrasting the hemodynamics of cyanotic and acyanotic heart disease.

CRITICAL EXPLORATION

Visit a neonatal intensive care unit and assess various infants. Identify heart sounds, differences in vital signs, and feeding problems.

PRACTICING FOR NCLEX

MULTIPLE-CHOICE QUESTIONS

Circle the letter that corresponds to the best answer for each question.

1. A child with coarctation of the aorta might require which of the following nursing interventions?

   a. Assisting the child and parents with coping with this terminal illness.

   b. Informing females with the condition that pregnancy seldom causes problems.

   c. Reassuring the child and parents that postoperative abdominal pain will subside.

   d. Scheduling the surgery during early infancy to prevent complications.

2. Nursing care of the child with an atrial septal defect would involve which of the following?

   a. Reporting splitting of the second heart sound immediately as a serious complication.

   b. Preparing the child and family for cardiac catheterization.

   c. Monitoring the diastolic murmur over the apical area that is diagnostic of the condition.

   d. Teaching parents about the lifelong medications required to control the condition.

3. Parents of a child with a pacemaker must be taught

   a. the procedure for cardiac defibrillation in case a dysrhythmia occurs.

   b. how to take the child's pulse accurately to determine pacemaker function.

   c. to change the pacemaker battery every year if symptoms indicate the need.

   d. that prolonged hiccuping is a harmless side effect from pacemaker leads.

4. Which of the following findings may be noted in a child with coarctation of the aorta?

   a. Low blood pressure in the upper extremities.

   b. High blood pressure in the lower extremities.

   c. A history of headaches and nosebleeds.

   d. A capillary refill of less than 5 seconds.

5. Which of the following would be most effective in reducing the workload of the heart of a child with heart failure?

   a. Bed rest in a semi-Fowler's position.

   b. Digoxin administration daily, intravenous or orally.

   c. Oxygen therapy by mask, cannula, or tent.

   d. Intravenous infusion of 2000 to 3000 mL/day.

6. Which of the following is true about congestive heart failure?

   a. Edema is an early symptom of heart failure in children.

   b. Irritability and restlessness may indicate abdominal pain from hepatomegaly.

   c. Left heart failure initially presents with jugular vein distention.

   d. Right heart failure results in pulmonary edema as an initial sign.

7. Reduction of complications from rheumatic fever can be accomplished through which of the following interventions?

   a. Administration of penicillin to children with strep throat or impetigo.

   b. Beginning speech therapy to reverse damage after antibiotics are completed.

   c. Pushing children with chorea to perform activities requiring fine motor movement to strengthen muscles.

   d. Withholding salicylates to prevent joint hemorrhage.

8. Nursing interventions for a child with Kawasaki disease may include which of the following?

   a. Maintaining heavy bed coverings and clothing to keep the child warm and comfortable.

   b. Palpating skin temperature and assessing capillary filling in fingers and toes.

   c. Performing range-of-motion exercises to joints hourly to prevent contractures.

   d. Withholding all aspirin-containing medications to prevent platelet agglutination.

9. Hypertension in children most commonly

   a. manifests frequent severe symptoms.

   b. cannot be treated with diet and daily exercise.

   c. results as a secondary manifestation of another disease.

   d. will resolve before adolescence without treatment if it is primary hypertension.

ALTERNATE FORMAT QUESTIONS

Multiple-Answer Multiple-Choice Questions

Circle the letter(s) corresponding to the appropriate answer(s). Select all that apply.

1. Which of the following would be appropriate for a child with a cardiovascular disorder?

   a. Assessing the skin surface of all black children to determine if cyanosis is present.

   b. Loosening the dressing on the cardiac catheter site to promote comfort.

   c. Bringing the parents of a child awaiting open heart surgery to the intensive care unit before surgery to prepare them.

   d. Administering intravenous fluids liberally and rapidly to a child after open heart surgery to replace massive blood loss.

   e. Reassuring the parents of a child with a ventricular septal defect that surgical repair is rarely required, even in large defects.

   f. Preparing an infant who has just been diagnosed with pulmonic stenosis, as well as his parents, for immediate surgery.

2. A child with heart failure is receiving medications to decrease afterload. Which of the following would the nurse expect to administer as ordered?

   a. Furosemide.

   b. Sprinolactone.

   c. Digoxin.

   d. Hydralazine.

   e. Nifedipine.

   f. Nitroprusside.

3. After teaching a group of nursing students about the different congenital heart defects, the instructor determines that teaching was successful when the students identify which of the following as examples of disorder with increased pulmonary blood flow?

   a. Ventricular septal defect.

   b. Aortic stenosis.

   c. Patent ductus arteriosus.

   d. Transposition of the great arteries.

   e. Total anomalous pulmonary venous return.

   f. Truncus arteriosis.

Nursing Care of a Family When a Child has an Immune Disorder

CHAPTER OVERVIEW

Chapter 42 discusses the immune process as it relates to childhood illness. Immune disorders noted in childhood are reviewed. The use of the nursing process to plan and provide care for the child and the family coping with an immune disorder is explored.

LEARNING OBJECTIVES

After mastering the contents of this chapter, you should be able to do the following:

1. Describe the immune process as it relates to childhood illnesses.

2. Identify National Health Goals related to immune disorders in children that nurses could help the nation achieve.

3. Use critical thinking to analyze ways that nursing care for a child with an immune disorder can be more family centered.

4. Assess a child with a disorder of the immune system.

5. Formulate nursing diagnoses for a child with a disorder of the immune system.

6. Establish outcomes for a child with a disorder of the immune system.

7. Plan nursing care pertinent to a child with an immune system disorder.

8. Implement nursing care for a child with an immune disorder such as teaching about environmental control.

9. Evaluate expected outcomes for achievement and effectiveness of care.

10. Identify areas related to care of a child with an immune disorder that could benefit from additional nursing research or application of evidence-based practice.

11. Integrate knowledge of immune disorders and the nursing process to achieve quality maternal and child health nursing care.

KEY TERMS

allergen	hyposensitization
anaphylaxis	immune response
antigen	immunity
autoimmunity	immunogen
cell-mediated immunity	immunoglobulins
chemotaxis	lymphokines
complement	lysis
cytotoxic response	macrophage
delayed hypersensitivity	phagocytosis
environmental control	tolerance
humoral immunity	
hypersensitivity response	

MASTERING THE INFORMATION

FILL IN THE BLANKS

Supply the missing term or the information requested.

1. Provide the type of primary immunodeficiency for each description.
   a. Cellular immune response remains adequate; child has resistance to viral, fungal, and parasitic infections, but all levels of immunoglobulins are abnormally low. _____
   b. Infection of surfaces exposed to the external environment and normally protected by mucus are common along with atopic diseases. _____

2. Human immunodeficiency virus (HIV) is spread by two primary routes in the adult population: _____ contact and _____ contact.

3. _____ results from an inability to distinguish self from nonself, causing the immune system to carry out immune responses against normal cells and tissue.

4. Assessment of the exact symptoms of an allergy is important in helping to identify the underlying _____.

5. The three goals for therapy in childhood allergy situations are to _____, _____, and _____.

6. The best way to identify the specific allergies in a child with food allergies is the use of a _____ _____ or an elimination diet.

7. Congenital immunodeficiencies usually manifest after the first _____ months of life.

8. When a child is stung by a bee, the immediate action should be to apply _____ to the site to minimize the absorption of the venom.

MATCHING

Match the terms in Column I with a definition, example, or related statement from Column II. Place the letter corresponding to the answer in the space provided.

Column I

1. ___ Antigen
2. ___ Cell-mediated immunity
3. ___ Hapten formation
4. ___ Immunocompetent cells
5. ___ Immunogen
6. ___ Lymphokines
7. ___ Memory cell
8. ___ Phagocytosis
9. ___ Serum sickness
10. ___ Suppressor cells

Column II

a. The neutralization of pathogens through ingestion by white blood cells.
b. Secretion by cytotoxic cells that contain or prevent migration of antigens.
c. Foreign substance capable of stimulating an immune response.
d. Responsible for retaining the formula or ability to produce specific immunoglobulins.
e. A hypersensitivity reaction to a foreign serum antigen or drug.
f. A nonantigenic substance that becomes antigenic when combined with a higher-weight molecule.
g. T cells that reduce the production of immunoglobulins against a specific antigen.
h. An antigen that can be readily destroyed by an immune response.
i. When antibodies are formed in response to a particular antigen; acquired through T-lymphocyte activity.
j. Cells capable of resisting foreign invaders.

SHORT ANSWER

Supply the missing term or the information requested.

1. State two measures a parent can take to decrease allergies in the bedroom, living room, and at school.

   _____

   _____

2. Compare seborrheic dermatitis and infantile eczema in terms of the presence of itching, age of onset, length of disease, and mood of the child.

   _____

   _____

3. Differentiate between congenital and acquired immunodeficiency disorders.

   _____

   _____

4. Discuss the purpose and use of skin testing when assessing allergies in children.

   _____

   _____

APPLYING YOUR KNOWLEDGE

CASE STUDY

José is a 4-year-old child with a primary B cell, IgA type immune deficiency disorder. He is admitted to your unit with an upper respiratory tract infection. His parents are concerned that his brothers and sisters will also contract the immune deficiency, so they would not let their other children play with José.

1. What is the most important concept you must include in a teaching plan for José's parents?

   _____

   _____

2. How would you approach his parents regarding their fears about José's siblings?

   _____

   _____

3. What areas would be a priority when caring for José?

   _____

   _____

CRITICAL INQUIRY EXERCISE

1. Prepare a teaching plan on the diagnosis of allergic rhinitis for a child and his or her family.

2. What would your response be to a fellow nurse who refuses to care for a client with contact dermatitis because the nurse fears becoming infected?

CRITICAL EXPLORATION

During a clinical experience, monitor care provided to a client with AIDS. Note the precautions used in care and the client's emotional response to the care and care providers. Note the care that you felt was particularly good, as well as ways in which care—physical and emotional—might have been improved.

PRACTICING FOR NCLEX

MULTIPLE-CHOICE QUESTIONS

Circle the letter that corresponds to the best answer for each question.

1. Nurses can help the nation achieve health goals related to human immunodeficiency virus by doing which of the following?

   a. Instructing young people that intravenous drugs are safer than oral drugs, although both are bad.

   b. Encouraging drug addicts to share needles primarily with friends, if they must use drugs.

   c. Educating children about the importance of using condoms or practicing abstinence.

   d. Avoiding discussions related to sex around adolescents younger than 18 years old.

2. Janice has a deficiency that affects her humoral immunity. The nurse prepares to teach Janice about this condition as resulting from inadequate

   a. B cells.

   b. antigens.

c. T cells.

d. allergens.

3. When teaching a group of parents about atopic disorders, which of the following would the nurse be least likely to include in the discussion?

a. Asthma.

b. Hay fever.

c. Atopic dermatitis.

d. Serum sickness.

4. Which of the following actions would be appropriate when providing care to a child with a hypersensitivity condition?

a. Having a syringe filled with a 1:5 dilution of the antigen on hand to counteract an unexpected anaphylactic reaction from skin testing.

b. Keeping the child at the health care setting for 30 minutes after the hyposensitization process.

c. Excluding the child with allergies from planning methods of environmental control to avoid resistance to the changes.

d. Encouraging parents who know of familial allergy patterns to bottlefeed infants.

ALTERNATE FORMAT QUESTIONS

Multiple-Answer Multiple-Choice Questions

Circle the letter(s) corresponding to the correct answer(s). Select all that apply.

1. Which of the following interventions would be appropriate when caring for the child with an immune disorder?

a. Anticipate treating child who faints but does not respond to amyl nitrate for possible anaphylaxis.

b. Administer a smaller-than-normal dosage of foreign serum to a child known to manifest serum sickness.

c. Do not allow children who develop urticaria as a result of exposure to extreme temperatures to swim in cold water.

d. Instruct parents of children with atopic dermatitis to cover the area with wet dressings containing Burow's solution.

e. Teach parents that all of the solution in an Epi-Pen must be ejected on injection.

2. A nurse is preparing a presentation about primary and secondary immunodeficiencies. Which of the following would the nurse include as examples of primary immunodeficiencies?

a. T-lymphocyte deficiencies.

b. Human immunodeficiency virus.

c. Severe combined immunodeficiency syndrome.

d. Hypogammaglobulinemia.

e. B-lymphocyte deficiencies.

3. Which of the following statements by the parents of a child who has an insect sting allergy indicates effective teaching?

a. "She needs to wear socks when walking outside."

b. "We won't let him take out the trash."

c. "We will make sure she doesn't use any scented products."

d. "He can mow the lawn as long as he does it after dusk."

e. "We'll tell him to avoid drinking from an open soda can when outside."

43

Nursing Care of a Family When a Child has an Infectious Disorder

CHAPTER OVERVIEW

Chapter 43 discusses common infectious disorders of childhood. The nursing techniques required to address the needs of children and their families when coping with an infectious disease are reviewed. The use of the nursing process to plan and provide care for the child with an infectious disease and his or her family is explored.

LEARNING OBJECTIVES

After mastering the contents of this chapter, you should be able to do the following:

1. Describe the causes and course of common infectious disorders of childhood.

2. Identify National Health Goals related to infectious disorders in children that nurses could help the nation achieve.

3. Use critical thinking to analyze ways that care of a child with an infectious disorder could be more family centered.

4. Assess a child with an infectious disorder.

5. Formulate nursing diagnoses for a child with an infectious disorder.

6. Establish outcomes for the care of a child with an infectious disorder.

7. Plan nursing care for a child with an infectious disorder.

8. Implement nursing care specific to the child with an infectious disorder, such as helping alleviate the pruritus of a rash.

9. Evaluate expected outcomes for achievement and effectiveness of care.

10. Identify areas of nursing care related to children with infectious diseases that could benefit from additional nursing research or application of evidence-based practice.

11. Integrate knowledge of infectious diseases and nursing process to achieve quality maternal and child health nursing care.

KEY TERMS

catarrhal stage	Koplik's spots
chain of infection	means of transmission
convalescent period	portal of entry
enanthem	portal of exit
exanthem	prodromal period
exotoxin	reservoir
fomites	septicemia
incubation period	susceptible host
interferon	

MASTERING THE INFORMATION

FILL IN THE BLANKS

Supply the missing term or the information requested.

1. _____ is the time between the invasion of an organism and the onset of symptoms of infection.

2. _____ is a common rickettsial disease transmitted by a tick.

3. _____ enters the body through the skin, migrates to the intestinal tract, and thrives on blood, causing severe anemia.

4. _____ is highly contagious viral infection that spreads by direct or indirect contact of saliva or vesicles, possibly being reactivated at a later time.

5. _____, caused by the papillomavirus, represents one of the most common dermatologic diseases in children.

6. A serious complication from mumps occurring in males over the age of puberty is _____.

MATCHING

Match the terms in Column I with a definition, example, or related statement from Column II. Place the letter corresponding to the answer in the space provided.

Column I

1. ___ Pathogen
2. ___ Prodromal period
3. ___ Chain of infection
4. ___ Reservoir
5. ___ Fomites
6. ___ Herpes labialis
7. ___ Exanthem
8. ___ Illness
9. ___ Interferon
10. ___ Furuncle
11. ___ Vector

Column II

a. A rash on the skin.

b. Organisms that cause disease in children.

c. A time between the beginning of nonspecific symptoms and specific symptoms.

d. The stage during which specific symptoms are evident.

e. The method by which organisms spread and enter a new individual to cause disease.

f. The container or place in which organisms grow and reproduce.

g. Inanimate objects such as soil, food, or water.

h. Living carriers such as insects.

i. A cold sore, representing a type 1 herpesvirus invasion.

j. A lymphokine; prevent cells from being host to more than one virus at a time.

k. An infection of the hair follicle; a boil.

SHORT ANSWER

Supply the missing term or the information requested.

1. Name the five types of microorganisms that can cause disease or illness.

   _____

   _____

2. Identify the most likely outcome once the rabies disease process begins.

   _____

   _____

3. State the incubation period and period of communicability for mumps.

   _____

   _____

4. Discuss the method through which organisms are spread, listing the elements necessary to complete the chain of infection.

   _____

   _____

5. Discuss circumstances that cause a child to be susceptible to infection.

   _____

   _____

6. Describe the universal precautions health care providers should take in all clinical settings.

_____

_____

7. List the signs and symptoms of scarlet fever.

_____

_____

APPLYING YOUR KNOWLEDGE

CASE STUDY

Petro Juan, age 17, is admitted to your unit with infectious mononucleosis. Petro is complaining of tiredness but his parents are encouraging him to be more active to regain his strength.

1. What are some factors that contributed to Petro being a susceptible (at risk) host for infection?

_____

_____

_____

2. What would be your response to Petro's parents regarding their approach to Petro's treatment?

_____

_____

_____

3. What factors should be included in the nutritional plan of care?

_____

_____

_____

CRITICAL INQUIRY EXERCISE

1. If your patient was on infection control precautions and you observed another health care professional entering the patient's room without wearing protective items, what would you do?

2. A patient is admitted to your unit, and you suspect from his history that he has had a recent

exposure to a person with an active case of varicella. Your hospital requires a physician's order before placing a patient on respiratory isolation. What actions would you take?

CRITICAL EXPLORATION

While on a clinical unit, provide care for a child on various types of transmission-based precautions. Compare precautions taken with each patient when emptying urine, providing the bedpan, or collecting and testing a blood specimen.

PRACTICING FOR NCLEX

MULTIPLE-CHOICE QUESTIONS

Circle the letter that corresponds to the best answer for each question.

1. Belinda, age 6, has been diagnosed with infectious mononucleosis. The nurse should do which of the following?

a. Encourage Belinda to return to school and normal physical activity after 10 days.

b. Limit Belinda's fluids to decrease the workload of the spleen.

c. Keep Belinda in bed for a week or more with quiet games and books.

d. Deeply palpate Belinda's upper stomach daily and report any complaints of tenderness.

2. When a child is scratched by a cat, the parents should be instructed to do which of the following?

a. Destroy the animal to prevent subsequent attacks.

b. Submit the animal for a blood test to diagnose cat scratch disease.

c. Monitor the child for irritability and changes in level of consciousness.

d. Place ice on enlarged nodes to control and decrease swelling.

3. To prevent exposure to Lyme disease, an individual should do which of the following?

a. Wear dark-colored clothing to avoid attracting ticks.

b. Inspect the skin of children exposed to wooded areas for tick bites.

c. Apply calamine lotion to tick bite areas immediately to remove poison.

d. If a tick is noted on the skin, remove it quickly using your fingernails.

ALTERNATE FORMAT QUESTIONS

Multiple-Answer Multiple-Choice Questions

Circle the letter(s) corresponding to the appropriate answer(s). Select all that apply.

1. Which of the following interventions would be appropriate for a child with an infectious disorder?

   a. _____ Instruct parents to wash impetigo skin crusts daily with half-strength peroxide.

   b. _____ Explain to parents that the child with pertussis (whooping cough) must be watched closely for airway obstruction.

   c. _____ Inform parents that a temperature of 101°F to 102°F is an expected symptom in children with tetanus.

   d. _____ Instruct parents to monitor children with possible tick bites for signs and symptoms of Rocky Mountain spotted fever.

   e. _____ Instruct parents of school-aged children with head lice that lice infestation can occur regardless of personal hygiene.

   f. _____ Examine a child's oral area to detect the presence of pinworms.

2. After teaching a group of students about the chain of infection, the instructor determines that the teaching was successful when the students identify which of the following as a component?

   a. Reservoir.

   b. Prodromal period.

   c. Means of transmission.

   d. Exit portal.

   e. Exanthem.

   f. Incubation.

3. A nurse is preparing a presentation for a local parent–teacher group on common fungal infections occurring in children. Which of the following would the nurse include?

   a. Lyme disease.

   b. Tinea capitis.

   c. Impetigo.

   d. Candidiasis.

   e. Scabies.

Nursing Care of a Family When a Child has a Hematologic Disorder

CHAPTER OVERVIEW

The disease process of some blood disorders in children may be insidious; presenting symptoms in the early stage of the disease may not alert parents. However, many of these illnesses can become life-threatening. The nurse must be able to synthesize knowledge of findings from systems assessments with the signs and symptoms of hematologic disorders. Chapter 44 provides the student with the knowledge to care for the child and family with a hematologic disorder. The case study addresses the altered hematologic processes in a sickle-cell crisis.

LEARNING OBJECTIVES

After mastering the contents of this chapter, you should be able to do the following:

1. Describe the major hematologic disorders of childhood.

2. Identify National Health Goals related to children with hematologic disorders that nurses could help the nation achieve.

3. Use critical thinking to analyze ways that nursing care for a child with a hematologic disorder could be more family centered.

4. Assess a child with a hematologic disorder.

5. Formulate nursing diagnoses for a child with a hematologic disorder such as sickle-cell anemia.

6. Identify expected outcomes for a child with a hematologic disorder.

7. Plan nursing care for a child with a hematologic disorder.

8. Implement nursing care related to a child with a hematologic disorder, such as reducing the possibility of infection.

9. Evaluate expected outcomes for achievement and effectiveness of care.

10. Identify areas related to care of children with hematologic disorders that could benefit from additional nursing research or application of evidence-based practice.

11. Integrate knowledge of hematologic disorders in children with nursing process to achieve quality maternal and child health nursing care.

KEY TERMS

agranulocytes
allogeneic transplantation
autologous transplantation
blood dyscrasias

erythroblasts
erythrocytes
erythropoietin
granulocytes

hemochromatosis
hemolysis
hemosiderosis
hypodermoclysis
leukocytes
leukopenia
megakaryocytes
normoblasts
pancytopenia
petechiae

plethora
poikilocytic
priapism
purpura
reticulocytes
synergeneic
    transplantation
thrombocytes
thrombocytopenia

MASTERING THE INFORMATION

FILL IN THE BLANKS

Supply the missing term or the information requested.

1. The ultimate therapy for treating acquired aplastic anemia is _____ _____ _____.

2. _____ is excessive destruction of red blood cells.

3. _____ __ _____ _____ is a potentially lethal immunologic response of donor T cells against the tissue of the recipient.

4. _____ are round nonnucleated bodies formed by bone marrow; normal range in count is 150,000 to 300,000 cm.

5. _____ are cells used to transport oxygen to body cells and carry carbon dioxide away from body cells.

MATCHING

Match the terms in Column I with a definition, example, or related statement from Column II. Place the letter corresponding to the answer in the space provided.

Column I

1. ___ Heinz bodies

2. ___ Leukopenia

3. ___ Disseminated intravascular coagulation

4. ___ Plethora

5. ___ Allogeneic transplantation

6. ___ Purpura

7. ___ Normochromic anemia

8. ___ Hypochromic anemia

9. ___ Erythropoietin

10. ___ Poikilocytic

Column II

a. Acquired disorder of blood clotting that results from excessive trauma.

b. Transfer of bone marrow from an immune-compatible donor via intravenous infusion to the recipient.

c. Odd-shaped particles in red blood cells.

d. Impaired production of erythrocytes by the bone marrow or loss of circulatory red blood cells.

e. Marked reddened appearance of the skin.

f. Red blood cells that are irregular in shape.

g. Results from a reduced number of white blood cells.

h. A hormone produced by the kidneys that stimulates the formation of red blood cells.

i. Hemorrhagic rash or small hemorrhages occurring in the superficial layer of the skin.

j. Inadequate hemoglobin synthesis accompanied by a reduction in the diameter of cells when hemoglobin synthesis is inadequate.

APPLYING YOUR KNOWLEDGE

CASE STUDY

Phyllis, age 12, has been experiencing problems from sickle-cell anemia since she was 1-year old. She has been admitted to the pediatric ward of a children's hospital with an admitting diagnosis of sickle-cell crisis.

1. Since Phyllis has previously been diagnosed with sickle-cell anemia, what characteristics would most likely be assessed?

   _____

   _____

   _____

2. What are the primary nursing goals when caring for Phyllis?

   _____

   _____

   _____

3. What precautionary measures would you need to consider when administering intravenous fluids to Phyllis?

_____

_____

_____

4. What findings on the assessment would suggest that Phyllis needs oxygen supplementation?

_____

_____

_____

CRITICAL INQUIRY EXERCISE

1. Develop a nursing care plan that addresses the nursing process to care for the patient with aplastic anemia.

2. Create a list of foods that would be most appropriate for a school-aged child with iron-deficiency anemia.

CRITICAL EXPLORATION

Attend a camp for children with sickle-cell anemia. Assess the program's objectives and goals for camp participants.

PRACTICING FOR NCLEX

MULTIPLE-CHOICE QUESTIONS

Circle the letter that corresponds to the best answer for each question.

1. Which of the following foods supplies the better source of iron for the infant?
   a. Human breast milk.
   b. Iron-fortified cereals.
   c. Vegetables.
   d. Fruit.

2. Which of the following drugs is contraindicated for a child who is diagnosed as deficient in glucose 6-phosphate dehydrogenase (G-6PD)?
   a. Acetylsalicylic acid.
   b. Acetaminophen.
   c. Ampicillin.
   d. Tetracycline.

3. Mrs. Hill brings her 10-month-old son, Keith, to the emergency room with a temperature of 104.6°F. He is dehydrated and has edema of the right ankle. He is admitted to the pediatric unit. The assessment revealed a diagnosis of sickle-cell crisis. The nurse explains to Mrs. Hill that Keith's signs and symptoms are a result of a(n)
   a. pain in the joints of the hands.
   b. amino acid deficiency.
   c. inborn error of metabolism.
   d. stasis of abnormal red blood cells in vessels.

4. Which of the following might the nurse assess in a child experiencing sickle-cell crisis?
   a. Elevated serum sodium and decreased WBCs.
   b. Dry mucous membranes and priaprism.
   c. Loss of appetite and diarrhea.
   d. Hematuria and flank pain.

5. A mother of a 9-month-old child diagnosed with sickle-cell anemia asks why the disorder had not diagnosed earlier. The nurse would integrate an understanding of which of the following when responding to the mother?
   a. The child had increased protection from maternal antibodies.
   b. The liver was immature and not fully functioning.
   c. The child still had fetal hemoglobin present.
   d. Circulatory blood volumes were increases for the first 6 to 8 months.

ALTERNATE FORMAT QUESTIONS
Multiple-Answer Multiple-Choice Questions

Circle the letter(s) corresponding to the appropriate answer(s). Select all that apply.

1. Which of the following would the nurse expect to find in a child with idiopathic thrombocytopenia?
   a. Epistaxis.
   b. Asymmetrical ecchymoses on the legs.
   c. Increased megakaryocytes.
   d. Leukocytosis.
   e. Hemolysis.
   f. More than two petechiae with the tourniquet test.

2. When reviewing the laboratory test results of a child diagnosed with DIC, which of the following would the nurse expect to find?

   a. Thrombocytosis.

   b. Fragmented large platelets on blood smear.

   c. Prolonged prothrombin time.

   d. Significantly low serum fibrinogen levels.

   e. Decreased fibrin split products.

   f. Shortened partial thromboplastin time.

3. After teaching the parents of a 5-year-old child diagnosed with iron deficiency anemia about the disorder and its management, which of the following statements indicates that the parents have understood the instructions?

   a. "Since she doesn't like meat, we'll try to get her to eat some eggs or cheese."

   b. "We will give her the iron with milk to increase its effectiveness."

   c. "She'll need to eat some more green leafy vegetables now that she's taking iron."

   d. "We'll have her play actively before meals so that she is hungry and wants to eat."

   e. "We have an appointment for a blood test in about a week to check her count."

45

Nursing Care of a Family When a Child has a Gastrointestinal Disorder

CHAPTER OVERVIEW

Chapter 45 describes the child with a disorder of the gastrointestinal system. The chapter addresses the importance of the gastrointestinal system to the entire body's ability to grow and develop in a healthy manner. The use of the nursing process to plan and provide care for the child and family coping with a gastrointestinal disorder is explored.

LEARNING OBJECTIVES

After mastering the contents of this chapter, you should be able to do the following:

1. Describe common gastrointestinal disorders seen in children.

2. Identify National Health Goals related to gastrointestinal disorders and children that nurses could help the nation achieve.

3. Analyze ways that nursing care of a child with a gastrointestinal disorder could be more family centered.

4. Assess a child with a gastrointestinal disorder.

5. Formulate nursing diagnoses for a child with a gastrointestinal disorder.

6. Develop expected outcomes for a child with a gastrointestinal disorder.

7. Plan nursing care for a child with a gastrointestinal disorder.

8. Implement nursing care for a child with a gastrointestinal disorder, such as preparing the child for surgery.

9. Evaluate expected outcomes for achievement and effectiveness of care.

10. Identify areas of care related to gastrointestinal disorders and children that could benefit from additional nursing research or application of evidence-based practice.

11. Integrate knowledge of gastrointestinal disorders with nursing process to achieve quality maternal and child health nursing care.

KEY TERMS

beriberi	McBurney's point
celiac disease	Meckel's diverticulum
dehydration	necrotizing
gastroesophageal reflux	enterocolitis
hiatal hernia	nutritional marasmus
inguinal hernia	overhydration
insensible loss	pellagra
intussusception	rickets
irritable bowel syndrome	scurvy
keratomalacia	steatorrhea
kwashiorkor	volvulus
liver transplantation	xerophthalmia

MASTERING THE INFORMATION

FILL IN THE BLANKS

Supply the missing term or the information requested.

1. Metabolic _____ is indicated when the arterial blood pH is less than 7.35 and HCO_3 is below 22 mEq/L.

2. A patient who is dehydrated with an arterial blood pH >7.45 and a bicarbonate level greater than 28 mEq/L is experiencing metabolic _____.

3. Fluid loss that occurs from evaporation from the skin and lungs is called _____ fluid loss.

MATCHING

Match the terms in Column I with a definition, example, or related statement from Column II. Place the letter corresponding to the answer in the space provided.

Column I

1. ____ Gastroesophageal reflux

2. ____ Aganglionic megacolon

3. ____ Hiatal hernia

4. ____ Isotonic dehydration

5. ____ Kwashiorkor

6. ____ Marasmus

7. ____ Celiac disease

8. ____ Hypertonic dehydration

Column II

a. Loss of body water and salt in proportion to each other.

b. Hirschsprung's disease, the absence of nerve cells and peristaltic waves in a section of the bowel.

c. Disorder due to a neuromuscular disturbance that causes a lax cardiac sphincter and lower esophagus.

d. A disease caused by protein deficiency seen more frequently in children ages 1 to 3 years.

e. A disease caused by deficiency of all food groups.

f. Loss of body water out of proportion to salt.

g. Intermittent protrusion of the stomach through the esophageal opening in the diaphragm.

h. Sensitivity or abnormal immunologic response to protein, usually the gluten factor.

SHORT ANSWER

Supply the missing term or the information requested.

1. Describe the "spitting up" associated with infants experiencing gastroesophageal reflux.

_____

_____

2. Identify the most common cause of abdominal surgery in children.

_____

_____

3. Name the most reliable diagnostic test used to confirm peptic ulcer disease.

_____

_____

APPLYING YOUR KNOWLEDGE

CASE STUDY

Aaron is 8 months old. His birth was uneventful and he has exhibited no previous health problems. Today his mother brings him to the emergency room exhibiting symptoms of dehydration.

1. What would be the major sources and minor sources of fluid loss for Aaron?

_____

_____

_____

2. What are the major history and physical assessments you would make for Aaron?

_____

_____

_____

CRITICAL INQUIRY EXERCISE

1. Create a teaching plan for the parents of a child with pyloric stenosis. Include preparation for hospitalization, surgery, and the recovery period.

2. Describe a process for determining if a patient's dehydration is isotonic, hypotonic, or hypertonic.

CRITICAL EXPLORATION

Visit a day-care center. Ask what the rules are regarding care of the child with diarrhea, fever, or vomiting. Observe the staff as they implement the infection control guidelines, and determine if these techniques are sufficient.

PRACTICING FOR NCLEX

MULTIPLE-CHOICE QUESTIONS

Circle the letter that corresponds to the best answer for each question.

1. A mother brings her 12-year-old daughter to the clinic for evaluation of complaints of a gnawing epigastric pain before meals. When questioned further, the child reports that the pain subsides after eating and she has had some episodes of vomiting. Examination reveals epigastric tenderness. The nurse interprets these findings as suggesting which of the following?

    a. Peptic ulcer disease.

    b. Inflammatory bowel disease.

    c. Hepatitis.

    d. Pyloric stenosis.

2. Which of the following laboratory results would lead the nurse to suspect a child is experiencing liver problems?

    a. Bile pigments present in stool specimen.

    b. Decreased serum albumin levels.

    c. Total serum bilirubin level of 1.5 mg/100 mL.

    d. Urine negative for bilirubin.

3. Which of the following nursing interventions might allay any guilt felt by the parents of a child with gastroesophageal reflux?

    a. Suggest the parents step outside the room while you feed the child so they do not view the "spitting up."

    b. Offer suggestions in positioning, since success through this measure builds confidence.

    c. Tell the parents that they were preparing the formula wrong and that this caused the condition.

    d. Reassure parents that this condition is usually due to dysentery and is not their fault.

4. When assessing an infant suspected of having pyloric stenosis, which of the following would the nurse expect to find?

    a. Periodic nonprojective vomiting.

    b. Moist mucous membranes.

    c. Sour-smelling emesis without bile.

    d. Bulging fontanelles.

ALTERNATE FORMAT QUESTIONS

Multiple-Answer Multiple-Choice Questions

Circle the letter(s) corresponding to the appropriate answer(s). Select all that apply.

1. Warren is a 6-month-old infant presenting in the ED with poor intake over last 3 days and severe diarrhea. Which of the following would the nurse expect to assess?

    a. Rapid respirations.

    b. Bulging fontanel.

    c. Dependent edema.

    d. Dry mucous membranes.

    e. Rapid thready pulse.

    f. Poor skin turgor.

2. Which of the following are glands denoted to secrete saliva?

    a. Parotid.

    b. Apocrine.

    c. Pituitary.

    d. Sublinqual.

    e. Submandibular.

3. When discussing the differences between Crohn's disease and ulcerative colitis to a parental support group, which of the following would the nurse include when describing Crohn's disease?

    a. Rectum primarily affected.

    b. Intermittent lesions.

    c. Severe anorexia.

    d. Anal lesions common.

    e. Commonly associated with cancer.

    f. Severe bloody diarrhea.

Nursing Care of a Family When a Child has a Renal or Urinary Tract Disorder

CHAPTER OVERVIEW

Chapter 46 discusses common renal and urinary tract disorders that occur in children and the nursing care needed for these children and their families. The normal function of the renal system is reviewed. The use of the nursing process to plan and provide care for the child and family with a renal or urinary tract disorder is explored.

LEARNING OBJECTIVES

After mastering the contents of this chapter, you should be able to do the following:

1. Describe common renal and urinary disorders that occur in children.

2. Identify National Health Goals related to renal or urinary tract disorders in children that nurses can help the nation achieve.

3. Analyze methods for making nursing care of the child with a renal or urinary disorder more family centered.

4. Assess a child for a renal or urinary tract disorder.

5. Formulate nursing diagnoses related to renal or urinary disorders in children.

6. Establish expected outcomes for a child with a renal or urinary disorder.

7. Plan nursing care related to urinary or renal disorders in children, such as preparing a child for peritoneal dialysis.

8. Implement nursing care for a child with a renal or urinary disorder, such as preparing a child for dialysis.

9. Evaluate expected outcomes for achievement and effectiveness of care.

10. Identify areas related to care of the child with a renal or urinary disorder that would benefit from additional nursing research or application of evidence-based practice.

11. Integrate knowledge of renal and urinary tract disorders with the nursing process to achieve quality maternal and child health nursing care.

KEY TERMS

Alport's syndrome
azotemia
Bowman's capsule
dialysis
enuresis
epispadias
exstrophy of the bladder
glomerular filtration rate
glomerulonephritis

hydronephrosis
hypospadias
nephrosis
patent urachus
polycystic kidney
postural proteinuria
prune belly
   syndrome
vesicoureteral reflux

MASTERING THE INFORMATION

FILL IN THE BLANKS

Supply the missing term or the information requested.

1. Glomerulonephritis involves the obstruction of the glomeruli because of complement fixation activated by an _____-_____ reaction, stimulated most often by a streptococcal infection.

2. The four characteristic symptoms of nephrotic syndrome are _____, _____, _____ , and _____.

3. Children with hemolytic–uremic syndrome usually have _____ skin coloring as well as the major symptoms of _____ with proteinuria, _____, and urinary casts in urine.

4. A _____ kidney is a condition involving abnormal development of the collecting tubules in which fluid-filled cysts, instead of kidney tissue, form in utero; it may be unilateral or bilateral.

5. An increase in blood levels of the products of cell metabolism such as _____ may indicate poor kidney function.

6. _____ refers to a retrograde flow of urine from the bladder into the ureters that may lead to a urinary tract infection.

MATCHING

Match the terms in Column I with a definition, example, or related statement from Column II. Place the letter corresponding to the answer in the space provided.

Column I

1. ___ Prune belly syndrome
2. ___ Azotemia
3. ___ Cystoscopy
4. ___ Cryptorchidism
5. ___ Enuresis
6. ___ Hypospadias
7. ___ Dialysis
8. ___ Acute transplant rejection
9. ___ Alport's syndrome
10. ___ Patent urachus

Column II

a. An autosomal dominant inherited disorder with chronic renal failure.
b. A fistula between the bladder and the umbilicus.
c. The opening of the urethra onto the ventral or lower surface of the penis.
d. Direct viewing of the bladder or ureter openings for examination.
e. Undescended testes often noted with hypospadias.
f. Involuntary voiding past the age when a child is expected to have attained bladder control.
g. Condition manifested by fever, proteinuria, oliguria, weight gain, and hypertension developing within 3 months following transplant.
h. Urethral obstruction in utero from abnormal urethral valves.
i. Separation and removal of solutes from body fluid by diffusion through a semipermeable membrane.
j. The accumulation of nitrogen waste in the bloodstream, often due to oliguria.

SHORT ANSWER

Supply the missing term or the information requested.

1. Explain why girls are at higher risk for urinary tract infections than are boys.

   _____

   _____

2. Compare and contrast the symptoms and treatment for nephrotic syndrome and acute glomerulonephritis.

_____

_____

3. Discuss the primary difference in the etiology of acute and chronic renal failure.

_____

_____

4. Discuss the dietary restriction of salt in a child with chronic renal failure.

_____

_____

APPLYING YOUR KNOWLEDGE

CASE STUDY

Rebecca, age 2, is admitted to your unit with dehydration and acute strep throat. After 3 days of treatment and intravenous fluids, you notice that Rebecca's urine output has remained low and her blood levels of nitrogen and creatinine are elevated.

1. What type of renal failure has Rebecca probably developed? What other symptoms of renal failure might you notice?

_____

_____

_____

2. How would you explain Rebecca's renal condition to her parents?

_____

_____

_____

3. What activity level would you expect to be ordered for Rebecca, and how would you help her maintain it?

_____

_____

_____

CRITICAL INQUIRY EXERCISE

1. Prepare a teaching plan for a child discharged on continuous ambulatory peritoneal dialysis.

2. Your patient, admitted after an automobile accident, has just been diagnosed as being brain dead. What would your response be if the doctor asked you to approach the family regarding donating the patient's kidneys? When and how would you choose to approach the family?

CRITICAL EXPLORATION

Visit a dialysis unit; review three or four charts and note the various causes of renal failure.

PRACTICING FOR NCLEX

MULTIPLE-CHOICE QUESTIONS

Circle the letter that corresponds to the best answer for each question.

1. Which of the following interventions might be most effective in preventing glomerulonephritis?
   a. Daily administration of children's multivitamins and iron.
   b. An increase in all children's fluid intake to 3 L daily.
   c. Prompt evaluation of childhood complaints of sore throat.
   d. Teaching children to void promptly when the urge is felt.

2. Which of the following would the nurse expect to assess in a child with acute glomerulonephritis?
   a. Blood pressure of 90/40.
   b. Hypovolemia and signs of dehydration.
   c. Hematuria and pulmonary edema.
   d. Severe, foul-smelling diarrhea.

3. The nurse could implement which of the following measures for a child who demonstrated enuresis with no apparent organic cause?
   a. Encourage the child to discuss concerns relative to changes in his environment or life.
   b. Instruct the parents never to let the child drink after dinner.

c. Limit the fluids of children with sickle-cell anemia since they are most prone to this condition.

d. Teach parents to strictly enforce bladder training with the child.

4. Bobby, age 10, has a diagnosis of acute nephrotic syndrome. Which of the following nursing interventions would be most appropriate?

a. Administering liberal intravenous and oral fluids to offset the accompanying dehydration.

b. Discussing the cushingoid effects of prescribed steroid therapy with the child and parents.

c. Reassuring the child and parents that diuretics will quickly reduce the edema.

d. Preparing the child and parents for the frequently terminal outcome of the disease.

5. Which of the following would be an appropriate explanation to provide to the parents of a child with severe hypertension who is awaiting a renal transplant?

a. After the child's nonfunctioning kidneys are removed, the child will have no food restrictions.

b. Removal of only one kidney is necessary to provide room for the new kidney.

c. Reluctant younger siblings can still serve as a kidney donor as long as the parent signs both surgery consent forms.

d. The transplanted kidney will be placed in the abdomen, not in the usual kidney space.

ALTERNATE FORMAT QUESTIONS

Multiple-Answer Multiple-Choice Questions

Circle the letter(s) corresponding to the appropriate answer(s). Select all that apply.

1. De'Anya is a nursing student preparing a clinical plan of care for her next day of practice in the hospital. She has been assigned several patients hospitalized with altered functioning of the urinary system. Which of the following would be appropriate to include De'Anya's plan of care for her patients?

a. Instruct the parents of the child with exstrophy of the bladder to give the infant a tub bath daily to remove sediment and maintain good hygiene.

b. Stress the importance repairing hypospadias before the child's maturity to prevent fertility problems.

c. Prepare the parents of the infant with urinary tract infections for diagnostic procedures to rule out urethral stenosis or bladder reflux.

d. Teach girls to wipe from back to front after voiding or stooling.

e. Encourage a child with a urinary tract infection to drink liberal amounts of fluids.

2. When caring for the patient with chronic renal failure undergoing hemodialysis, which of the following would be appropriate?

a. Instruct the parents of the child with chronic renal failure how to prepare a diet low in protein and phosphorus.

b. Administer aluminum hydroxide, alternating with milk, to prevent ulcer formation.

c. Encourage the child receiving corticosteroids to discuss angry feelings regarding their change in appearance.

d. Monitor the child frequently during hemodialysis to detect changes in cerebral tissue perfusion.

e. Encourage the parents to seek out time for themselves and voice frustrations and fears.

3. The mother of a 6-year-old girl diagnosed with a urinary tract infection asks the nurse what she can do to help prevent a recurrence. Which of the following would be important for the nurse to include in the teaching?

a. "Have your daughter wipe from front to back after urinating or moving her bowels."

b. "Buy the child synthetic underwear to decrease perineal irritation."

c. "Make sure that she doesn't use any bubble baths for bathing."

d. "Check to make sure your daughter drinks plenty of fluids especially if it's warm outside."

e. "Encourage her to use the bathroom to urinate every 6 to 8 hours."

f. "Help your daughter to wash her perineal area every day."

CHAPTER 47

Nursing Care of a Family When a Child has a Reproductive Disorder

CHAPTER OVERVIEW

Reproductive disorders in children range from mild infection to serious anatomic malformations. All require prompt treatment to prevent later disruption in sexual or reproductive health. Sensitive and careful questioning when assessing children with reproductive system dysfunction is essential. This chapter addresses the illnesses affecting external reproductive structures and reproductive organs. The case study affords the student the opportunity to plan the nursing care for a male adolescent with concerns about possible alteration in his reproductive system.

LEARNING OBJECTIVES

After mastering the contents of this chapter, you should be able to do the following:

1. Describe common reproductive disorders in children.

2. Identify National Health Goals related to reproductive disorders that nurses can help the nation achieve.

3. Analyze ways that nursing care for a child with a reproductive disorder can be more family centered.

4. Assess a child with a reproductive disorder.

5. Formulate nursing diagnoses for a child with a reproductive illness.

6. Develop expected outcomes for a child with a reproductive disorder.

7. Plan nursing care related to reproductive disorders in children.

8. Implement nursing care for a child with a reproductive disorder, such as teaching about normal menstruation.

9. Evaluate expected outcomes for achievement and effectiveness of care.

10. Identify areas related to the care of children with reproductive disorders that could benefit from additional nursing research or application of evidence-based practice.

11. Integrate knowledge of reproductive disorders in children with the nursing process to achieve quality maternal and child health nursing care.

KEY TERMS

amenorrhea	orchiectomy
anovulatory	orchiopexy
cryptorchidism	pelvic inflammatory
dysmenorrhea	disease (PID)
endometriosis	premenstrual
fibrocystic breast disease	dysphoric disorder
gynecomastia	pseudohermaphrodite
hermaphrodite	sexually transmitted
hydrocele	infection (STI)
menorrhagia	toxic shock syndrome
metrorrhagia	varicocele
mittelschmerz	vulvovaginitis

MASTERING THE INFORMATION

FILL IN THE BLANKS

Supply the missing term or the information requested.

1. A _____ is abnormal dilation of the veins of the spermatic cord.

2. _____ is an enlargement of the male breast.

3. _____ is failure of both testes to descend from the abdominal cavity to the scrotum.

4. Testicular cancer has symptoms of heaviness of the _____. It is _____ and _____ rapidly.

5. _____ is defined as experiencing abdominal pain during ovulation. The discomfort is felt on either side of the _____, near an ovary.

6. _____ is an inflammation of the glands and prepuce of the penis.

MATCHING

Match the terms in Column I with a definition, example, or related statement from Column II. Place the letter corresponding to the answer in the space provided.

Column I

1. ___ Endometriosis

2. ___ Amenorrhea

3. ___ Anovulatory

4. ___ Hydrocele

5. ___ Metrorrhagia

6. ___ Orchiectomy

7. ___ Pseudohermaphrodite

8. ___ Toxic shock syndrome

9. ___ Imperforate hymen

10. ___ Pelvic inflammatory disease

11. ___ Menorrhagia

Column II

a. An abnormally heavy menstrual flow.

b. Removal of the testes.

c. Menstrual cycles that occur without the release of an egg.

d. Infant with some external features of both sexes, although only ovaries or testes are present.

e. Condition most frequently caused by gonorrheal infections or chlamydia.

f. Abnormal growth of extrauterine endometrial cells.

g. An infection caused by toxin-producing strains of staphylococcus.

h. Fluid collection in the space called the processus vaginalis.

i. A membranous ring of tissue totally occluding the vagina.

j. Absence of menstrual flow; may suggest pregnancy.

k. Bleeding between menstrual periods.

APPLYING YOUR KNOWLEDGE

CASE STUDY

Peter, age 14, is seen in your clinic. He states he had sex with a girl who recently told him that she was diagnosed with syphilis. He insists that nobody else know about his visit to the clinic since he can pay for the medicine himself.

1. What symptoms would you question Peter about, and what diagnostic procedures would you prepare him for?

_____

_____

_____

2. What information would you include in your teaching plan for Peter?

_____

_____

_____

3. What obligations would you, as a health care provider, have to keep Peter's condition strictly confidential?

_____

_____

_____

CRITICAL INQUIRY EXERCISE

1. Create a poster board illustrating the female and male reproductive systems. Indicate the reproductive disorders common to both sexes and those specific to one gender or the other.

2. Write a teaching plan addressing the learning needs of a 13-year-old who indicates a desire to become sexually active. What difference, if any, would the gender of the adolescent make in the plan?

CRITICAL EXPLORATION

Arrange with your instructor to visit a health clinic that provides health care for adolescents who are sexually active. Note the health problems presented by the clients and identify the preventive measures provided by the professionals as they teach and counsel these clients.

PREPARING FOR NCLEX

MULTIPLE-CHOICE QUESTIONS

Circle the letter that corresponds to the best answer for each question.

1. Baby J., 1-day-old, is born with ambiguous genitalia. The nurse would incorporate teaching to help the parents as their child undergoes which of the following tests to determine gender?

 a. Blood cultures.

 b. Colposcopy.

 c. Karyotyping.

 d. Sedimentation rate.

2. A young female who has trichomonisis may exhibit which of the following?

 a. Greenish vaginal discharge.

 b. Cream cheese-like vaginal discharge.

 c. Patchy white lesions on vaginal wall.

 d. Frothy white or grayish-green vaginal discharge.

3. Which of the following would the nurse interpret as a symptom of the final stage of syphilis?

 a. Blindness.

 b. Chancre.

 c. Low-grade fever.

 d. Lymphadenopathy.

4. After teaching an adolescent with fibrocystic breast disease about measures to reduce discomfort, the nurse determines that the client needs additional teaching when she states which of the following would be a helpful measure?

 a. Acetaminophen.

 b. Oral contraceptives.

 c. Caffeine.

 d. Danocrine.

5. When talking to a group of adolescents about toxic shock syndrome, the nurse would include damage to which of the following as the most common method by which the organisms enter the body?

 a. Deep buccal tissue.

 b. Vaginal wall tissue.

 c. Urethral meatus.

 d. Nasal mucous membranes.

ALTERNATE FORMAT QUESTIONS
Multiple-Answer Multiple-Choice Questions

Circle the letter(s) corresponding to the appropriate answer(s). Select all that apply.

1. When preparing a teaching plan for a group of adolescents about pelvic inflammatory disease, the nurse would include which anatomical structures as being involved?

 a. Fallopian tubes.

 b. Vagina.

    c. Uterus.

    d. Ovaries.

    e. Ovarian support structures.

2. Which of the following are possible theories about the cause of premenstrual dysphoric disorder?

    a. Drop in progesterone.

    b. Vitamin B complex deficiency.

    c. Decreased ovarian blood supply.

    d. Hyperglycemia.

    e. Low calcium levels.

3. An adolescent is diagnosed with endometriosis. Which of the following would the nurse include as conservative treatment for this condition?

    a. Estrogen only oral contraceptives.

    b. Synthetic androgen.

    c. Gonadotropin-releasing hormone agonist.

    d. Larparotomy for excision.

    e. Intrauterine device.

    f. Prostaglandin inhibitor.

Nursing Care of a Family When a Child has an Endocrine or Metabolic Disorder

CHAPTER OVERVIEW

Chapter 48 reviews the care of the child with an endocrine or metabolic disorder. The chapter addresses the function of each hormone, the result of altered endocrine function, and a plan for nursing intervention. The case study helps the student understand the principles of assessing a child with an endocrine disorder.

LEARNING OBJECTIVES

After mastering the contents of this chapter, you should be able to do the following:

1. Describe the structure and function of the endocrine glands and why metabolic illnesses occur.

2. Identify National Health Goals related to childhood endocrine or metabolic disorders that nurses could help the nation achieve.

3. Analyze ways that care of the child with altered endocrine or metabolic function can be made more family centered.

4. Assess a child with a disorder of endocrine or metabolic function.

5. Formulate nursing diagnoses for a child with altered endocrine or metabolic function.

6. Develop expected outcomes for a child with endocrine or metabolic dysfunction.

7. Plan nursing care for a child with altered endocrine or metabolic function.

8. Implement nursing care, such as teaching medicine administration, to a child with an endocrine or metabolic disorder.

9. Evaluate expected outcomes for achievement and effectiveness of care.

10. Identify areas related to care of children with endocrine or metabolic disorders that could benefit from additional nursing research or application of evidence-based practice.

11. Synthesize knowledge of endocrine and metabolic dysfunctions and the nursing process to ensure quality maternal and child health nursing care.

KEY TERMS

carpal spasm   latent tetany
exophthalmos   manifest tetany
glycosuria   pedal spasm
hormones   polydipsia
hyperglycemia   polyuria
hypoglycemia   sella turcica
hypothalamus   Somogyi
ketoacidosis   phenomenon

MASTERING THE INFORMATION

FILL IN THE BLANKS

Supply the missing term or the information requested.

1. Type 1 (insulin-dependent) diabetes is characterized by almost no _____ secretion. The lack of insulin secretion contributes to a buildup of _____ in the bloodstream. If exogenous insulin is not administered, this person will develop _____ and _____.

2. Humulin-R insulin begins to work approximately _____ minutes after administration.

3. Hypertrophy of the thyroid gland in response to TSH secretion is called _____.

MATCHING

Match the terms in Column I with a definition, example, or related statement from Column II. Place the letter corresponding to the answer in the space provided.

Column I

1. ____ Cushing's syndrome

2. ____ Latent tetany

3. ____ Polydipsia

4. ____ Galactosemia

5. ____ Graves' disease

6. ____ Kussmaul breathing

7. ____ PKU

8. ____ Aldosterone

Column II

a. Excessive thirst.

b. Oversecretion of thyroid hormones.

c. Substance secreted in response to renin-angiotensin.

d. Overproduction of the adrenal hormone cortisol.

e. Deep and rapid respirations.

f. Neuromuscular irritability.

g. Metabolic disease inherited as an autosomal recessive trait.

h. Disorder of carbohydrate metabolism.

SHORT ANSWER

Supply the missing term or the information requested.

1. What is the primary function of the endocrine system?

   _____

   _____

2. For each hormone listed, identify the gland that secretes it.

   a. Thyroxine _____

   b. Somatotropin _____

   c. Insulin _____

   d. Antidiuretic hormone _____

   e. Aldosterone _____

   f. Corticotropin _____

3. State the onset of action and time to peak effect for Humulin N (NPH) insulin.

   _____

   _____

APPLYING YOUR KNOWLEDGE

CASE STUDY

Ashley, age 5, is admitted to the children's hospital after her mom reports to the pediatrician that she has been urinating very frequently and has lost weight. Her mom also reports that she had several incidents of incontinence while playing on the playground. A careful history taken by the nurse revealed that Ashley's appetite had also increased. On admission to the hospital, laboratory studies were ordered. The results revealed a blood glucose level of 400 mg/dL. Ashley's mother states, "I should have never let her eat all those sweets."

1. Based on the mother's comment, what teaching would the nurse need to do?

_____

_____

_____

2. What measures can be taken to lessen the discomfort for the diabetic child when frequent blood samples are needed?

_____

_____

_____

CRITICAL INQUIRY EXERCISE

1. Create a blood glucose monitoring flow sheet. Be sure to include the date, blood glucose before each meal and bedtime, insulin dosage (both regular and NPH taken daily), and an explanation column where the patient can identify the reason for fluctuation in blood glucose.

2. Role-play what it is like to check your blood glucose four times a day and record the amounts on your monitoring sheet. On the next day, change the numbers to indicate hyperglycemia all day. Indicate what may have contributed to the problem.

CRITICAL EXPLORATION

1. Attend a diabetes camp and offer to be a counselor in one of the cabins. Be sure to tell the camp director that diabetes is new to you and that you will need guidance.

2. Attend a meeting of the American Association of Diabetes Educators. Ask one of the certified diabetes educators about his or her job. How was certification obtained? Visit a diabetes education program that has been nationally recognized by the American Diabetes Association Advisory Council. Observe patient instructions and follow-up visits.

PRACTICING FOR NCLEX

MULTIPLE-CHOICE QUESTIONS

Circle the letter that corresponds to the best answer for each question.

1. The nurse explains the purpose of insulin to a child who is a newly diagnosed diabetic and her parents, stating that it causes the blood glucose to
   a. increase.
   b. decrease.
   c. remain the same throughout.
   d. increase, then decrease.

2. The nurse checks a child's glucose level before bedtime and finds it to be 50 mg/dL. The nurse would assess Shajun for which of the following?
   a. Thirst.
   b. Flushing.
   c. Dehydration.
   d. Sweating.

3. A child is to begin using an insulin pump. The nurse instructs the child's parent to test the child for hypoglycemia at 2 AM based on the understanding that a drop in blood glucose at this time may be related too little
   a. food.
   b. exercise.
   c. fluid.
   d. sodium.

4. A child who receives a split dose of regular and NPH insulin twice a day is planning to play soccer at 3:00 in the afternoon. It would be best to
   a. take no insulin that morning.
   b. decrease regular insulin dosage in the morning.
   c. decrease NPH insulin dosage in the morning.
   d. increase the NPH insulin dosage in the morning.

5. After teaching a newly diagnosed diabetic child and her parents about causes of hypoglycemia, the nurse determines that the teaching was effective when they state which of the following as a cause?

    a. Missing an insulin injection.

    b. Missing a meal or a snack.

    c. Too small an insulin dosage.

    d. Too large a meal or snack.

ALTERNATE FORMAT QUESTIONS

Multiple-Answer Multiple-Choice Questions

Circle the letter(s) corresponding to the appropriate answer(s). Select all that apply.

1. Which of the following reflects accurate information about endocrine disease processes.

    a. Growth hormone deficiency is a pituitary disorder.

    b. Hashimotos's disease interferes with thyroid gland function.

    c. Cushing syndrome is an underproduction of cortisol by the adrenal gland.

    d. The most frequent occurring pancreatic disorder in children in type 2 diabetes.

    e. Dysfunction of the parathyroid gland can cause calcium imbalances.

2. Diabetes Insipidus is a disease described as involving which of the following?

    a. An excessive release of the antidiuretic hormone (ADH).

    b. Trauma to the pituitary gland as a possible cause.

    c. Polydispsia.

    d. High urine specific gravity (1.001 to 1.005).

    e. Polyuria.

3. A nurse is preparing a presentation for a group of middle school students about the endocrine system, glands, and associated hormones. The nurse would include which of the following hormones as being secreted by the pituitary gland?

    a. Growth hormone.

    b. Corticotropin.

    c. Antidiuretic hormone.

    d. Insulin.

    e. Cortisol.

    f. Aldosterone.

49

Nursing Care of a Family When a Child has a Neurologic Disorder

CHAPTER OVERVIEW

Chapter 49 discusses the care of the child with a neurologic disorder. The physiologic and psychological impact of common neurologic conditions on children at various stages of growth and development is discussed. The use of the nursing process to plan and provide care for the child with a neurologic disorder and his or her family is explored. The case study explores the nursing care of the child with a potentially life-threatening neurologic infection.

LEARNING OBJECTIVES

After mastering the contents of this chapter, you should be able to do the following:

1. Describe common neurologic disorders in children.

2. Identify National Health Goals related to neurologic disorders and children that nurses could help the nation achieve.

3. Analyze ways in which care of a child with a neurologic disorder can be optimally family centered.

4. Assess a child with a neurologic disorder.

5. Formulate nursing diagnoses for a child with a neurologic disorder.

6. Establish expected outcomes for a child with a neurologic disorder.

7. Plan nursing care for a child with a neurologic disorder.

8. Implement nursing care, such as monitoring medicine effectiveness, for a child with a neurologic disorder.

9. Evaluate expected outcomes for achievement and effectiveness of care.

10. Identify areas related to care of children with neurologic disorders that could benefit from additional nursing research or application of evidence-based practice.

11. Integrate knowledge of neurologic disorders and the nursing process to achieve quality maternal and child health nursing care.

KEY TERMS

astereognosis	graphesthesia
automatisms	hemiplegia
autonomic dysreflexia	infantile spasms
choreoathetosis	kinesthesia
choreoid	paraplegia
decerebrate posturing	pulse pressure
decorticate posturing	quadriplegia
diplegia	status epilepticus
dyskinetic	stereognosis

MASTERING THE INFORMATION

FILL IN THE BLANKS

Supply the missing term or the information provided.

1. The nervous system consists of two separate systems, the _____ and the _____ nervous systems.

2. Tests for cerebellar function involve testing for normal _____ and _____.

3. Signs of _____, in which a child is unsure of time and place, may be the first indication of increased intracranial pressure.

4. Cerebral perfusion pressure is calculated by subtracting the mean intracranial pressure from the mean _____ pressure.

5. The major cause of meningitis in newborns is the group B hemolytic _____ organism.

6. The treatment for infant botulism consists of _____ _____.

7. Convulsions associated with high fever are most common in _____-aged children.

8. Indicate if the following actions test sensory, motor, or cerebellar function.

   a. Asking a child to touch each finger on one hand with the thumb of that hand in rapid succession. _____

   b. Asking a child to resist your action as you push down or up on his or her hands.
   _____

   c. Touching the child's elbow with a vibrating tuning fork. _____

9. Identify the seizure described below as psychomotor, absence, tonic–clonic, or simple partial.

   a. Generalized seizures with a prodromal, aural, tonic, and clonic stages.
   _____

   b. Involves only one area of the brain; no altered level of consciousness.
   _____

   c. May begin with a sudden change in posture, circumoral pallor, a 5-minute loss of consciousness without a postictal stage.
   _____

   d. "Petit mal," generalized seizures involving a staring spell lasting for a few seconds.
   _____

MATCHING

Match the terms in Column I with a definition, example, or related statement from Column II. Place the letter corresponding to the answer in the space provided.

Column I

1. ___ Electroencephalogram

2. ___ Graphesthesia

3. ___ Kinesthesia

4. ___ Ataxic

5. ___ Neurofibromatosis

6. ___ Diplegia

7. ___ Stereognosis

8. ___ Decorticate posture

9. ___ Decerebrate posture

10. ___ Myelography

Column II

a. Awkward wide-base gait.

b. Subcutaneous tumors along nerve pathways, with excessive skin pigmentation and possible optic or acoustic nerve degeneration.

c. The ability to recognize a shape that has been traced on the skin.

d. Depiction of electrical patterns of the brain.

e. The ability to distinguish movement.

f. Child's arms are abducted and flexed on the chest with wrists flexed.

g. Spastic cerebral palsy involvement affecting primarily the lower extremities.

h. The ability to recognize an object by touch.

i. Indication of nonfunctional midbrain with rigid extension and adduction of arms and wrist pronation.

j. Radiographic study of spinal cord involving the use of a contrast medium.

APPLYING YOUR KNOWLEDGE

CASE STUDY

Mrs. Vereen has brought Shawn to the emergency room with an elevated temperature. Shawn is 4 years old and has had a cold for several days. Shawn's temperature on assessment was 104°F orally. He began to have a seizure during admission and was immediately taken to the treatment room. After some initial testing, he was diagnosed with H. influenzae meningitis.

1. How was the diagnosis confirmed?

_____

_____

_____

2. What treatments would the nurse expect to administer? What might occur if this condition is left untreated?

_____

_____

_____

3. Should there be a concern for siblings and family members of the child with bacterial meningitis?

_____

_____

_____

CRITICAL INQUIRY EXERCISE

1. Develop an abbreviated assessment for a soccer coach to assess an injured child with a mobility problem. Include advice the coach must give the persons who may want to assist him or her before professional help arrives.

2. Prepare a teaching plan stressing the importance of health care to prevent accidents; customize this plan to teach a parent group in a day-care setting. Include the National Health Goals as they relate to upper respiratory infections, the relationship of a disease and age frequency, and bike riding on streets.

CRITICAL EXPLORATION

1. While on a pediatric clinical unit, perform a neurologic assessment on a client with no known neurologic conditions and on a client with a neurologic condition affecting neuromuscular or cerebral function. Note the differences in findings.

2. Observe the room of a client who has a history of seizures, or areas in which

precautions should be taken, and note the seizure precautions taken for that client's safety.

PRACTICING FOR NCLEX

MULTIPLE-CHOICE QUESTIONS

Circle the letter that corresponds to the best answer for each question.

1. Melle, age 7, is admitted to your unit after an automobile accident. You would suspect increased intracranial pressure if your assessment revealed which of the following?

   a. Bradycardia.

   b. Decreased pulse pressure.

   c. Hypotensive blood pressure.

   d. Tachypnea.

2. A doll's eye reflex

   a. can be used to assess a comatose child who cannot respond to a light.

   b. indicates increased intracranial pressure if present.

   c. results when a child turns his or her eyes to the left as his or her head is turned to the left rapidly.

   d. represents an abnormal neurologic finding.

3. Billy, age 2, has been diagnosed with cerebral palsy. The nurse should explain which of the following to Billy's parents?

   a. Cerebral palsy involves a progressive nerve degeneration.

   b. Contractures are unavoidable since ambulation is impossible.

   c. The brain damage that occurred at birth can be repaired with surgery when the child is older.

   d. Two children with cerebral palsy may exhibit totally different symptoms and abilities.

4. A child with Guillain-Barré syndrome will require which of the following nursing interventions?

   a. Feeding the child orally to maintain the muscles of mastication.

b. Explaining to parents that steroids will be effective in halting the paralysis.

c. Immobilizing extremities to decrease stimulation of muscle spasm.

d. Inserting an indwelling catheter into the bladder to monitor urine output.

5. To decrease the incidence of spinal cord injury in children and adolescents, the nurse should do which of the following?

   a. Caution children and adolescents against diving into shallow water.

   b. Encourage the intake of vitamins A and C to minimize spinal cord injury.

   c. Instruct adolescents to ride motorcycles instead of driving cars.

   d. Teach back exercises to children to strengthen their weak vertebrae.

6. A child with a cervical spinal injury should be watched very carefully for which of the following?

   a. Hypoactive bowel sounds during the second recovery phase.

   b. Hyperreflexia of the bladder during the first recovery phase.

   c. Profuse diaphoresis during the second recovery phase.

   d. Respiratory distress during the first recovery phase.

7. Which of the following would lead the nurse to suspect that a child with a spinal cord injury is developing autonomic dysreflexia?

   a. Bradycardia and flushed face.

   b. Headache and hypertension.

   c. Hypotension and pallor.

   d. Pale skin and dizziness.

8. Which of the following is true about the third phase of spinal cord recovery?

   a. Autonomic dysreflexia is a common occurrence.

   b. Spasticity of muscles and reflexes is noted.

   c. Flaccid paralysis of the diaphragm and skeletal muscles is present.

   d. Permanent limitation of motor and sensory function can be assessed.

9. Benje, age 7, is admitted to the emergency room with suspected spinal cord injury after an automobile accident. Which of the following nursing interventions would be appropriate?

   a. Move the child from the admission stretcher to a firm-examining table on admission.

   b. Hyperextend the head if respiratory resuscitation is necessary.

   c. Remove any hard head coverings and replace with a support neck brace.

   d. Maintain spinal immobilization during neurologic assessments.

10. Nursing care of the child who has suffered a spinal cord injury may include which of the following interventions?

    a. Pushing carbonated beverages during the first phase of recovery to acidify urine.

    b. Using Credé's maneuver to establish a defecation pattern.

    c. Helping the child and family adjust to permanent mobility loss during the first recovery phase.

    d. Supporting the child and family during the grieving process after the second recovery phase.

ALTERNATE FORMAT QUESTIONS

Multiple-Answer Multiple-Choice Questions

Circle the letter(s) that corresponds to the best answer(s) for each question. Select all that apply.

1. Which of the following would the nurse expect to assess in a child with migraine headaches?

   a. Bilateral pain under both eyes.

   b. Pain aggravated by routine activity.

   c. Family history of migraine headaches.

   d. Report of blurred vision prior to headache.

   e. Relief commonly obtained with acetaminophen.

2. Which of the following agents would a nurse expect could be prescribed for a child with tonic–clonic seizures?

   a. Phenobarbital.

   b. Valproic acid.

   c. Phenytoin.

   d. Dexamethasone.

   e. Carbamazepine.

3. Which of the following would indicate to the nurse that a child has increased intracranial pressure?

   a. Dilated pupil.

   b. Hypertension.

   c. Tachycardia.

   d. Tachypnea.

   e. Oriented to time.

   f. Decreased deep tendon reflexes.

50

Nursing Care of a Family When a Child has a Vision or Hearing Disorder

CHAPTER OVERVIEW

Chapter 50 discusses the eyes and ears as essential sensory organs. Disorders involving these organs in childhood may retard normal growth and development and, if untreated, may lead to long-term illness. This chapter addresses the structure of the eyes and ears, the physiology of vision and hearing, and common vision and hearing disorders, as well as the nurse's role in health promotion and management of vision and hearing disorders.

LEARNING OBJECTIVES

After mastering the contents of this chapter, you should be able to do the following:

1. Describe the structure and function of the eyes and ears and disorders of these organs as they affect children.

2. Identify National Health Goals related to vision and hearing disorders of children that nurses could help the nation achieve.

3. Use critical thinking to analyze ways that nursing care of children with a disorder of vision or hearing could be more family centered.

4. Assess a child who has a disorder of vision or hearing.

5. Formulate nursing diagnoses related to a child with a disorder of vision or hearing.

6. Establish expected outcomes for a child with a disorder of vision or hearing.

7. Plan nursing interventions for a child with a disorder of vision or hearing.

8. Implement nursing care to meet the specific needs of a child who has a disorder of the eyes or ears, such as educating parents about the symptoms of otitis media.

9. Evaluate expected outcomes for achievement and effectiveness of care.

10. Identify areas related to care of children with vision or hearing disorders that could benefit from additional nursing research or application of evidence-based practice.

11. Integrate knowledge of childhood disorders of the eyes or ears with the nursing process to achieve quality maternal and child health nursing care.

KEY TERMS

accommodation	myopia
amblyopia	nystagmus
astigmatism	orthoptics
diplopia	photophobia

enucleation
fovea centralis
goniotomy
hyperopia
light refraction

ptosis
stereopsis
strabismus
tympanocentesis

g. Chief function of cleaning the external ear.

h. Constriction of the pupil as it adjusts from focusing on a distant point to a near point.

i. Low-grade granulation tissue tumor of the meibomian or tarsal gland on the eyelid.

j. Reduction in vision due to disuse of a structurally normal eye; "lazy eye."

MASTERING THE INFORMATION

FILL IN THE BLANKS

Supply the missing term or the information requested.

1. _____ is the ability to locate an object in space relative to other objects.

2. Eye exercises are referred to as _____.

3. _____ is a refractive error (farsightedness) in which vision is blurry at close range.

4. _____ is a congenital incomplete closure of the facial cleft.

MATCHING

Match the terms in Column I with a definition, example, or related statement from Column II. Place the letter corresponding to the answer in the space provided.

Column I

1. ___ Accommodation

2. ___ Chalazion

3. ___ Dacryostenosis

4. ___ Cerumen

5. ___ Ptosis

6. ___ Blepharitis marginalia

7. ___ Amblyopia

8. ___ Nystagmus

9. ___ Convergence

10. ___ Dacryocystitis

Column II

a. Turning of both eyes medially.

b. Infection of the eyelid margin.

c. Inflammation of the nasolacrimal duct.

d. Rapid, irregular eye movements.

e. The inability to raise the upper eyelid normally.

f. Interruption of the tear flow; blockage of the lacrimal drainage system.

APPLYING YOUR KNOWLEDGE

CASE STUDY

Ms. Jones's foster daughter Sally, age 6, was admitted to the hospital for surgery on the left eye. The presurgical diagnosis was a cataract of the left eye. The history and physical examination revealed that Sally's mother is a teenager and Sally has been in foster care since age 2. There was no medical history, and the laboratory and examination report stated that the lens of the left eye was opaque at the edges.

1. What might the nurse suspect as the etiology of the cataract?

_____

_____

_____

2. Postoperatively, Sally complains of thirst; the postoperative orders read, "may have fluids when fully awake." When would the nurse allow Sally to have fluids, and why?

_____

_____

_____

3. When teaching Ms. Jones postoperative care, what preventive measures would you want to address?

_____

_____

_____

CRITICAL INQUIRY EXERCISE

1. Prepare an interaction program for a school-aged child who is hospitalized for a scheduled eye surgery. Focus on anticipatory guidance, before and after surgery. Incorporate measures to reduce anxiety, promote independence, and use parental participation.

2. Prepare a list of key points for parents to remember when interacting with their school-aged child in the hospital environment.

CRITICAL EXPLORATION

1. Make an appointment to visit the local support chapter for citizens who are deaf. Identify the support groups organized in cooperation with this agency. Note the teaching materials and classes made available to support the parents of the child with a hearing disability.

2. Visit a health clinic and participate in the hearing and vision screening for children entering school. Observe the steps taken when a child is found to have a vision or hearing problem.

PRACTICING FOR NCLEX

MULTIPLE-CHOICE QUESTIONS

Circle the letter that corresponds to the best answer for each question.

1. The nurse should expect which of the following findings when assessing a child with acute otitis media?
   a. Excessive cerumen in the outer ear.
   b. Recent respiratory tract infection.
   c. Increased mobility on the pneumatic examination.
   d. Copious amount of tenacious fluid.

2. The primary cause of visual impairment in children is
   a. ocular trauma.
   b. exposure to elevated oxygen levels during infancy.
   c. congenital malformations.
   d. eye infection.

3. To visualize the inner surface of a child's lower eyelid and most of the bottom globe, the nurse would
   a. pull the top eyelid outward and up.
   b. invert the top eyelid with a special apparatus.

   c. press on the lower lid with a finger tip.
   d. use a cotton tipped applicator to flip the lower lid.

4. If the ciliary body of the eye is involved with a penetration injury, sympathetic iritis may occur. This is described as
   a. a hemorrhagic paralysis.
   b. inflammation of the opposite eye.
   c. a global contusion.
   d. an infectious process of the globe.

5. The nurse would suspect which of the following if a child is scheduled for tonometry?
   a. Cataracts.
   b. Diplopia.
   c. Retinal detachment.
   d. Glaucoma.

6. A child is to undergo a goniotomy procedure to provide an opening to the canal of Schlemm. Preoperatively, which of these drugs would the nurse expect to administer to this child?
   a. Ampicillin (Amoxil).
   b. Cefazolin (Ancef).
   c. Acetazolamide (Diamox).
   d. Atropine.

7. Which of the following conditions is likely to occur as a sequela to untreated cataracts in infants?
   a. Amblyopia.
   b. Dacryostenosis.
   c. Astigmatism.
   d. Keratitis.

8. Which of the following would be important for the nurse to include in the plan of care for a child who is being prepared to undergo eye surgery?
   a. Showing the child a doll with patches over both eyes.
   b. Restraining the child at the wrist bilaterally for 24 hours.
   c. Avoiding discussion of the impending surgery.
   d. Introducing the child to other children on the unit.

ALTERNATE FORMAT QUESTIONS

Multiple-Answer Multiple-Choice Questions

Circle the letter(s) corresponding to the appropriate answer(s). Select all that apply.

1. Which of the following statements about ear disorders is accurate.

   a. _____ In the assessment of swimmer's ear, Pseudomonas and Candida are often found to be agents involved in the infection.

   b. _____ An internal ear canal altered by a fungal disease may appear brown or black.

   c. _____ There is a higher incidence of otitis media in infants who are breastfed than in those who are formula-fed.

   d. _____ A myringotomy is a surgical procedure used to drain purulent fluids from an infected middle ear.

   e. _____ The inner ear canal should be cleaned regularly with a cotton-tip swab to prevent the accumulation of drainage and cerumen.

2. Which of the following would a nurse suspect as a possible cause of conductive hearing loss?

   a. Impacted cerumen.

   b. Immobile tympanic membrane.

   c. Drug therapy.

   d. Meningitis.

   e. Serous otitis media.

3. The nurse is providing anticipatory guidance about preventing hearing loss to parents of a young child. Which of the following would the nurse include?

   a. "Try to avoid exposing the child to loud noises, like the television or radio."

   b. "Clean the child's ears daily with a cotton swab."

   c. "Get the child treated quickly if he develops a sore throat and fever."

   d. "Make sure that the child's immunizations are kept up-to-date."

   e. "Instill full strength hydrogen peroxide at least weekly into the ear canal."

Nursing Care of a Family When a Child has a Musculoskeletal Disorder

CHAPTER OVERVIEW

Chapter 51 discusses the common musculoskeletal disorders experienced in childhood and the potential effects of these disorders on the child's growth and development. The use of the nursing process to plan and provide age-appropriate nursing care addressing the physiologic and psychological needs of the child with musculoskeletal disorders and of family members is explored.

LEARNING OBJECTIVES

After mastering the contents of this chapter, you should be able to do the following:

1. Describe common musculoskeletal disorders in children.

2. Identify National Health Goals related to musculoskeletal disorders and children that nurses can help the nation achieve.

3. Use critical thinking to analyze ways that care of a child with a musculoskeletal disorder can be more family centered.

4. Assess a child with a musculoskeletal disorder.

5. Formulate nursing diagnoses related to a child with a musculoskeletal disorder.

6. Establish expected outcomes for a child with a musculoskeletal disorder.

7. Plan nursing care for a child with a musculoskeletal disorder.

8. Implement nursing care, such as supplying age-appropriate diversional activities, for a child with a musculoskeletal disorder.

9. Evaluate expected outcomes for achievement and effectiveness of care.

10. Identify areas related to care of a child with a musculoskeletal disorder that could benefit from additional nursing research or application of evidence-based practice.

11. Integrate knowledge of musculoskeletal disorders with nursing process to achieve quality maternal and child health nursing care.

KEY TERMS

apposition	metaphysis
arthroscopy	myopathy
cartilage	periosteum
compartment syndrome	remodeling
diaphysis	resorption
distraction	sequestrum
epiphyseal plate	sprain
epiphysis	strain
fracture	traction
malleoli	

MASTERING THE INFORMATION

FILL IN THE BLANKS

Supply the missing term or the information requested.

1. A bone injury occurring at the _____ _____ of the long bone may result in irregular or abnormal bone length, and injury to the _____ or the bone may result in irregular bone width.

2. Proper fitting of crutches requires a space of ___ to ____ inches between the axilla crutch pad and the child's axilla and elbow flexion of about ____ degrees.

3. Osgood–Schlatter disease is a _____ and _____ of the tibial tuberosity occurring in children who are athletic and at the _____ or _____ stage of development.

4. Apophysitis occurs most commonly in _____ who are growing rapidly. Pain produced by this condition can be treated by adding a _____ to the shoe heel to reduce tension on the heel cord.

5. During the periods of acute inflammation in juvenile arthritis, joints should be _____, but children may do _____ exercise.

6. A _____ is a muscle-tendon injury; a _____ is a ligament injury.

MATCHING

Match the terms in Column I with a definition, example, or related statement from Column II.

Place the letter corresponding to the answer in the space provided.

Column I

1. ____ Apposition
2. ____ Diaphysis
3. ____ Epiphyseal plate
4. ____ Genu varum
5. ____ Metaphysis
6. ____ Metatarsus adductus
7. ____ Myopathy
8. ____ Osteogenesis imperfecta
9. ____ Skeletal traction
10. ____ Striated muscle
11. ____ Smooth muscle
12. ____ Periosteum

Column II

a. Acquired or inherited disease of the muscular system.
b. The type of muscle responsible for gastrointestinal peristalsis.
c. The predominant type of muscle in the body.
d. The cartilage segment at which increase in long bone length occurs.
e. The thin area between the long bone shaft and the rounded end of the bone.
f. The long central shaft of the long bone.
g. Evident when there is over an inch between the medial surfaces of the knees when standing with the malleoli of the ankles touching.
h. The passing of a pin or wire through the skin into the end of the long bone to immobilize a fracture.
i. Outer sensitive layer of the bone.
j. The amount of end-to-end contact of the bone fragments.
k. Connective tissue disorder characterized by the formation of brittle bones.
l. Turning in of the forefoot; can be corrected with stretching exercises.

SHORT ANSWER

Supply the missing term or the information requested.

1. Discuss why a child with a condition requiring a leg brace might have a nursing diagnosis of "Disturbed body image."

   _____

   _____

2. What nursing measures could be taken to help a school-aged child on complete bed rest with traction meet his developmental tasks?

   _____

   _____

3. Discuss two measures for managing itching underneath a cast and two measures that should not be used.

   _____

   _____

4. Discuss three exercises used to strengthen the foot arches of a child with flat feet.

   _____

   _____

5. Compare and contrast the causes of and the treatment for structural and functional scoliosis.

   _____

   _____

6. Describe the following types of braces and traction and the appropriate use of each: Milwaukee brace, Halo traction, Bryant's traction, Buck's traction, and Skeletal traction.

   _____

   _____

APPLYING YOUR KNOWLEDGE

CASE STUDY

Evelyn Demark, 10 years old, has osteogenesis imperfecta and is admitted to your unit with a fracture of the right forearm due to an injury in gymnastics class.

1. What would you need to discuss during your teaching session with Evelyn and her parents related to activity choices?

   _____

   _____

   _____

2. How would Evelyn's plan of care differ if she did not have osteogenesis imperfecta?

   _____

   _____

   _____

CRITICAL INQUIRY EXERCISE

1. Write a care plan for a school-aged child hospitalized with bilateral leg traction after an accident. Include age-appropriate activities.

2. What safety and development issues would you include in a teaching plan for a 7-month-old child with a broken femur due to a fall down the stairs at home?

CRITICAL EXPLORATION

Walk through your home and the home of a friend. Note any circumstances that could represent a danger to a child.

PRACTICING FOR NCLEX

MULTIPLE-CHOICE QUESTIONS

Circle the letter that corresponds to the best answer for each question.

1. Benji, age 11, has been diagnosed with osteomyelitis after a right leg injury 2 months ago. He and his parents were told that he must be admitted to the hospital for treatment. The nurse should explain which of the following to Benji and his parents?

   a. Benji will need to ambulate immediately after surgery, although it may be uncomfortable.

   b. Blood will be drawn for culture to determine the specific medication for treatment of the infection.

c. Infection control measures are necessary to prevent the spread of this condition to the entire family.

d. The antibiotic therapy Benji will need must be administered intravenously and will be complete before discharge.

2. Amy, 3 years old, has been diagnosed with osteogenesis imperfecta. When planning her care, the nurse should consider which of the following?

a. Active range-of-motion and weight-lifting exercises will be necessary to strengthen weak long bone shafts.

b. Amy's parents should be encouraged to facilitate her development by not restricting her activities.

c. Genetic counseling will be appropriate if Amy's condition is congenital or late occurring.

d. The treatment for this condition requires lifelong oral intake of calcium supplements.

3. When teaching Sheila, 13 years old, to walk with crutches, the nurse should instruct her to

a. move one crutch forward at a time when using a three-point swing-through gait.

b. rest the crutch pad on the upper arm to bear her weight on the axilla crutch pad.

c. carry books and other items in a backpack to keep her hands free.

d. use a two-point gait when no weight bearing is allowed.

4. Marla, age 12, has a cast on her left leg. During a follow-up phone call, Marla states she is experiencing occasional numbness in her left foot and the foot feels cool. The nurse should respond in which of the following ways?

a. Explain to Marla that she needs to wiggle her toes frequently to prevent the return of the numbness and coolness.

b. Inform Marla and her mother of the need to elevate the extremity to promote good circulation.

c. Instruct Marla and her mother to return to the doctor for possible removal of the cast.

d. Teach Marla isometric exercises to use when numbness and coolness occur.

5. The nurse would determine that the plan of care for a child with juvenile arthritis had been effective if which of the following findings was noted?

a. The parents state the need to avoid aspirin administration to prevent Reye's syndrome.

b. Eighty percent of meals are eaten when offered after periods of rest and administration of pain medication.

c. Splints are applied during the day and removed at night by parents to promote sleep.

d. Ice baths are applied to the affected joints by parents twice daily.

6. A plan of care for a girl suspected of having myasthenia gravis may include which of the following?

a. Administering cholinergic drugs to suppress the hyperactivity actions of acetylcholine.

b. Inquiring if the child has had difficulty in school recently due to difficulty in reading or in seeing the board.

c. Reassuring the adolescent female that myasthenia gravis will not affect her childbearing potential.

d. Scheduling medications after mealtime to decrease gastrointestinal symptoms, choking, and possible aspiration.

7. Congenital muscular dystrophy differs from Duchenne's disease and facioscapulohumeral muscular dystrophy in which of the following ways?

a. Congenital muscular dystrophy results in degeneration of muscle fibers.

b. Congenital muscular dystrophy can result in problems with parental bonding.

c. In facioscapulohumeral muscular dystrophy, the predominant symptom is facial weakness.

d. Victims of Duchenne's disease experience periods of exacerbation and remission.

ALTERNATE FORMAT QUESTIONS

Multiple-Answer Multiple-Choice Questions

Circle the letter(s) corresponding to the appropriate answer(s). Select all that apply.

1. A child has had spinal instrumentation for treatment of scoliosis. Which of the following nursing interventions would be appropriate?

   a. _____ Maintain the head of the bed at a 45° elevation.

   b. _____ Logroll the child to a side-lying position every 2 hours unless Luque or segmented rods are used.

   c. _____ Monitor the neurologic and vascular functions of the extremities every hour for the first 24 hours.

   d. _____ Explain the need to keep the child NPO until bowel sounds are audible.

   e. _____ Instruct the parents not to touch the child during the early postoperative period.

   f. _____ Explain to parents that even severe scoliosis can be completely corrected with surgery.

2. A child is diagnosed with polyarticular arthritis. When assessing this child, which of the following would the nurse expect to find?

   a. High spiking fever.

   b. Nodules on pressure sensitive body areas.

   c. Affected finger and hand joints.

   d. Iridocyclitis.

   e. Enlarged lymph nodes.

3. After teaching the parents of an 11-year-old girl with myasthenia gravis about the disorder and treatment with neostigmine, which of the following statements indicates successful teaching?

   a. "We need to notify her health care provider if her weakness suddenly increases."

   b. "We should give the drug with food or milk so her stomach doesn't get upset."

   c. "Exposing her to stress will actually help her muscles from becoming weak."

   d. "We can expect her muscle weakness to become progressively worse as time goes on."

   e. "We will talk to her school to see if we can get her a modified schedule to allow her to rest."

Nursing Care of a Family When a Child has an Unintentional Injury

CHAPTER OVERVIEW

Accidents are a major cause of childhood morbidity and mortality, and prevention is a goal that nurses and other health care providers always strive for. However, not all accidents can be prevented. Chapter 52 describes the principles of nursing care for the child with an unintentional injury. The uses of the nursing process to assess, plan, and provide appropriate nursing care and to address the physiologic and psychological needs of the child and family involved with an unintentional injury are discussed.

LEARNING OBJECTIVES

After mastering the contents of this chapter, you should be able to do the following:

1. Describe the causes and consequences of common accidents and injuries in childhood and measures to prevent them.

2. Identify National Health Goals related to children who have experienced trauma that nurses can help the nation achieve.

3. Use critical thinking to analyze ways that care of children with unintentional injuries can be more family centered.

4. Assess a child who is unintentionally injured from an accident.

5. Formulate nursing diagnoses related to an unintentionally injured child.

6. Establish expected outcomes for an unintentionally injured child.

7. Plan nursing care related to an unintentionally injured child.

8. Implement nursing care for a child with an unintentional injury, such as providing pain relief.

9. Evaluate expected outcomes for achievement and effectiveness of nursing care.

10. Identify areas related to care of children with unintentional injuries that could benefit from additional nursing research or application of evidence-based practice.

11. Integrate knowledge of unintentional injuries in childhood with nursing process to achieve quality maternal and child health care.

KEY TERMS

allografting	homografting
autografting	near drowning
contrecoup injury	otorrhea
debridement	plumbism
drowning	rhinorrhea
escharotomy	stupor
heterografts	

MASTERING THE INFORMATION

FILL IN THE BLANKS

Supply the missing term or the information requested.

1. The extent of a child's injury depends on _____, the _____ that was injured, and the _____ the child received.

2. Full thickness or _____ degree burns are not extremely painful.

3. Equipment used to care for a severely burned child must be _____ to prevent wound infection.

4. Second- or third-degree burns may receive _____ treatment, which involves leaving the burned area exposed to air.

MATCHING

Match the terms in Column I with a definition, example, or related statement from Column II. Place the letter corresponding to the answer in the space provided.

Column I

1. ____ Allografting

2. ____ Chelating agents

3. ____ Contrecoup injury

4. ____ Contusion

5. ____ Escharotomy

6. ____ Heterografting

7. ____ Leptomeningeal cyst

8. ____ Plumbism

9. ____ Rhinorrhea

10. ____ Stupor

11. ____ Autografting

Column II

a. Cutting into the tough leathery scab over a burned area to release a tight band around an extremity.

b. Placing of skin from cadavers or a donor on a cleaned burn site.

c. A tearing or laceration of brain tissue, with symptoms specific to the brain area affected.

d. Grogginess from which an individual can be roused.

e. Lead poisoning; usually occurs in toddlers and preschool children.

f. Clear fluid draining from the nose; if it is cerebrospinal fluid it will be positive for glucose.

g. A concussion on the side of the brain opposite that which was struck; occurs as the brain recoils from the force of the blow.

h. Skin from a nonhuman source, such as porcine (pig), used to promote skin growth after a burn.

i. Skin taken from an unburned area of a burn victim's body and placed on a prepared burned area to facilitate healing.

j. Substances that act to remove lead from soft tissue and bone and eliminate it in the urine.

k. Results from projection of the arachnoid membrane into the fracture site; may cause symptoms of increased intracranial pressure.

SHORT ANSWER

Supply the missing term or the information requested.

1. Identify the three areas that assessed with the Glasgow Coma Scale.

   _____

   _____

2. Discuss the appropriate method for discharge teaching of parents of injured children discharged from the emergency room.

   _____

   _____

3. Explain why the "rule of nines" cannot be used to determine the extent of burns on infants and children.

_____

_____

4. Discuss the reason why burn injuries to the face and throat can be more hazardous than other burn injuries.

_____

_____

5. Describe the infection control measures used for burn victims.

_____

_____

6. Describe the appropriate emergency treatment for the indicated burn injuries: first-, second-, and third-degree burn; electrical burn.

_____

_____

APPLYING YOUR KNOWLEDGE

CASE STUDY

Mr. and Mrs. Chin come to your emergency room with their 3-year-old son, Jay. Jay is an active child who has broken his arm and sprained a wrist climbing on furniture. Jay likes to ride his tricycle around the house and yard and once nearly drank a liquid cleaner that was not placed out of reach in the kitchen. Jay's arm is placed in a cast.

1. What safety issues would you need to address with the Chin family, and what further assessments would you make?

_____

_____

_____

2. What age-appropriate activities would you suggest to the Chin family to facilitate Jay's development?

_____

_____

_____

CRITICAL INQUIRY EXERCISE

1. What safety suggestions could you give to a couple who have open fireplaces and space heaters in their home and three active children ages 18 months, 3 years, and 5 years?

2. Prepare a plan of care addressing outdoor summer activities and dress for parents of a child who lives on a ranch in the Southwest.

CRITICAL EXPLORATION

1. Visit a burn center and observe the care measures taken for clients at various ages and with various types and degrees of burns.

2. Locate the names and phone numbers of the emergency medical system and the poison control center in your neighborhood.

PRACTICING FOR NCLEX

MULTIPLE-CHOICE QUESTIONS

Circle the letter that corresponds to the best answer for each question.

1. Which of the following would be a serious danger sign if noted in a child after head trauma?
   a. Complaint of headache along the area of trauma.
   b. Blood pressure changing from 120/80 to 110/70.
   c. Memory deficit with inability to recall time or date.
   d. Pupils equal and briskly reactive to light.

2. Which of the following would the nurse include in the plan of care for a child in a coma?
   a. Encouraging parents to be positive since coma is often short term in children.
   b. Performing passive range-of-motion exercises to maintain muscle tone.
   c. Feeding the child with a spoon and fork to stimulate memories of normal activity.
   d. Maintaining the child in a flat, supine position to simulate normal sleeping position.

3. Jan, age 13, is admitted with third-degree burns over 25% of her body. Which of the following would be a priority concern in Jan's plan of care?

   a. Liberal medication to control Jan's severe pain.

   b. Arranging age-appropriate diversional activities.

   c. Preventing hypovolemia and circulatory collapse.

   d. Increasing oral intake of proteins to build tissue.

4. A realistic outcome for the parents of a child who is the victim of unintentional injury would be for the parents to

   a. admit responsibility for the child's trauma.

   b. allow the child to perform household chores without supervision to strengthen self-esteem.

   c. prevent all future accidental childhood injury.

   d. state measures they can take to prevent common accidents from occurring.

ALTERNATE FORMAT QUESTIONS

Multiple-Answer Multiple-Choice Questions

Circle the letter(s) corresponding to the appropriate answer(s). Select all that apply.

1. Which of the following would be appropriate interventions for a child who has experienced an unintentional injury?

   a. *Subdural hematoma*: Monitor for seizures, vomiting, or hyperirritability for up to 20 days after the trauma.

   b. *Acetaminophen poisoning*: Administer acetylcysteine in a carbonated drink.

   c. *Caustic poisoning*: Administer syrup of ipecac followed by cold water or milk.

   d. *Hydrocarbon ingestion*: Monitor the child for respiratory irritation.

   e. *Iron poisoning*: Monitor for initial nausea, diarrhea, and abdominal pain followed by melena and hematemesis and shock 12 hours later.

   f. *Plant poisoning*: Reassure parents that this is not serious and requires no treatment.

2. After teaching a group of students about unintentional injuries and their treatment, which of the following if described by the group as appropriate indicates successful teaching?

   a. *Concussion*: Instruct parents not to allow the child to sleep for 24 hours after the trauma.

   b. *Foreign body obstruction*: Irrigate the child's ear canal with saline to remove a peanut.

   c. *Frostbite*: Place the affected body part in hot water to restore circulation immediately.

   d. *Snake bite*: Apply a cold compress to the site immediately and keep the site in a dependent position to slow venom spread; monitor for bruising and bleeding.

   e. *Facial burn*: Monitor for stridor or other signs of respiratory tract obstruction.

   f. *Third-degree burn over 10% of the body*: Decrease fluid intake to aid kidneys in filtration of waste and concentration of urine.

3. A nurse is preparing a presentation for a local parent group about accidents and injuries in children. Which of the following would the nurse include as being a most common accident in children between the age of 10 to 14 years?

   a. Drowning.

   b. Poisoning.

   c. Burns.

   d. Motor vehicles.

   e. Firearms.

   f. Foreign object inhalation

Nursing Care of a Family When a Child has a Malignancy

CHAPTER OVERVIEW

The diagnosis of a malignancy (cancer) in a child can be devastating to a family. However, the prognosis for children is continually improving. Chapter 53 provides an overview of the special care needs of the child with a malignancy. The physical and psychological effects of various types of childhood cancers are discussed. The use of the nursing process to plan and provide care for the child and the family coping with a malignancy is explored.

LEARNING OBJECTIVES

After mastering the contents of this chapter, you should be able to do the following:

1. Describe normal cellular growth and theories that explain how cells alter to become malignant in children.

2. Identify National Health Goals related to the care of the child with a malignancy that nurses can help the nation to achieve.

3. Use critical thinking to propose ways that nursing care for a child with a malignancy can be more family centered.

4. Assess a child with a common malignant process, such as a rhabdomyosarcoma, neuroblastoma, nephroblastoma, or leukemia.

5. Formulate nursing diagnoses related to a child with a malignancy.

6. Establish expected outcomes for a child with a malignancy.

7. Plan nursing care specific to a child with a malignancy.

8. Implement nursing care for a child receiving cancer therapy, such as explaining why chemotherapy destroys malignant cells.

9. Evaluate expected outcomes for achievement and effectiveness of care.

10. Identify areas related to care of children with malignancies that could benefit from additional nursing research or application of evidence-based practice.

11. Integrate knowledge of abnormal cell growth in children with the nursing process to achieve quality maternal and child health nursing care.

KEY TERMS

biopsy	leukemia
chemotherapeutic agent	lymphoma
Ewing's sarcoma	metastasis

neoplasm
nephroblastoma
neuroblastoma
oncogenic virus

osteogenic sarcoma
rhabdomyosarcoma
sarcoma
tumor staging

MASTERING THE INFORMATION

FILL IN THE BLANKS

Supply the missing term or the information requested.

1. Because cells lining the stomach are fast growing, _____ and _____ are common side effects of chemotherapy.

2. _____ _____ is a malignant tumor occurring most often in the bone marrow of the midshaft of long bones.

3. _____ is a rare malignant tumor of the eye.

4. _____ may be required for a large malignant tumor of the eye.

MATCHING

Match the terms in Column I with a definition, example, or related statement from Column II. Place the letter corresponding to the answer in the space provided.

Column I

1. ____ Alopecia

2. ____ Allogeneic

3. ____ Astrocytoma

4. ____ Medulloblastoma

5. ____ Neoplasm

6. ____ Neuroblastoma

7. ____ Oncogenic

8. ____ Osteogenic sarcoma

9. ____ Rhabdomyosarcoma

10. ____ Staging

Column II

a. A term commonly used for a new abnormal growth that does not respond to growth control mechanisms.

b. Cancer-causing agent.

c. Hair loss; occurs secondary to almost all chemotherapeutic cancer drugs.

d. A transplant between a histocompatible person and a child with cancer.

e. Designating the extent of a malignant process.

f. Slow growing cystic tumor arising from the glial tissue of the neural cells.

g. Fast growing tumor found most commonly in the cerebellum.

h. A tumor of striated muscle.

i. A tumor arising from the cells of the sympathetic nervous system.

j. A malignant tumor of long bone involving rapidly growing bone tissue.

SHORT ANSWER

Supply the missing term or the information requested.

1. Name the three phases of chemotherapy for acute lymphocytic leukemia.

_____

_____

2. Identify how Hodgkin's disease is confirmed.

_____

_____

3. Describe five of the common categories of chemotherapeutic cancer agents.

_____

_____

4. Discuss factors that may contribute to decreased nutritional status in a child with cancer.

_____

_____

APPLYING YOUR KNOWLEDGE

CASE STUDY

Mr. and Mrs. Morrell have been advised that Joseph has a brain tumor. He was admitted 2 days ago for preoperative lab work. Today is the day of the surgery, and you are assigned as Joseph's operating room nurse. When reading the surgical checklist, you found that Joseph had not received an enema or any methods to evacuate the bowel.

1. What would be your response after learning of this situation?

_____

_____

_____

2. What would be the priority areas to address when providing postoperative care for Joseph?

_____

_____

_____

CRITICAL INQUIRY EXERCISE

1. Prepare a teaching plan for a child with a diagnosis of leukemia or her parents.

2. Develop a tool to contrast the presenting symptoms that may be seen on an assessment for a child presenting with leukemia. The tool should help you determine the type of malignancy based on the clinical picture.

CRITICAL EXPLORATION

Visit a pediatric cancer ward. Note the varied types of childhood cancer and the types of medical and nursing treatments being provided.

PRACTICING FOR NCLEX

MULTIPLE-CHOICE QUESTIONS

Circle the letter that corresponds to the best answer for each question.

1. Mrs. Peters states she's glad her son Tim's cancer was caught early and now he is safe from cancer in later life. The nurse should respond with which of the following principles in mind?
   a. Cancer is less likely to strike Tim again.
   b. Childhood cancer usually instills an immunity to cancer.
   c. Children surviving one cancer have a greater risk for a second cancer.
   d. Cancer onset is unpredictable and carries no pattern of recurrence.

2. Children with cancer would be most vulnerable for skeletal side effects from radiation therapy at which of the following ages?
   a. 2 years.
   b. 4 years.
   c. 6 years.
   d. 12 years.

3. Which of the following is true about radiation therapy?
   a. The skin areas at which the radiotherapy is directed should be washed daily with soap and water.
   b. Creams and lotions should not be applied to the radiation site until a radiation series is complete.
   c. Sedatives and analgesics should be withheld during radiotherapy.
   d. Radiation may result in excessive salivary gland function.

4. Which of the following nursing interventions is most important when caring for a child receiving vincristine?
   a. Administering salicylates to relieve nerve pain.
   b. Encouraging intake of high-fiber foods.
   c. Monitoring for frequent diarrheal stools.
   d. Planning age-appropriate coloring or drawing activities.

5. The decreased platelet production from leukemia's effect on a child's bone marrow would result in which of the following symptoms?
   a. Flushed skin.
   b. Epistaxis.
   c. Hyperthermia.
   d. Tachycardia.

6. Children who have a brain tumor will have which of the following symptoms?
   a. Abdominal pain.
   b. Diarrhea.
   c. Hypotension.
   d. Vomiting.

7. Which of the following interventions may be needed for the parents of a child diagnosed with a brain tumor?

   a. Allowing the parents to delay treatment for weeks if needed until the denial stage resolves.

   b. Explaining that removal of a small peripheral tumor is a minor surgical procedure.

   c. Reinforcing preoperative explanations about the nature of the child's diagnosis after surgery is over.

   d. Reassuring parents that radiation and chemotherapy can cure brain tumors and prevent metastasis.

ALTERNATE FORMAT QUESTIONS
Multiple-Answer Multiple-Choice Questions

Circle the letter(s) corresponding to the appropriate answer(s). Select all that apply.

1. Which of the following would be appropriate to include in the plan of care for a child with a malignancy?

   a. Encouraging children receiving chemotherapy to take clear fluids, even if they are nauseated, to prevent uric acid buildup in the kidney.

   b. Using ice packs to the scalp of children with leukemia to decrease alopecia.

   c. Placing a warm compress on a site of infiltration of a chemotherapeutic agent.

   d. Administering live virus vaccines to immunosuppressed children to achieve maximum protection against infection.

   e. Monitoring a child receiving chemotherapy for leukemia for nuchal rigidity, headache, irritability, and vomiting.

   f. Encouraging normal activity and regular school for children in the maintenance phase of leukemia therapy.

2. Which of the following would the nurse expect to assess in a child with osteogenic sarcoma?

   a. Progressively increasing pain in the abdomen.

   b. Onion skin like reaction on radiographic examination.

   c. Swelling of the affective extremity near the knee.

   d. Elevated level of serum alkaline phosphatase.

   e. Pathologic fracture.

3. The parents of a 17-year-old bring the adolescent to the clinic to evaluate a mole on the child's back. The parents are concerned that the child may have malignant melanoma. Which of the following would lead the nurse to suspect that the mole is benign rather than indicative of malignant melanoma?

   a. Symmetrical shape.

   b. Irregular border.

   c. Light brown pigmentation.

   d. Size of 3 mm.

   e. Ulcerated.

   f. Scaly white appearance.

Nursing Care of a Family When a Child has a Cognitive or Mental Health Disorder

CHAPTER OVERVIEW

Children who are cognitively impaired or have a mental health disorder have the same fundamental needs as other children. The nurse has a responsibility to provide the families of these children with skills to observe, solve problems, make decisions, and prevent illness. This chapter presents common illnesses, identifies behaviors, and explores methods of helping the family manage.

LEARNING OBJECTIVES

After mastering the contents of this chapter, you should be able to do the following:

1. Describe common cognitive and mental health disorders that occur in children.

2. Identify National Health Goals related to cognitive or mental health disorders that nurses can be instrumental in helping the nation achieve.

3. Analyze ways that care of a child with a cognitive or mental health disorder can be more family centered.

4. Assess a child for a cognitive or mental health disorder.

5. Formulate nursing diagnoses related to the cognitive or mental health disorders of childhood.

6. Establish expected outcomes for a child with a cognitive or mental health disorder.

7. Plan nursing care for a child with a cognitive or mental health disorder.

8. Implement nursing care for a child with a cognitive or mental health disorder, such as helping a parent reduce environmental stimuli.

9. Evaluate expected outcomes for achievement and effectiveness of care.

10. Identify areas related to cognitive or mental health that could benefit from additional nursing research or application of evidence-based practice.

11. Integrate knowledge of childhood cognitive and mental health disorders and nursing process to achieve quality maternal and child health nursing care.

KEY TERMS

anhedonia
binge eating
catatonia
choreiform movements
complex vocal tics
coprolalia
dyslexia
echolalia
flat affect

graphesthesia
hyperactivity
labile mood
motor tics
palilalia
purging
stereognosis
vocal tics

MASTERING THE INFORMATION

FILL IN THE BLANKS

Supply the missing term or the information requested.

1. _____ is the term that describes the eating of nonfood substances such as dirt, clay, and crayons.

2. _____ is a perplexing condition which parents may view as the child rejecting them.

3. Complex vocal tics include the repeated use of works or phrases out of context including _____ (use of socially unacceptable words) and _____ (repeating one's own words).

MATCHING

Match the terms in Column I with a definition, example, or related statement from Column II. Place the letter corresponding to the answer in the space provided.

Column I

1. ____ Encopresis

2. ____ Motor tics

3. ____ Catatonia

4. ____ Dyslexia

5. ____ Tourette's disease

Column II

a. Muscle movements such as rapid repetitive eye blinking or facial twitching.

b. Inherited syndrome of facial and complex vocal tics.

c. Passing feces in culturally unacceptable places.

d. A learning disorder involving a reading disability.

e. Behaviors seen in children with schizophrenia, characterized by withdrawal and stuporous depression.

SHORT ANSWER

Supply the missing term or the information requested.

1. List the criteria for mental retardation as described by DSM-IV-TR.

   _____

   _____

2. Define labile mood.

   _____

   _____

3. Describe graphesthesia, stereognosis, and choreiform movements.

   _____

   _____

4. Children with schizophrenia may reveal what type of affect?

   _____

   _____

APPLYING YOUR KNOWLEDGE

CASE STUDY

Stephen is 2.5 years old, his mother brings him to the health clinic with an ear infection. The history and physical exam reveal that Stephen's behavior is quite different from that of the other siblings. The mother reports that he hates to be held, only utters sounds when trying to talk, gets upset easily, and screams constantly. You notice that Stephen has excoriated lesions on his thumbs.

1. Based on the information, what would be a probable diagnosis for Stephen and why?

   _____

   _____

   _____

2. How can the nurse assist the parents in bonding with Stephen and providing developmental support?

_____

_____

_____

CRITICAL INQUIRY EXERCISE

1. Arrange with your instructor to invite to your classroom the mother of an 8-year-old or older child with a cognitive or mental health disorder. Ask her to explain how she prepares the child for health visits and what she does in the household to protect the child from injury.

2. Develop an assessment tool to be used in a clinical setting to help the health care professional recognize the signs and symptoms of teenage depression.

CRITICAL EXPLORATION

Attend a school that has an academic or vocational curriculum for the retarded student. Research the activities in the curriculum that will help the student become a functional member of his or her community and society.

PRACTICING FOR NCLEX

MULTIPLE-CHOICE QUESTIONS

Circle the letter that corresponds to the best answer for each question.

1. After teaching the parents of a child diagnosed with ADHD about the disorder, the nurse determines that more teaching is needed if the parents identify which of the following as a characteristic of this disorder?
   a. Hyperactivity.
   b. Inattentiveness.
   c. Impulsiveness.
   d. Conscientiousness.

2. When providing anticipatory guidance to parents of a hyperactive child, the nurse would encourage them to
   a. assign chores appropriate to the child's age.
   b. be flexible and lenient regarding limits.
   c. give instructions to this child in the group setting with the other siblings.
   d. delay punishing the child to allow the child time to think about mistakes.

3. Baby girl Franshon, 12 months old, is admitted to the hospital for electrolyte imbalance and to rule intestinal obstruction. After careful assessment it is determined that Baby Franshon is regurgitating her food after ingestion and then reswallowing it. Research postulates that this is a form of self-stimulation by the infant termed
   a. encopresis.
   b. rumination.
   c. anhedonia.
   d. bulimia.

4. Felicia is 15 years old and is admitted to the hospital with anorexia nervosa. She is a model and often spoken of as an overachiever. As the nurse interviews Felicia and her family, she may discover other findings such as
   a. early development of secondary sex characteristics.
   b. permissive parenting.
   c. amenorrhea.
   d. hyperglycemia.

5. Which of the following is commonly seen in children with an eating disorder?
   a. Morbid obesity.
   b. Ingesting copious amounts of water.
   c. Body mass index above 85% of expected.
   d. Binge eating and purging.

6. A child with an IQ of 44 would be categorized as having which type of mental retardation?
   a. Mild.
   b. Moderate.
   c. Severe.
   d. Profound.

ALTERNATE FORMAT QUESTIONS

Multiple-Answer Multiple-Choice Questions

Circle the letter(s) corresponding to the appropriate answer(s). Select all that apply.

1. Which of the following statement(s) about bulimia nervosa are correct?
   a. Girls with bulimia may be slightly underweight or at normal weight.
   b. Abuse of purgatives, laxatives, and diuretics are used to control weight.
   c. Counseling focuses on having the girl relinquish control.
   d. Erosion of tooth enamel from vomiting occurs less frequently.
   e. The individual with bulimia views food as revolting.

2. A child is diagnosed with Tourette's syndrome. While assessing the child, the nurse observes motor tics. Which of the following might the nurse observe?
   a. Eye blinking.
   b. Coughing.
   c. Throat clearing.
   d. Neck jerking.
   e. Facial grimacing.
   f. Snorting.

3. Which of the following would a nurse expect to assess in a child with schizophrenia?
   a. Flat affect.
   b. Hallucinations.
   c. Hyperactivity.
   d. Rambling speech.
   e. Vocal tics.
   f. Anhedonia.

Nursing Care of a Family in Crisis: Abuse and Violence in the Family

CHAPTER OVERVIEW

Abuse and violence are national problems with serious consequences for children. Chapter 55 describes the physiologic and psychological effects of abuse in the family. The use of the nursing process to identify, plan, and provide appropriate nursing care to help victims and their family members or significant others cope with the trauma of abuse and violence is discussed.

LEARNING OBJECTIVES

After mastering the contents of this chapter, you should be able to do the following:

1. Discuss the types of abuse seen in families and the theories explaining their occurrence.

2. Identify National Health Goals related to an abused family that nurses can help the nation achieve.

3. Analyze ways that nurses can help make care more family centered and so ideally help to prevent family abuse.

4. Assess a family that is physically or emotionally abused.

5. Formulate nursing diagnoses related to an abused family.

6. Develop expected outcomes for an abused family.

7. Plan nursing care for a family in which abuse has occurred.

8. Implement nursing care for an abused family such as ways to role model better parenting.

9. Evaluate expected outcomes for effectiveness and achievement of care.

10. Identify areas related to care of the abused family that could benefit from additional nursing research or application of evidence-based practice.

11. Integrate knowledge of family abuse with nursing process to achieve quality maternal and child health nursing care.

KEY TERMS

abuse	learned helplessness
failure to thrive	mandatory
incest	reporters
intimate partner abuse	molestation

Munchausen syndrome
  by proxy
pedophile
permissive reporters
rape trauma syndrome

shaken baby
  syndrome
silent rape
  syndrome

MASTERING THE INFORMATION

FILL IN THE BLANKS

Supply the missing term or the information requested.

1. _____ is often the first person to identify the symptoms of possible child abuse.

2. Excessive use of _____ by the abusive person is strongly associated with abuse.

3. When questioned about an injury, an abused child will usually _____ the parent's story.

MATCHING

Match the terms in Column I with a definition, example, or related statement from Column II. Place the letter corresponding to the answer in the space provided.

Column I

1. ___ Abuse

2. ___ Disorganization phase

3. ___ Incest

4. ___ Mandatory reporters

5. ___ Molestation

6. ___ Munchausen syndrome by proxy

7. ___ Pedophile

8. ___ Failure to thrive

9. ___ Shaken baby syndrome

10. ___ Reorganization phase

Column II

a. Severe activity between family members.

b. A form of child neglect occurring because of a disturbance in the parent–child relationship.

c. Parents who repeatedly bring a child to a health care facility reporting symptoms of illness when, in fact, the child is well.

d. Willful injury of one person by another.

e. The first stage of rape trauma syndrome; lasts about 3 days.

f. The second stage of rape trauma syndrome; may last months or years.

g. People who must notify the authorities of suspected abuse; nurses fall into this category.

h. Sexual abuse involving between an adult and child, such as oral–genital contact or viewing genitals.

i. An adult who seeks out children for sexual gratification.

j. Condition involving whiplash injury to the neck, edema to the brain stem, retinal hemorrhages, and potential respiratory arrest.

SHORT ANSWER

Supply the missing term or the information requested.

1. Identify the triad of circumstances that generally combine to result in child abuse.

_____

_____

2. Discuss why children in an abusive family situation might have other undiagnosed medical problems.

_____

_____

3. Discuss one major reason why victims of child abuse might grow to be abusers themselves.

_____

_____

4. Discuss one method of differentiating between organic and nonorganic failure to thrive.

_____

_____

5. List symptoms of infants demonstrating failure to thrive relative to physical and social development.

_____

_____

APPLYING YOUR KNOWLEDGE

CASE STUDY

Alissa, age 26, appears in your emergency room with her 4-year-old daughter, Daisy. She states, "He's hurting her. See, he's made her bleed." Alissa is pointing at Daisy's underpants, which are soiled with a dark-red stain.

1. What would your initial actions be?

_____

_____

_____

2. How would you proceed in your care planning for Daisy?

_____

_____

_____

CRITICAL INQUIRY EXERCISE

1. Describe your feelings about a report of rape made by a female child 5 years of age who says, "Daddy hurt me."

2. What would your response be to a male adolescent who reports that his coach sexually abused him, or to a wife who says her husband raped her?

CRITICAL EXPLORATION

Visit a rape crisis center in your neighborhood. Note three activities performed by the nurse in that setting.

PRACTICING FOR NCLEX

MULTIPLE-CHOICE QUESTIONS

Circle the letter that corresponds to the best answer for each question.

1. Because abuse involves and affects all the members of a family, the nurse should include which of the following as part of the expected outcomes?
   a. Disrupting the dysfunctional family.
   b. Improving overall family functioning.
   c. Punishing the abusive family member.
   d. Removing the abuse victim from the family.

2. When planning a strategy to address child and intimate partner abuse, the nurse should do which of the following?
   a. Lecture parents suspected of child abuse on the evils of violence.
   b. Report suspected child abuse whenever a child with bruises is admitted.
   c. Stop parental visitation immediately if child abuse is suspected.
   d. Work with pregnant teen groups to teach parenting skills.

3. At his first physical, Bob, 14 years old, stated that the multiple long whip-like scars on his back occurred as a result of falling backward against a rough bedroom floor when he was playing with a friend. The nurse should respond in which of the following ways?
   a. Ask additional questions regarding the cause of the injury and any other injuries noted.
   b. Discuss with Bob the fact that his clumsiness is probably a part of his adolescence and that he will outgrow it.
   c. Instruct Bob the importance of exercise and good nutrition to avoid easy bruising.
   d. Tell Bob you do not believe him and you want to know if his parents caused his injuries.

4. Sheila, 11 years old, is admitted with vaginal bleeding. The nurse notices that Sheila and her mother are very nervous but state that they are "sure it's just menstrual blood." The nurse should initially do which of the following?
   a. Accept the fact that Sheila is probably beginning menses; do not jump to conclusions.
   b. Explain to Sheila and her mother that menstrual bleeding does not occur at this early age.
   c. Insist that Sheila's mother tell if someone is abusing Sheila.
   d. Gently examine Sheila for torn perineal tissue or lacerations.

5. Which of the following would place a parent at high risk for being a child abuser?
   a. Being poor and a member of a minority group.
   b. Choosing to have a baby without being married.

c. Having less than a high school education.

d. Severe disappointment with the sex of a new baby.

6. Daryl, age 7, states he cannot tell about his father's beating him because the beating will get worse. The nurse should remember which of the following when replying to Daryl?

a. Daryl might be angry with his parents and making up this story.

b. Daryl's mother can protect him from the father if necessary.

c. Most institutions can hold a child for 72 hours for protection.

d. Seven-year-olds are not reliable witnesses of child abuse.

7. A realistic outcome for a woman admitted with a broken collarbone caused by a husband with a history of violence would be that the woman might do which of the following?

a. Fight back the next time he hurts her.

b. Identify what she does that causes her husband to become violent.

c. Leave the abusive man immediately and never see him again.

d. State the names of two shelters she can go to when necessary.

8. The nurse caring for an abused child or abused woman should do which of the following?

a. Allow the family members to remain alone together as much as possible, regardless of the situation, to facilitate family stability.

b. Assume that the abuse was malicious and isolate the victim from family members.

c. Refrain from becoming emotionally involved in the situation.

d. Stay with the child or abused woman throughout the examination process and questioning sessions to offer needed support.

9. Which of the following would be most accurate about abuse?

a. Neglect can be an unintentional form of child abuse.

b. Psychological abuse is not as damaging as physical abuse.

c. Keeping families together throughout therapy is essential.

d. Abuse victims experience guilt only if they caused the abuser to become violent.

ALTERNATE FORMAT QUESTIONS
Multiple-Answer Multiple-Choice Questions

Circle the letter(s) corresponding to the appropriate answer(s). Select all that apply.

1. Which of the following would be appropriate for a patient with abuse or violence in the family.

a. Inform the parents you suspect child abuse as soon as you note suspicious signs.

b. Interview the victim in front of the abuser to make the abuser confess to the crime.

c. Examine the child or suspected victim in a fully undressed state whenever possible.

d. Protect the child's or victim's modesty as much as possible.

e. Do not try to nurture the infant with failure to thrive since this will interfere with family–child bonding.

f. Take photographs of injuries and bruises.

2. Which of the following would characterize intimate partner abuse at level III?

a. Occasional episodes of violence.

b. Beatings sustained with fractures.

c. Daily events of abuse.

d. Use of a weapon for the abuse.

e. Resultant permanent disability.

3. The nurse is preparing a presentation for a community group about rape. Which of the following would the nurse expect to include in the discussion?

a. Rape victims typically experience symptoms that can last for several weeks.

b. Rape is considered a crime of violence.

c. A person can be accused of statutory rape even if the victim consented to the sexual activity.

d. The incidence of date rape is gradually decreasing.

e. The average rape victim is an adolescent female.

Nursing Care of a Family When a Child has a Long-Term or Terminal Illness

CHAPTER OVERVIEW

Chapter 56 discusses the physiologic and emotional concerns related to caring for a family coping with a long-term or fatal illness. The emotional effects of chronic and terminal illness on the entire family as well as on the nursing care provider are reviewed. The use of the nursing process to plan and provide care for the family involved with long-term or terminal illness is explored.

LEARNING OBJECTIVES

After mastering the contents of this chapter, you should be able to do the following:

1. Describe common concerns of parents of children with a long-term or terminal illness.

2. Identify National Health Goals related to children with long-term or terminal illnesses that nurses could help the nation achieve.

3. Use critical thinking to analyze ways that nursing care of a child with a long-term or terminal illness can be more family centered.

4. Assess adjustment of a child or family to a long-term or terminal illness.

5. Formulate nursing diagnoses for a child with a long-term or terminal illness.

6. Identify expected outcomes for a child with a long-term or terminal illness.

7. Plan nursing care for a child with a long-term or terminal illness.

8. Implement nursing care for a child with a long-term or terminal illness, such as helping parents with time management.

9. Evaluate expected outcomes for effectiveness and achievement of care.

10. Identify areas related to the care of children with long-term or terminal illnesses that could benefit from additional nursing research or application of evidence-based practice.

11. Integrate knowledge of long-term and terminal illness in children with nursing process to achieve quality maternal and child health nursing care.

KEY TERMS

anticipatory grief
death
grief process
vulnerable children

MASTERING THE INFORMATION

FILL IN THE BLANKS

Supply the missing term or the information requested.

1. The reactions a nurse may have to the terminal illness of a child include _____, a sense of failure and grief.

2. Most school-aged children _____ what is happening to them when their disorder has a fatal prognosis.

3. A parent's usual response to the diagnosis of a terminal illness in a child is _____.

MATCHING

Match the terms in Column I with a definition, example, or related statement from Column II. Place the letter corresponding to the answer in the space provided.

Column I

1. ____ Infant

2. ____ Toddler

3. ____ Preschooler

4. ____ School-ager

5. ____ Adolescent

Column II

a. View death as temporary early in this stage; later realize death is final; focus on how they will cope without parents.

b. See death as sleep and fear separation more than death.

c. Have no understanding of their impending death; comfort and security are their main focus.

d. Have adult concerns of death but view themselves as basically indestructible; need to remain as active as possible.

e. May have viewed the death of a relative but do not understand or relate this to their own death; need to maintain routines.

ADDITIONAL MATCHING QUESTIONS

Match the terms in Column I with a definition, example, or related statement from Column II. Place the letter corresponding to the answer in the space provided.

Column I

1. ____ Anticipatory grief

2. ____ Bargaining stage

3. ____ Depression

4. ____ Denial stage

5. ____ Anger stage

6. ____ Hospice

7. ____ Death

8. ____ Organ donation

9. ____ Autopsy

10. ____ Grief reaction

Column II

a. Absence of respirations, no heart sounds, absence of body movement or reflexes, and dilated fixed pupils.

b. The experience that occurs when news of chronic illness or impending death is received.

c. Action that may provide a comfort for parents to know a part of their child has helped another child to live.

d. Parents possibly promising to do good deeds so the terminally ill child will get well.

e. Parental problem solving skills impaired possibly leading nurse to be an ineffective.

f. Mandatory if homicide, suicide, or harmful death is suspected.

g. A third opinion regarding the disease or prognosis may be requested.

h. Option for children allowing them to die in a homelike setting.

i. Parents beginning to really think about the child's impending death.

j. Parents possibly criticizing the nurse or scolding the child frequently.

SHORT ANSWER

Supply the missing term or the information requested.

1. Describe the factors that affect how people cope with situations.

   _____

   _____

2. Briefly compare the effects of a chronic illness such as diabetes might have on a family with the effects of a chronic illness such as muscular dystrophy.

   _____

   _____

3. Discuss how the age of the parents might affect their ability to care for a disabled child.

   _____

   _____

4. Why would healthy parents of a chronically ill or disabled child need to have a will prepared?

   _____

   _____

5. How might evaluating the plan of care for a family with a terminally ill child after the child's death be beneficial for a nurse?

   _____

   _____

6. List three of the seven approaches to communicating with dying children.

   _____

   _____

APPLYING YOUR KNOWLEDGE

CASE STUDY

Patricia, age 10, is involved in an automobile accident that results multiple injuries including a spinal cord injury. Her parents arrived an hour ago and have been told that she will most likely be paralyzed from the waist down.

1. What reactions might you expect from Patricia's parents? What factors may affect their coping?

   _____

   _____

   _____

2. How might Patricia respond?

   _____

   _____

   _____

CRITICAL INQUIRY EXERCISE

1. How might you feel if a patient you cared for over several weeks died on your day off? How would those feelings differ, if at all, if the patient was elderly and terminally ill; a young adult automobile accident victim; a child; or recovering well when you left the day before?

2. How would your approach differ, if at all, when providing care for the family members of a patient who died suddenly, and providing care for family members of a patient who died after a long hospitalization during which the patient wasted away and experienced pain?

CRITICAL EXPLORATION

1. Spend a day with a chronically ill child and his or her family. Record interactions and determine if any maladaptive coping behaviors are present.

2. Spend a day with a terminally ill child and his or her family. Note the family dynamics (reactions of the child and parents). Record your reaction to the situation, the child, and the family.

PRACTICING FOR NCLEX

MULTIPLE-CHOICE QUESTIONS

Circle the letter that corresponds to the best answer for each question.

1. Bobby, age 10, has a diagnosis of type 1 diabetes. His mother has expressed plans to tutor Bobby at home and design a comfortable, quiet life to help him cope with his condition. Which of the following nursing diagnoses would best address this situation?

   a. Readiness for enhanced parenting related to chronic illness.

   b. Risk for complicated grieving related to loss of child's expected activity level.

   c. Risk for delayed growth and development related to lack of age-appropriate stimulation.

   d. Disabled family coping related to parent's inability to accept child's illness.

2. Polly, age 5, is admitted to the hospital with cystic fibrosis and pneumonia. Polly's mother tells the nurse that Polly must have pulmonary therapy before breakfast to eat a good meal. The nurse should respond in which of the following ways?

   a. Assure Polly's mother that the hospital staff is very competent and will take good care of the child.

   b. Inform Polly's mother of the visiting hours and insist she go home and rest since Polly is in good hands.

   c. Listen to the mother and note the schedule and procedures that Polly is accustomed to at home.

   d. Nod, and after the mother has gone plan Polly's care according to the hospital schedule.

3. Mr. and Mrs. Peters have a 4-year-old son, Bryan, who has been diagnosed with a terminal illness. The nurse would be concerned if which of the following plans were made by the family?

   a. Arrangements were being made to find a consistent sitter who could care for Bryan while Mrs. Peters works 4 hours a day.

   b. Mr. Peters states he plans to stay home with Bryan in the evenings so that Mrs. Peters can go to her exercise class.

   c. Mrs. Peters states she intends to care for Bryan around the clock and will need no assistance from anyone.

   d. The Peters family intends to take Bryan home and care for him there so he will die surrounded by family members.

4. David, 14, has leukemia and is in the hospital for the fourth time. When assessing his mother to determine if she is progressing through the stages of grief over her teenage son's terminal illness, the nurse would find which of the following to be signs of maladaptive coping?

   a. David's mother seems very sad at times and occasionally walks out of his room crying.

   b. David's mother shows the same signs of denial she showed when he was admitted to the hospital the first time.

   c. David's mother speaks of how good a son he was and how she is really going to miss him.

   d. David's mother spends a lot of time with David and brings him all his favorite foods from home.

5. The nurse notes that a terminally ill child's parents are not visiting very frequently or providing needed support. Which of the following could the nurse do?

   a. Call the parents in and have them explain to the child why they are not visiting as often as they should.

   b. Spend as much time with the child as possible, recognizing that the parents may need to withdraw temporarily to cope.

   c. Tell the child it is good to have time alone to think about death and to prepare for this new experience.

   d. Warn the parents that if they do not visit the child frequently now, they may experience intense guilt feelings after death.

ALTERNATE FORMAT QUESTIONS
Multiple-Answer Multiple-Choice Questions

Circle the letter(s) corresponding to the appropriate answer(s). Select all that apply.

1. Which of the following would be appropriate when caring for a child with a terminal illness?

   a. The nurse should encourage the parents of a child in the "dying phase" to stay close to the room because the child will not live more than 2 to 3 days.

b. The family living with a child who is dying should be provided time to talk about physical and emotional difficulties they might be having.

c. At the onset of death, metabolism increases and the child may become flushed because cardiac stoke volume increases.

d. Medications are best delivered intravenously as the child nears death to promote absorption and improve onset of drug action.

e. The nurse should avoid focusing on self-awareness when preparing to work with a dying child because the focus should be on the child and family.

2. The statements below represent the various stages of grief. Place the statements in the proper sequence from first to last.

a. "I'm sad that this is happening."

b. "It's okay that this is happening."

c. "I'll devote my life to volunteering if he gets well."

d. "This is just not fair that he is so sick."

e. "How can this be? He's such a healthy child."

3. The nurse is preparing a plan of care for the parents of a toddler who is diagnosed with a terminal illness and is dying. The nurse would need to integrate an understanding of which of the following into the plan of care?

a. Toddlers understand death as a separation.

b. They realize that death is final.

c. Toddlers have a need for routines.

d. Toddlers need to feel comfortable and secure.

e. They have difficulty relating death to what they are experiencing.

f. They feel sad about being away from their parents.

Answers

CHAPTER 1

MASTERING THE INFORMATION

FILL IN THE BLANKS

1. neonatal nurse practitioner
2. scope
3. rehabilitation
4. promotion

MATCHING

1. f **2.** e **3.** c **4.** a **5.** g **6.** h **7.** b **8.** d

SHORT ANSWER

1. Any two of the following would be accurate: families are not as extended so are smaller than previously; single parents have become the most common type of parent in the United States; 90% of women work outside the home, at least part time; families are more mobile than previously and there is an increase in the number of homeless women and children; incidence of both child and intimate partner abuse is increasing; families are more health conscious than ever before; health care must respect cost containment. (See Table 1.2 in text for possible implications.)
2. Nursing staff will be required to provide intensive health teaching with follow-up by home care nurses. Patients and parents must be prepared to recognize danger signs that warrant immediate attention and to respond appropriately. Parents should be allowed to do as much for the child or the newborn as they wish to prepare them to care for the child or the newborn on discharge.
3. The following are methods for promoting empowerment: respecting the views of the children and parents; regarding parents as important participants in their own or their child's health, and keeping them informed of the child's status and including them in the decision-making process; and making each client feel important by showing a warm manner and keen interest.

APPLYING YOUR KNOWLEDGE

CASE STUDY

1. Suggested answers may include but are not limited to the following: earlier detection of possible complications; education about possible complications with emphasis on the need for evaluation if any occur; education about healthy nutrition and ways to foster fetal growth and development.
2. Suggested answers may include but are not limited to the following: determination of client's family situation, family structure, cultural beliefs, and individual circumstances such as client's preferences about individuals to include.
3. Suggested answers may include but are not limited to the following: client's view, meaning, or interpretation of the pregnancy; person(s) who is(are) considered the primary decision-maker(s); extent of involvement of other family members; specific health beliefs, practices or rituals associated with pregnancy, labor, and birth.

PRACTICING FOR NCLEX

MULTIPLE-CHOICE QUESTIONS

1. b **2.** d **3.** d **4.** b **5.** c

ALTERNATE FORMAT QUESTIONS

Multiple-Answer Multiple-Choice Questions

1. a, b, c **2.** a, d

CHAPTER 2

MASTERING THE INFORMATION

FILL IN THE BLANKS

1. Hispanic
2. Chinese Americans
3. murder
4. Prejudice

MATCHING

1. e **2.** a **3.** f **4.** d **5.** b **6.** c

TRUE OR FALSE

1. T **2.** T

APPLYING YOUR KNOWLEDGE

CASE STUDY

1. Suggested answers may include but are not limited to the following: assessing the client's nutritional status; evaluating diet including typical foods consumed; identifying cultural influences on food choices (specific foods to be avoided, preferred foods, cooking methods for the food, person responsible for purchasing and cooking the food); determining the availability of appropriate foods such as client's ability to purchase food and transportation to get to the grocery stores.

2. Suggested answers may include but are not limited to the following: determining the client's likes and dislikes and evaluating the nutritional content of the foods that the client likes; offering suggestions about combining foods that client likes to increase nutritional value; ensuring that suggestions are available in the local store for the client to purchase; asking the client to have the person responsible for purchasing and/or cooking the food (if not the client) to come with the client so that they can work together to develop appropriate solutions; referring the client to local community services that assist with nutrition or transportation if necessary; ensuring compliance with the use of prenatal vitamins; checking with the health care provider about possible additional supplementation.

PRACTICING FOR NCLEX

MULTIPLE-CHOICE QUESTIONS

1. a **2.** b **3.** c

ALTERNATE FORMAT QUESTIONS

Multiple-Answer Multiple-Choice Questions

1. a, b, c, e **2.** a, b, e

CHAPTER 3

MASTERING THE INFORMATION

FILL IN THE BLANKS

1. foster
2. communal
3. function
4. gay or lesbian
5. procreation

MATCHING

1. b **2.** c **3.** d **4.** e **5.** a

APPLYING YOUR KNOWLEDGE

CASE STUDY

1. Suggested answers may include but are not limited to the following: the need to establish a baseline for health information on the child and identify potential problems; identify possible illnesses or lacking immunizations if child was born in another country; determine stage of parenting of parents; assess siblings' responses to child.

2. Suggested answers may include but are not limited to the following: time spent in planning, typically 9 months for biologic parents, but for adoptive parents it may be much longer; possible sudden appearance of a child becoming available along with suddenly becoming parents; conflict between trying to preserve child's native culture and socializing child into the community with foreign adoption; adopted adolescent seeking out birth parents possibly causing adoptive parents to feel rejected.

3. Suggested answers may include but are not limited to the following: telling child around age 3 years on considered less stressful than having child stumble onto information when school-aged or adolescent; promotion of trust and security for the child.

4. Suggested answers may include but are not limited to the following: child's behavior reflects testing to see if parents will "keep" the child; child has passed honeymoon behavior stage where child behaved perfectly for fear of being given away again.

PRACTICING FOR NCLEX

MULTIPLE-CHOICE QUESTIONS

1. c **2.** a **3.** c

ALTERNATE FORMAT

Multiple-Answer Multiple-Choice Questions

1. a, b, d, e **2.** e, f **3.** b, d, e, f

CHAPTER 4

MASTERING THE INFORMATION

FILL IN THE BLANKS

1. family routines
2. 30
3. indirect
4. privacy, confidentiality
5. leave
6. handwashing

MATCHING

1. b **2.** a **3.** d **4.** c **5.** e

SHORT ANSWER

1. Nurses can encourage women to seek prenatal care and can educate women about the signs and

symptoms of preterm labor so that women can get help at a point at which labor can be halted.

2. Children requiring acute care or surgery often need follow-up home visits. Those with chronic conditions such as bronchial pulmonary dysplasia, cystic fibrosis, and childhood cancer are often cared for at home rather than in hospital settings when at all possible so they are not separated from their family. Many children in terminal stages of disease are also cared for at home, receiving hospice care.

APPLYING YOUR KNOWLEDGE

CASE STUDY

1. Suggested answers may include but are not limited to the following: rationale for care at home; determination of knowledge level and understanding of condition; reinforcement of instructions and recommendations for staying at home, such as bedrest and activity level; identification of available resources including family and finances; possible need for assistant to help with client's care and home management; diversional activities to occupy time; possible ways for client to stay in contact with work within activity restrictions.

2. Suggested answers may include but are not limited to the following: reinforcement of activity restrictions; self-monitoring of contractions, fetal movements, fetal heart rate; measures to cope with activity restrictions; medication teaching as appropriate; warning signs that require notification; need for continued adequate nutrition and fluid intake; promotion of elimination.

PRACTICING FOR NCLEX

MULTIPLE-CHOICE QUESTIONS

1. b **2.** c **3.** d **4.** d

ALTERNATE FORMAT QUESTIONS

Multiple-Answer Multiple-Choice Questions

1. a, c, d, f **2.** a, b, d, e, f **3.** c, d, f

CHAPTER 5

MASTERING THE INFORMATION

FILL IN THE BLANKS

1. gonad
2. Menopause
3. Thelearche

MATCHING

1. k **2.** f **3.** j **4.** c **5.** a **6.** d **7.** g **8.** h **9.** b **10.** i **11.** e

TRUE OR FALSE

1. T **2.** T

APPLYING YOUR KNOWLEDGE

CASE STUDY

1. Suggested answers may include the following but are not limited to: Education about sexuality, conception (prevention or promotion); role-modeling for gender roles; interventions to strengthen sense of maleness or femaleness.

2. Suggested answers may include the following but are not limited to: Synthesis and release of gonadotropin-releasing hormone; anterior pituitary secretion of follicle-stimulating hormone (FSH) and luteinizing hormone (LH); role of central nervous system in directing action of hypothalamus; triggering of estrogen by FSH at puberty and first phase of menstrual cycle; LH direction of secretion of progesterone after ovulation.

3. Suggested answers may include the following but are not limited to: Menopausal changes; use of medications to treat underlying disorders; decreased sperm production, erectile power, achievement of orgasm and sex drive in males beginning in the middle adult years; decreased erectile firmness or ejaculatory forces with possible prolongation of erection for older adult males; decreased vaginal secretions in older adult females.

4. Suggested answers may include the following but are not limited to: Education about safe sex practices, prevention of sexually transmitted infections, reduction of adolescent sexual activity, recommended screenings, HPV vaccination, breast self-examination.

PRACTICING FOR NCLEX

MULTIPLE-CHOICE QUESTIONS

1. d **2.** c **3.** a

ALTERNATE FORMAT QUESTIONS

Multiple-Answer Multiple-Choice Questions

1. a, b, d **2.** a, c, d **3.** a, b, c, e

CHAPTER 6

MASTERING THE INFORMATION

FILL IN THE BLANKS

1. Condom
2. diaphragm
3. estrogen, progesterone

MATCHING

1. d **2.** c **3.** a **4.** b **5.** e

SHORT ANSWER

1. Estrogen content of the pill suppresses follicle-stimulating hormone (FSH) and luteinizing hormone (LH). The progesterone constituent decreases the

permeability of cervical mucus, limiting sperm mobility and access to the ova. Progesterone interferes with tubal transport and endometrial proliferation, making implantation unlikely.

2. The "minipill differs from the traditional oral contraceptive in that it is composed of progestins only. Ovulation occurs, but implantation will not.

3. Intrauterine devices (IUDs) are rarely selected as a method of contraception for adolescents because teens tend to have variable sexual partners and no prior pregnancies, both contraindications for IUD use. Spermicides and condoms, barrier methods, are commonly used by the adolescent population. They are economical and require no parental consent. However, spermicides have a failure rate of 20%. Adolescents should be cautioned carefully about the use of condoms. They are most effective when applied before any penile–vulvar contact. The self-lubricated type breaks less frequently. The condom should fit loosely enough to allow the penis tip to collect the ejaculate without undue pressure. Condom efficiency is lessened by body heat when carried for some time in pockets and wallets. The use of a vaginally inserted spermicide further enhances the efficiency of the condom.

APPLYING YOUR KNOWLEDGE

CASE STUDY 1

1. Suggested answers may include but are not limited to the following: starting contraceptive on the first Sunday closest to 2 weeks after birth; using a second form of contraception during the initial 7 days; taking the pill consistently each day; having the pill in plain sight as an aid to remembering to take the pill (keeping the pills out of reach of small children); informing of possible side effects and when to notify her health care provider.

2. Suggested answers may include but are not limited to the following: once daily administration; time not important but consistency such as with a meal or at bedtime; menstrual flow beginning during the 7 days she is taking the placebo tablets or if a 21-day pack, during the 7 days when she is not taking any pills.

3. Suggested answers may include but are not limited to the following: importance of consistent daily administration; time of day not as important as consistency in taking the pill; possible administration with meals or at bedtime to help remember to take the pill; having pill in sight to (but out of reach of young children) to aid as a reminder.

CASE STUDY 2

1. Suggested answers may include but are not limited to the following: need for menstrual cycles to be established for at least 2 years; possible suppression of pituitary-regulating activity if started too early; early closure of epiphyses and halting of growth if started too early.

2. Suggested answers may include but are not limited to the following: estrogen content of pills leading to closure of epiphyses of long bones; subsequent halting of growth and preadolescent growth spurt.

CASE STUDY 3

1. Suggested answers may include but are not limited to the following: nonjudgmental attitude; avoidance of imposing personal beliefs and values on woman; support for the woman's contraceptive decision; sensitivity to woman's religious, cultural, and moral beliefs; need for nurse's self-awareness.

2. Suggested answers may include but are not limited to the following: laminaria causing cervical dilation increasing woman's risk for infection; antibiotic prophylaxis for prevention of possible infection.

PRACTICING FOR NCLEX

MULTIPLE-CHOICE QUESTIONS

1. b 2. a 3. b 4. b

ALTERNATE FORMAT QUESTIONS

Multiple-Answer Multiple-Choice Questions

1. a, c, d 2. a, d, e 3. d, e, f

CHAPTER 7

MASTERING THE INFORMATION

FILL IN THE BLANKS

1. ethical
2. inherit
3. genotype

MATCHING

1. d 2. h 3. f 4. b 5. g 6. a 7. i 8. e 9. c

SHORT ANSWER

1. Genetic testing allows the couple to make informed choices about future reproduction.

2. If the disease is dominantly inherited, two out of four children could inherit the disease; if the disease is recessively inherited, one out of four children could inherit the disease. (See text, Figures 7.2 and 7.4.)

3. Any two of the following: provide concrete, accurate information about the process of inheritance and inherited disorders; reassure people who are concerned that their children will inherit a disorder that the disorder will not occur; allow people who are affected by inherited disorders to make informed choices about future reproduction; offer support to people who are affected by genetic illness.

4. In both situations, the couple would most likely not be ready for or amenable to counseling. At this point, they are probably experiencing disbelief, shock, and/or grief.

APPLYING YOUR KNOWLEDGE

CASE STUDY

1. Suggested answers may include but are not limited to the following: X-linked recessive disorders require inheritance of recessive gene; female with affected gene heterozygous for disorder; male with the gene would manifest disorder; Bennie without the disorder, so therefore, does not have the gene. However, a 50% chance that male child will have disease and 50% chance that female child will carry gene.
2. Suggested answers may include but are not limited to the following: explanation of disorder, including what to expect related to growth and development of the child; referral to supportive services; coping strategies; involvement of family members appropriate if couple agrees to share information with them; importance of maintaining the couple's privacy and confidentiality while ensuring couple has necessary support and guidance.

PRACTICING FOR NCLEX

MULTIPLE-CHOICE QUESTIONS

1. b **2.** a **3.** d **4.** b **5.** b **6.** c

ALTERNATE FORMAT QUESTIONS

Multiple-Answer Multiple-Choice Questions

1. a, b, c, e, f **2.** c, d **3.** b, d

CHAPTER 8

MASTERING THE INFORMATION

FILL IN THE BLANKS

1. biopsy
2. allergic
3. cryptoorchidism

MATCHING

1. e **2.** h **3.** f **4.** c **5.** i **6.** j **7.** a **8.** b **9.** g
10. d

SHORT ANSWER

1. relief, grief
2. surrogate mother
3. acidic
4. Therapeutic insemination
5. In vitro

APPLYING YOUR KNOWLEDGE

CASE STUDY

1. Suggested answers may include but are not limited to the following: increasing age leading to an increased risk for subfertility in females; deferring pregnancy to late thirties possibly increasing difficulty in conceiving.

2. Suggested answers may include but are not limited to the following: culture and use of alternative therapies impacting conception; cultural attitudes toward sexual relations, pregnancy, and parenting; effect of culture on pattern of sexual relations (i.e., Orthodox Jewish law); forbiddence of therapeutic insemination by some cultures to preserve male lineage; cultural influences on how couple may react to diagnosis of subfertility and meaning of diagnosis to them.

PRACTICING FOR NCLEX

MULTIPLE-CHOICE QUESTIONS

1. b **2.** c **3.** c

ALTERNATE FORMAT QUESTIONS

Multiple-Answer Multiple-Choice Questions

1. b, c **2.** a, b, d, e **3.** a, d

CHAPTER 9

MASTERING THE INFORMATION

FILL IN THE BLANKS

1. amniotic membrane
2. Hydraminos
3. zygote

MATCHING

1. d **2.** h **3.** j **4.** b **5.** f **6.** i **7.** a **8.** g **9.** e
10. c

CHRONOLOGICAL ORDER

1. End of 8 gestation weeks: Heart has septum and valves. Facial features are definitely discernible.
2. End of 12 gestation weeks: Nail beds forming on toes and fingers; tooth buds present; heart sounds audible by Doppler instrument.
3. End of 16 gestation weeks: Formation of lanugo; liver and pancreas are functioning; fetus demonstrates swallowing reflex.
4. End of 20 gestation weeks: Quickening experienced by the mother; beginning of vernix caseosa.
5. End of 24 gestation weeks: Average weight is 550 g; passive antibody transfer from mother to fetus.
6. End of 28 gestation weeks: Average weight is 1200 g; lung alveoli begin maturing with surfactant.
7. End of 32 gestation weeks: Average weight is 1600 g; assumes delivery position; store iron.
8. End of 36 gestation weeks: Additional deposits of subcutaneous fat and lanugo start to diminish.

SHORT ANSWER

1. Oxygen and other nutrients such as glucose, amino acids, fatty acids, minerals, vitamins, and water diffuse from the maternal blood through the cell layers of the chorionic villi to the villi capillaries. From there, nutrients are transported back to the developing embryo. There is no direct exchange of

blood between the embryo and mother; the exchange is carried out only by selective osmosis through the chorionic villi.

APPLYING YOUR KNOWLEDGE
CASE STUDY

1. Suggested answers may include but are not limited to the following: five parameters (fetal reactivity, fetal breathing movements, fetal body movement, fetal tone, and amniotic fluid volume); each parameter scored as 0, 1, or 2 with a maximum score of 2 for each leading to a possible high score of 10.
2. Suggested answers may include but are not limited to the following: considered more accurate in predicting fetal well-being than any other single assessment; similar in scoring to Apgar score at birth, thus sometimes called fetal Apgar.
3. Suggested answers may include but are not limited to the following: assisting with obtaining information for scoring; educating woman and partner about the test, rationale for use; explaining scoring and what it means about the fetus.

PRACTICING FOR NCLEX
MULTIPLE-CHOICE QUESTIONS

1. b **2.** b **3.** b **4.** a **5.** c

ALTERNATE FORMAT QUESTIONS
Multiple-Answer Multiple-Choice Questions

1. a, b, e, f **2.** a, b, c, d, e **3.** b, c, d, e

CHAPTER 10

MASTERING THE INFORMATION
FILL IN THE BLANKS

1. Multipara
2. Primigravida
3. Goodell's sign

MATCHING

1. b **2.** c **3.** a **4.** b **5.** a **6.** c **7.** b **8.** a **9.** b **10.** c **11.** b

SHORT ANSWER

1. The nurse can play an important role in promoting health during pregnancy by providing preconception counseling especially related to nutrition and safe sex practices so they can enter intended pregnancies in good health.
2. The lateral recumbent position would help prevent pressure on the vena cava that could impair circulation, and also help assist the kidneys to function at maximum efficiency.
3. The kidneys are taxed heavily to filter an increased blood volume. The glomerular filtration rate is increased, filtrating glucose faster than the renal tubules can reabsorb it, and therefore, accidentally spilling glucose into the urine. In addition, lactose, the sugar of breast milk, will be spilled in the urine during pregnancy.
4. After confirmation of pregnancy, most women are more conscious about their diets, the use of over-the-counter medicines, and cigarette smoking. Also, if the woman desires to voluntarily terminate the pregnancy, the risk of complications from an abortion is minimized.

APPLYING YOUR KNOWLEDGE
CASE STUDY

1. Suggested answers may include but are not limited to the following: emotions will depend on psychological aspects such as the environment raised, messages about pregnancy from the family; current culture and societal views; and timing of pregnancy; client's current status of being alone and anxious and timing of pregnancy, planning of pregnancy and degree of emotional support from others; client's ability to adapt to stress; symptoms for past 5 months suggesting knowledge deficit, possible denial; possible upset, worry, disbelief due to current situation of being alone.
2. Suggested answers may include but are not limited to the following: response dependent on personal beliefs and values related to pregnancy termination; questions as to the current length of client's gestation and availability of methods for termination; possible other options in lieu of termination due to current status.

PRACTICING FOR NCLEX
MULTIPLE-CHOICE QUESTIONS

1. d **2.** c **3.** b **4.** b **5.** a

ALTERNATE FORMAT QUESTIONS
Multiple-Answer Multiple-Choice Questions

1. a, b, c, d, e **2.** a, b, e **3.** a, b, d

CHAPTER 11

MASTERING THE INFORMATION
FILL IN THE BLANKS

1. gynecoid
2. anthropoid
3. platypelloid
4. android

MATCHING

1. b **2.** c **3.** a

TRUE OR FALSE

1. T **2.** F **3.** F **4.** F **5.** T

APPLYING YOUR KNOWLEDGE

CASE STUDY

1. Suggested answers may include but are not limited to the following: lithotomy position; on back with thighs flexed and feet resting in examining table stirrups; buttocks extending slightly beyond end of examining table; pillow under head.
2. Suggested answers may include but are not limited to the following: speculums; spatula for cervical scraping; clean examination glove; lubricant; glass slide or liquid collection device for Pap smear; culture tube; two or three sterile cotton-tipped applicators or cytobrushes for cervical cultures; good examining light; stool at correct sitting height.
3. Suggested answers may include but are not limited to the following: allow woman time to talk before exam and before assuming position; having support person at head of the table during exam; talking with woman throughout exam, explaining what will be happening; holding woman's hand; encouraging slow deep breaths to relax; draping to protect privacy and prevent chilling; pillow under head to help abdominal muscles relax.

PRACTICING FOR NCLEX

MULTIPLE-CHOICE QUESTIONS

1. d   2. c   3. b   4. d   5. c

ALTERNATE FORMAT QUESTIONS

Multiple-Answer Multiple-Choice Questions

1. a, b, d   2. a, b, c   3. a, c, d, e

CHAPTER 12

MASTERING THE INFORMATION

FILL IN THE BLANKS

1. teratogens
2. first
3. Hemorrhoids

MATCHING

1. i   2. f   3. g   4. a   5. h   6. b   7. j   8. e   9. c
10. d

SHORT ANSWER

1. Education
2. *Bathing*: tub baths are permitted unless membranes are ruptured, cervical dilation is present, or balance is disturbed. *Breast care*: firm bra with wide straps, wash colostrum away with clean water, use pads inside bra to keep nipples dry and change pads frequently. *Perineal hygiene*: douching is contraindicated; wipe from front to back. *Dressing*: common sense and comfort, moderate to low-heeled shoes, avoid restrictive clothing, including garters, tight girdles, and knee high stockings. *Sexual activity*:

permitted as tolerated, except when membranes have ruptured or vaginal spotting is noted; if history of spontaneous abortion, refrain from sex until after the time of prior abortion; use of condom with nonmonogamous partners, use caution with oral–genital contact. *Exercise*: individualized, moderate activity, walking encouraged, jogging, or body contact sports may be contraindicated. *Sleep*: increased amounts encouraged, relaxation exercises, afternoon naps in late pregnancy. *Travel*: no restrictions in early pregnancy, late in pregnancy arrange for emergency care in case of early labor; frequent stretching on long trips.
3. Refer to Box 12.8 of the text.
4. Refer to Box 12.6, Focus on Family Teaching in text.
5. Prolonged anxiety produces physiological changes leading to vasoconstriction, including constriction of the uterine vessels that could interfere with blood and nutrient supply to the fetus.

APPLYING YOUR KNOWLEDGE

CASE STUDY

1. Suggested answers may include but are not limited to the following: increased blood volume due to pregnancy; sudden movement causing necessary circulatory adjustments to accommodate increased blood supply leading to palpitations; expanding blood volume increasing pressure on cerebral arteries causing headache.
2. Suggested answers may include but are not limited to the following: encouraging woman to talk about work and tension-related issues; assisting woman in developing appropriate measures to reduce stress; teaching positive coping strategies; encouraging woman to ask for help if needed at work.

PRACTICING FOR NCLEX

MULTIPLE-CHOICE QUESTIONS

1. b   2. a   3. b   4. a   5. c   6. c   7. b

ALTERNATE FORMAT QUESTIONS

Multiple-Answer Multiple-Choice Questions

1. a, b, e   2. b, c, e   3. a, b, c, d

CHAPTER 13

MASTERING THE INFORMATION

FILL IN THE BLANKS

1. 11.2 kg, 15.9 kg (25 to 35 lb)
2. D, B_{12}, calcium
3. 500, 1000

MATCHING

1. d   2. e   3. b   4. i   5. a   6. h   7. j   8. c   9. f
10. g

SHORT ANSWER

1. Inadequate maternal dietary intake could result in fetal deprivation with premature birth, stillborn, small-for-gestational age newborn, functional immaturity, or birth anomalies.
2. High parity, short intervals between pregnancies, or rigorous dieting for weight loss may deplete nutritional reserves. (See text for additional factors.)
3. Foods with caffeine should be avoided because caffeine stimulates the central nervous system and is associated with low birth weight. Artificial sweeteners should be avoided as much as possible, since safety is not completely established; saccharine is eliminated slowly from the fetus; alcoholic beverages should not be ingested because of their potentially teratogenic effects on the fetus.
4. *Protein.* Source: meat, eggs, milk. Significance: supplies needed B vitamins (B_{12}) and essential amino acids. *Calcium.* Source: milk, milk products. Significance: necessary for fetal skeletal and tooth formation. *Fat.* Source: vegetable oils are preferred. Significance: supplies essential fatty acid needed for new cell growth. *Folic acid.* Source: fresh fruits and vegetables. Significance: necessary for red blood cell formation. Iodine. Source: iodized salt, seafood. Significance: essential for the formation of thyroxine and proper thyroid gland function. *Iron.* Source: organ meats, eggs, green leafy vegetables, whole grains, enriched breads, dried fruit. Significance: needed to build hemoglobin and increased red cell volume.

APPLYING YOUR KNOWLEDGE

CASE STUDY

1. Suggested answers may include but are not limited to the following: usual dietary intake (dietary recall) including snacks; person responsible for cooking; level of activity; food likes and dislikes; level of knowledge about nutrition and pregnancy; possible psychosocial issues related to pregnancy, such as acceptance, extent of support.
2. Suggested answers may include but are not limited to the following: rejection of food sources identified by adults as nutritious; intake of "fast foods" and "junk foods"; nutrients often lacking such as calcium, iron, folic acid, and total calories.
3. Suggested answers may include but are not limited to the following: for both the need for intake of a nutritious diet adapting instructions to their developmental stage and lifestyle. For adolescent: food sources high in calcium, iron, folic acid, and total calories; respect for right to reject traditional foods as long as nutrient intake sufficient; need for nutritious snacks instead of "junk foods"; assistance with preparation of nutritious foods by adolescent or support person or parents. For woman over age 40: high fluid intake to remove waste products; adequate calcium to prevent bone density loss; suggestions based on woman's lifestyle and demands.

PRACTICING FOR NCLEX

MULTIPLE-CHOICE QUESTIONS

1. c **2.** a **3.** c **4.** b

ALTERNATE FORMAT QUESTIONS

Multiple-Answer Multiple-Choice Questions

1. a, d, e **2.** a, c **3.** a, b, c

CHAPTER 14

MASTERING THE INFORMATION

FILL IN THE BLANKS

1. psychosexual method
2. Effleurage
3. Kegel
4. psychoprophylactic

MATCHING

1. d **2.** f **3.** b **4.** a **5.** e **6.** c

SHORT ANSWER

1. **a.** *Distraction*: If brain cells of the body that register pain are all preoccupied with stimuli other than pain, these cells will not register pain. Therefore, focusing on other stimuli will divert attention and reduce pain.
   b. *Reduction of anxiety*: Pain impulses to the brain are enhanced in the presence of anxiety. Reducing anxiety will reduce pain perception.
2. **a.** *Hospital settings*: Advantages: attended by skilled professionals during labor, birth, and the postpartal period; encouraged to be prepared to control the discomfort of birthing through nonmedication measures; encouraged to consider breastfeeding; emergency care and extended high-risk care are immediately available. Disadvantages: mother does not feel totally in control of the birthing process; possible separation from the family; possible fragmentation of care.
   b. *Alternative birth center*: Advantages: extended high-risk care is easily arranged; woman encouraged to control discomfort of labor through nonmedication measures; woman encouraged to be knowledgeable about labor process and participate in decision making; woman encouraged to breastfeed; family presence; attendance by skilled professions during labor and birth. Disadvantages: extended high-risk care not immediately available; woman may be fatigued following birth and she must independently monitor her postpartal status.
   c. *Home birth*: Advantages: the woman has more control over the childbirth experience and may avoid nosocomial infections; she has the greatest freedom to express her individuality and there is no separation from family; allows for family integrity. Disadvantages: adequate equipment other than first line

emergency equipment unavailable; abrupt change in goals possible if hospitalization needed; woman and support person may become exhausted because of responsibility placed on them; possible interference with "taking-in phase"; woman must independently monitor her postpartal status.

APPLYING YOUR KNOWLEDGE

CASE STUDY

1. Suggested answers may include but are not limited to the following: level of health; ability to adapt to changing circumstances; availability of adequate support persons during labor and for several days after birth.
2. Suggested answers may include but are not limited to the following: encouragement of family integrity; no separation of woman and family; immediate integration of newborn into family.
3. Suggested answers may include but are not limited to the following: outcomes for abdominal contraction–reduction of constipation, effective second-stage pushing, restoration of abdominal tone after pregnancy—use of standing or lying position; demonstration of tightening and relaxing muscles; ability to repeat exercises throughout day; demonstration of "blowing out candle" technique (deep inspiration, normal exhalation, forceful exhalation); outcomes of pelvic floor contractions–reduction of postpartal pain, promotion of perineal healing—use of sitting position or ambulating; demonstration of tightening muscles of perineum (like stopping flow of urine, holding for 3 seconds and then relaxing) with repetition of sequence 10 times; demonstration of rapid contraction and relaxation of muscles surrounding vagina 10 to 25 times; outcomes for pelvic rocking—relief of backache during pregnancy and early labor, increased flexibility—use of different positions (hands and knees, lying, sitting, standing); demonstration of arching of back holding for 1 minute, then hollowing back.

PRACTICING FOR NCLEX

MULTIPLE-CHOICE QUESTIONS

1. a 2. b 3. c

ALTERNATE FORMAT QUESTIONS

Multiple-Answer Multiple-Choice Questions

1. b, d 2. a, d 3. a, b, e

CHAPTER 15

MASTERING THE INFORMATION

FILL IN THE BLANKS

1. minus (negative), plus (positive)
2. preparatory (latent)
3. ripening

MATCHING

1. d 2. k 3. h 4. b 5. a 6. c 7. f 8. e 9. g 10. j 11. i

ADDITIONAL MATCHING QUESTIONS

1. e 2. d 3. f 4. c 5. a

SHORT ANSWER

1. temperature
2. uterus, cervix, vagina, external perineum
3. Any three of the following are correct: lightening, increased level of activity, slight weight loss, Braxton Hicks contractions, ripening of the cervix, uterine contractions, show, and rupture of the membranes
4. Passenger, passage, powers, psyche
5. inspection, palpation, vaginal examination, fetal heart tones, sonography
6. Any three of the following would be correct: uterine muscle stretching, pressure on cervix, oxytocin stimulation, change in ratio of estrogen and progesterone, placental age and deterioration, rising fetal cortisol levels, and fetal membrane production of prostaglandin.
7. Diaphoresis serves to cool and limit warming of the woman through the evaporation process.
8. Labor is longer due to ineffective descent of the fetus, ineffective dilation of the cervix, and irregular and weak uterine contractions.
9. Leopold's maneuvers are a systematic method of observation and palpation to determine fetal presentation and position. Four maneuvers are performed with the woman in a supine position with her knees flexed and her bladder empty. (Refer to Text Box 15.6 for more information.)
10. Labor can result in emotional distress, fatigue, and fear in the woman. The nurse should provide culturally sensitive support and stress-reduction measures, promote the presence of a significant other, explain all actions, and not be judgmental or have high expectations of the woman's performance.
11. The mother's pulse and blood pressure both increase during contractions. The fetal pulse may slow slightly during contractions with a return to baseline levels.
12. The father or significant other can provide an important support to the mother during the labor process and may serve as a labor coach.
13. Fetal tachycardia indicates fetal distress (severe due to hypoxia, maternal fever, drugs, fetal arrhythmia, or maternal anemia, or hyperthyroidism). Fetal bradycardia when moderate is not considered serious and is probably due to a vagal response; if severe, it signifies fetal hypoxia. Late deceleration suggests uteroplacental insufficiency or decreased uterine blood flow during contractions. Variable pattern indicates compression of the cord. Sinusoidal pattern indicates fetal anemia or hypoxia.

APPLYING YOUR KNOWLEDGE

CASE STUDY

1. Suggested answers may include but are not limited to the following: explaining that each labor is different and that this is woman's first labor experience; providing frequent updates about progress and condition; focusing on positive aspects; ensuring continuous support by nurse and woman's sister; encouraging woman and husband to talk about husband's work and making a mutual decision.
2. Suggested answers may include but are not limited to the following: holding woman's hand; providing frequent updates on condition; encouraging sister to participate if woman allows; checking on woman frequently; offering comfort measures; staying with the woman as she enters the second stage.
3. Suggested answers may include but are not limited to the following: address previous learning and experience to determine knowledge level; assessment of previous labor pattern and what was done; providing continuous encouragement with frequent explanations and updates on progress.

PRACTICING FOR NCLEX

MULTIPLE-CHOICE QUESTIONS

1. b **2.** d **3.** d **4.** b **5.** d **6.** b **7.** a **8.** c **9.** c
10. d **11.** b **12.** a **13.** c **14.** b **15.** b

ALTERNATE FORMAT QUESTIONS

Multiple-Answer Multiple-Choice Questions

1. b, c, e **2.** a, b, e **3.** b, c, a, e, d, f

HOT SPOT QUESTIONS

1. a **2.** a
3.

−4 (floating)
−3
−2
−1
0 (engaged)
+1
+2
+3
+4 (at outlet)

CHAPTER 16

MASTERING THE INFORMATION

MATCHING

1. i, **2.** c **3.** g **4.** j **5.** e **6.** b **7.** a **8.** d **9.** f
10. h

SHORT ANSWER

1. Enduring a painful labor.
2. Educating women about the advantages of prepared childbirth; helping women to use breathing patterns or other comfort techniques during labor so that they need a minimum of analgesia and anesthesia; conscientious monitoring of women who receive analgesics and anesthesia during labor and birth.
3. anoxia due to uterine contractions, stretching of the cervix and perineum
4. systemic, T10, L1
5. Knowledge allows the woman to make the best choices for herself and her child; it also decreases fear and anxiety related to the labor experience.
6. Knowledge reduces anxiety and decreases the amount of pain medication that may be required.
7. Pain medications given too early in the labor experience tend to slow or even stop contractions, which will delay dilation of the cervix and prolong labor. Once labor is well under way, however, pain medication could speed the progress of labor because the woman is able to work with, not against, contractions.
8. The significant other could provide support and decrease the woman's anxiety and pain.

APPLYING YOUR KNOWLEDGE

CASE STUDY

1. Suggested answers may include but are not limited to the following: impact —increased anxiety on both woman and partner leading to increased anxiety for the woman and increased pain sensation; couple's view of pain and pain relief; couple's expectations about pain; actions—instructions in methods for coping and nonpharmacologic methods; information about progress of labor and status; encouragement of partner to support woman; use of partner to assist woman in feeling in control; additional support from nursing personnel.
2. Suggested answers may include but are not limited to the following: all medications crossing placenta with some effect on fetus; avoidance of testing woman to limit of her endurance; effective use balancing relaxation and relief with minimal systemic effects; administration of medication as early as woman needs it; medications variable in duration (meperidine given if birth greater than 3 hours away); safety and risks associated with each type of analgesia or anesthesia so couple can make informed choice.
3. Suggested answer may include but are not limited to the following: use of medications if appropriate; position changes; use of prepared childbirth method.

PRACTICING FOR NCLEX

MULTIPLE-CHOICE QUESTIONS

1. b **2.** b **3.** c **4.** a **5.** c

ALTERNATE FORMAT QUESTIONS
Multiple-Answer Multiple-Choice Questions

1. b, c, d, e, f **2.** a, c, f **3.** b, c

CHAPTER 17

MASTERING THE INFORMATION
FILL IN THE BLANKS
1. Kegel (perineal)
2. lochia serosa
3. Afterpains
MATCHING
1. f **2.** i **3.** c **4.** d **5.** a **6.** h **7.** b **8.** j **9.** e
10. g
ADDITIONAL MATCHING QUESTIONS
1. a **2.** c **3.** d **4.** b
SHORT ANSWER
1. Taking-in phase
2. Lactation
3. Episiotomy
4. During the taking-in phase, the woman is passive and wishes to be ministered to; during the taking-hold phase, the woman begins to initiate actions and takes more, but not all, responsibility for herself and her child; during the letting-go phase, the woman redefines and assumes her new role.
5. A sitz bath supplies moist heat, which increases circulation to the perineum, thereby reducing edema, and promotes healing and comfort. An ice bag during the first 24 hours postpartum will aid in reducing edema and possible hematoma formation and promote healing and comfort.
6. *Fundus*: Immediately postpartum, it can be found halfway between the umbilicus and symphysis pubis; it will decrease one fingerbreadth per day (1 cm/day in size) from the umbilicus until no longer palpable.
  Cervix: Immediately after delivery, it is soft and malleable with the internal and external os open; 7 days postpartum, the external os is narrowed to a pencil-sized opening and is firm. The external os assumes a permanent starlike or slitlike pattern.
  Vagina: The hymen is permanently torn. The vagina is soft with few rugae, a large diameter and a thin wall early postpartum. The wall may thicken and involute to prepregnancy size by 6 weeks postpartum with exercise and if proper hormone release resumes.

APPLYING YOUR KNOWLEDGE
CASE STUDY
1. Suggested answers may include but are not limited to the following: impact on adjustment—change in father's expectation; disappointment due to female sex impacting ability to feel positively immediately after birth; feelings of inadequacy in not producing a son; actions—role-modeling positive behaviors; pointing out child's good points; offering positive reinforcement for interaction with newborn; allowing father to verbalize feelings.
2. Suggested answers may include but are not limited to the following: lack of comfort with touching genital area; possible lack of knowledge related to need for care; discussion of female genitalia or sexual organs considered taboo by culture; exhaustion from labor.

PRACTICING FOR NCLEX
MULTIPLE-CHOICE QUESTIONS
1. b **2.** c **3.** c **4.** c **5.** a **6.** b **7.** c **8.** c **9.** b
10. c **11.** d **12.** d **13.** a **14.** b **15.** b **16.** d
ALTERNATE FORMAT QUESTIONS
Multiple-Answer Multiple-Choice Questions

1. a, c **2.** a, b **3.** a, b, e

CHAPTER 18

MASTERING THE INFORMATION
FILL IN THE BLANKS
1. neonatal period
2. 120 to 140 beats per minute
3. acrocyanosis
MATCHING
1. c **2.** f **3.** b **4.** e **5.** g **6.** d **7.** h **8.** a **9.** j
10. i
TRUE OR FALSE
1. T **2.** F **3.** F **4.** T
SHORT ANSWER
1. 30–50
2. convection, conduction, radiation, evaporation
3. Habituation, orientation, motor maturity, self-quieting ability, social behavior, and variation.
4. *Bottlefed*: stools are bright yellow, have a more foul odor. *Breastfed*: stools are light yellow, sweet smelling.
5. Neonates who have not passed a stool in 24 hours past birth should be evaluated for meconium ileus, imperforate anus, or bowel obstruction.
6. *First period of reactivity*: Rapid heartbeat and respiration, alert behavior, searching activity. *Second period of reactivity*: Occurs between 2 and 6 hours of life; baby wakes again after quiet resting period, often gagging and choking on mucus that has accumulated in the mouth. He or she is again alert and responsive and interested in the surroundings. (See also Table 18.1 in the textbook.)
7. A child of 20 lb or less should be placed with the seat facing the back of the car; car seat should have a five-point harness with broad straps; parents

should not use sack sleepers or papoose clothing. Seat should face backward until the infant can sit without support (approximately 21 lb). When the infant can sit without support, he may be transferred to a toddler car seat.

8. Hemorrhage, infection, or urethral fistula may occur.
9. Cold sores may be indicative of herpes simplex; the infant's immature immune system may render him or her vulnerable to a serious illness.

APPLYING YOUR KNOWLEDGE
CASE STUDY

1. Suggested answers may include but are not limited to the following: reflexes including blink, rooting, sucking, extrusion, swallowing, palmar grasp, step-in-place, placing, plantar grasp, tonic neck, moro, Babinski, magnet, crossed extension, trunk incurvation, Landau, and deep tendon reflexes. (See Figs. 18.4 to 18.9 in the textbook.)
2. Suggested answers may include but are not limited to the following: passage of meconium; normal finding; indicative of anal patency and no meconium ileus.
3. Suggested answers may include but are not limited to the following: most likely physiologic jaundice due to break down of red blood cells and immature liver; testing of indirect bilirubin levels; if values higher, possible pathologic jaundice possibly leading to kernicterus if untreated.

PRACTICING FOR NCLEX
MULTIPLE-CHOICE QUESTIONS

1. a 2. d 3. c 4. d 5. b

ALTERNATE FORMAT QUESTIONS
Multiple-Answer Multiple-Choice Questions

1. d, e 2. b, c, d, e 3. a, c, d, f

CHAPTER 19

MASTERING THE INFORMATION
FILL IN THE BLANKS

1. Breast, mammary
2. sucking on the breast
3. 110 to 120

MATCHING

1. b 2. n 3. e 4. o 5. h 6. c 7. a 8. f 9. i
10. g 11. d 12. l 13. m 14. j 15. k

TRUE OR FALSE

1. T 2. T 3. F 4. F 5. T 6. T 7. F 8. F

SHORT ANSWER

1. Delivery of the placenta.
2. anterior pituitary, prolactin

3. Colostrum a thin, watery, yellow fluid composed of protein, sugar, fat, water, minerals, vitamins, and maternal antibodies for the first 3 to 4 days; then transitional milk on 2nd to 4th day, and eventually mature or true milk by the 10th day.

APPLYING YOUR KNOWLEDGE
CASE STUDY

1. Suggested answers may include but are not limited to the following: for mother—a protective function in preventing breast cancer; aid in uterine involution; empowering empowering effect, because it is a skill only a woman can master; cost and preparation time reduction; opportunity for true symbiotic bond between mother and child; for newborn—anti-infective properties; ideal electrolyte and mineral composition for human infant growth; ease in digestibility; improved ability to regulate calcium or phosphorus levels; prevention of excess weight gain.
2. Suggested answers may include but are not limited to the following: frequent breast emptying via infant sucking; pain relief; breast support; warm packs to breasts or warm shower with massage to promote milk flow; manual expression or breast pumping; assurance that symptoms of engorgement are healthy and temporary usually subsiding 24 hours after it first becomes apparent.
3. Suggested answers may include but are not limited to the following: football hold or maternal positioning (lying on side with pillow); stimulation of rooting reflex; grasping nipple; releasing from nipple when breastfeeding completed.

PRACTICING FOR NCLEX
MULTIPLE-CHOICE QUESTIONS

1. b 2. a 3. c 4. c 5. d 6. a 7. c

ALTERNATE FORMAT QUESTIONS
Multiple-Answer Multiple-Choice Questions

1. a, c, e 2. d, e 3. a, b, e

CHAPTER 20

MASTERING THE INFORMATION
FILL IN THE BLANKS

1. Poor placental perfusion
2. stasis of blood, hypercoagulability, blood vessel damage
3. *Escherichia coli* (*E. coli*)

MATCHING

1. c 2. h 3. d 4. a 5. i 6. f 7. g 8. e 9. b
10. j

ADDITIONAL MATCHING EXERCISES

1. b **2.** c **3.** d **4.** e **5.** a

SHORT ANSWER

1. Refer to Table 20.1 in the textbook for examples.
2. Pregnancy results in dilated ureters and stasis of urine, which predisposes a woman to urinary tract infection.
3. *Diet*: 1800 to 2200 calorie diet, evenly distributed over three meals and three snacks. *Exercise*: begin exercise regime before pregnancy, maintain consistent daily exercise, and eat a protein or complex carbohydrate snack before exercise. *Insulin*: dosage and type may need adjustment—less early in pregnancy, more late in pregnancy. *Glucose monitoring*: blood testing is preferred, use milk to treat hypoglycemia.

APPLYING YOUR KNOWLEDGE

CASE STUDY

1. Suggested answers may include but are not limited to the following: between weeks 28 to 32 with peak of increased blood volume; severe symptoms possibly occurring any time during pregnancy.
2. Suggested answers may include but are not limited to the following: impact—increased demands of small children; inability to obtain adequate rest or nutrition; possible forgetfulness with taking medications if ordered due to demands of children; possible increased risk of infection due to small children especially if in day care or other activities where they may be exposed; interventions—planning ways to obtain rest; getting woman help with children and household; offering suggestions for ways to ensure adequate nutrition; assisting with planning and scheduling medications if ordered to ensure compliance.

PRACTICING FOR NCLEX

MULTIPLE-CHOICE QUESTIONS

1. d **2.** b **3.** a **4.** d **5.** a **6.** d **7.** b **8.** a **9.** a
10. d **11.** b **12.** c **13.** c

ALTERNATE FORMAT QUESTIONS

Multiple-Answer Multiple-Choice Questions

1. c, e **2.** b, c, d **3.** a, d, e

CHAPTER 21

MASTERING THE INFORMATION

FILL IN THE BLANKS

1. gestational trophoblastic disease, premature cervical dilatation
2. abruptio placenta
3. isoimmunization

MATCHING

1. d **2.** g **3.** f **4.** i **5.** j **6.** h **7.** k **8.** a **9.** e
10. c **11.** b

IDENTIFICATION

1. c **2.** a **3.** b **4.** c **5.** b **6.** a

SHORT ANSWER

1. Spontaneous abortion.
2. Ectopic pregnancy.
3. HELLP syndrome.
4. Mild preeclampsia.
5. Hydramnios.
6. The time during pregnancy at which bleeding occurs helps in the identification of the cause of the bleeding.
7. A woman with an ectopic pregnancy may experience the same initial symptoms of early pregnancy. However, if tubal rupture occurs, the woman may experience a sharp, stabbing, lower abdominal pain; vaginal spotting; and possibly signs of shock.
8. Heparin is used in disseminated intravascular coagulation (DIC) to stop blood coagulation so that coagulation factors will be available to restore normal clotting throughout the body.
9. A woman with multiple gestation may be instructed to do the following: maintain bedrest the last 2 to 3 months of the pregnancy; refrain from coitus during the last 2 to 3 months of pregnancy; plan extra rest time during the day; eat six small meals per day instead of three large ones; report any abnormal bleeding or swelling, since the risk for eclampsia, hydramnios, placenta previa, and anemia are higher in multiple gestation. Counseling and support to help the woman work through two role changes instead of one should also be a part of the teaching plan.

APPLYING YOUR KNOWLEDGE

CASE STUDY

1. Suggested answers may include but are not limited to the following: proteinuria and blood pressure rises to 140/90 mm Hg, taken on two occasions at least 6 hours apart; systolic blood pressure greater than 30 mm Hg and a diastolic pressure greater than 15 mm Hg above prepregnancy values; edema not just the typical ankle edema of pregnancy but also edema in the upper part of the body; weight gain of more than 2 lb per week in the second trimester or 1 lb per week in the third trimester. Teaching involving looking for these signs, especially edema and weight gain.
2. Suggested answers may include but are not limited to the following: antiplatelet therapy; bedrest; nutrition; emotional support; more frequent follow up; compliance with instructions and therapy.

PRACTICING FOR NCLEX

MULTIPLE-CHOICE QUESTIONS

1. c **2.** d **3.** d **4.** a **5.** c **6.** c **7.** c **8.** a **9.** c
10. c

ALTERNATE FORMAT QUESTIONS

Multiple-Answer Multiple-Choice Questions

1. c, e **2.** b, d **3.** a, c, e

CHAPTER 22

MASTERING THE INFORMATION

FILL IN THE BLANKS

1. emancipated minor
2. engagement, prolonged, fetal descent
3. postpartum hemorrhage

MATCHING

1. e **2.** f **3.** d **4.** j **5.** c **6.** i **7.** h **8.** a **9.** b
10. g

SHORT ANSWER

1. Early age of menarche in girls, an increase in the rate of sexual activity among teenagers, and a lack of knowledge of (or inability to use) contraceptive information among sexually active teenagers and desire by teens to have a baby.
2. Any three of the following would be correct: increased incidence of pregnancy-induced hypertension, iron-deficiency anemia, preterm labor, and cephalopelvic disproportion, inability to adapt postpartally, lack of knowledge about infant care.
3. The nurse can teach adolescents about the dangers of substance abuse and the complications, both psychological and physical, of teenage pregnancy. In addition, nurses can research effective birth control measures for adolescents (that they might actually use).
4. The nurse has a legal obligation to help devise a safe plan of care for the child while protecting the cognitively challenged mother's right to maintain control of her child.
5. Any of the following would be accurate: fear of discovery and being reported to authorities for drug abuse, need for frequent drug doses and inability to wait for services, insufficient finances to support both her drug habit and medical care and nutritious food.

APPLYING YOUR KNOWLEDGE

CASE STUDY

1. Suggested answers may include but are not limited to the following: modifications for antepartal care, pregnancy, labor and birth; mobility level; sensory capabilities; adaptations; safety; transportation; elimination; knowledge level and educational needs; support persons; plans for postpartum care of self and newborn; feeding choices for newborn; postpartum contraception.

2. Suggested answers may include but are not limited to the following: adolescent nutritional issues; adolescent developmental stage; support persons available; meaning of pregnancy to adolescent.
3. Suggested answers may include but are not limited to the following: suggestions dependent on adolescent's lifestyle (i.e., frequency of sexual activity), motor and sensory limitations (limited upper extremity function may interfere with using diaphragm), and any other underlying medical problems such as history of thrombophlebitis (would contraindicate use of oral contraceptives); emphasis on need for safe sex practices.

PRACTICING FOR NCLEX

MULTIPLE-CHOICE QUESTIONS

1. a **2.** c **3.** b **4.** a **5.** a **6.** a **7.** d **8.** d **9.** a

ALTERNATE FORMAT QUESTIONS

Multiple-Answer Multiple-Choice Questions

1. a, b, c, e **2.** a, c, e, f **3.** b, c, d

CHAPTER 23

MASTERING THE INFORMATION

FILL IN THE BLANKS

1. Vacuum extraction
2. knee-chest, Trendelenburg
3. Inertia, dysfunctional

MATCHING

1. h **2.** i **3.** e **4.** j **5.** g **6.** c **7.** a **8.** d **9.** b
10. f

DYSFUNCTION AND THE STAGES OF LABOR

1. a **2.** a **3.** b **4.** b **5.** a **6.** a

SHORT ANSWER

1. pathologic retraction ring, rupture
2. heart, kidney
3. cord compression, hypoxia/anoxia
4. The power (force that propels the fetus, uterine contractions), the passenger (the fetus), and the passageway (the birth canal).
5. Fetal and uterine monitoring.
6. Hypotonic uterine contractions, hypertonic uterine contractions, and uncoordinated contractions.
7. Prolonged latent phase, prolonged deceleration phase, protracted active phase, and secondary arrest of dilatation.
8. Small-for-gestational age (SGA) infants; cord prolapse; cord compression, intracranial hemorrhage, abnormal fetal presentation.
9. Any two: dysfunctional labor, early rupture of membranes, higher risk of anoxia from prolapsed cord; traumatic injury to the aftercoming head, fracture of the spine or arm.

10. Occipitoposterior position, breech presentation, face presentation, brow presentation, and transverse lie.
11. Woman is unable to push with contractions, cessation of progress in the second stage of labor, fetus in abnormal position, or fetus is immature.
12. Any two: complete, frank, double footing, and single footing.

APPLYING YOUR KNOWLEDGE

CASE STUDY

1. Suggested answers may include but are not limited to the following: anxiety about multiple births; anxiety related to preterm labor; fear/anxiety related to breech positioning of one twin; anxiety/fear related to status of twins currently; worry/concern/fear related to history of previous problems with multiple birth (death of one twin) and similar things happening now.
2. Suggested answers may include but are not limited to the following: maternal status, including vital signs, uterine contractions, cervical effacement and dilatation; fetal heart rates and patterns; maternal and fetal responses to labor; maternal complaints of pain; couple's ability to cope; couple's understanding of the current situation; couple's level of anxiety and fear; laboratory test results.

PRACTICING FOR NCLEX

1. b 2. c 3. a 4. c 5. d

ALTERNATE FORMAT QUESTIONS

Multiple-Answer Multiple-Choice Questions

1. a, c, d, f 2. b, c, e, f 3. b, c, e

CHAPTER 24

MASTERING THE INFORMATION

MATCHING

1. b 2. c 3. d 4. a

TRUE OR FALSE

1. T 2. F 3. F 4. F

SHORT ANSWER

1. A well-informed support person will be able to help minimize the client's experiences of anxiety.
2. A sonogram aids in locating the placenta to avoid an accidental incision of this organ during the surgical procedure. It also helps to determine fetal presentation and maturity.
3. Urinary output must be assessed to determine the presence of urinary retention, overextension of bladder capacity, and potential for permanent bladder damage, and to avoid interference with uterine contractions that may lead to postpartal hemorrhage. Voiding also provides evidence of adequate urinary and circulatory function.

4. *Pneumonia*: Pain minimizes activity, allowing secretions in lung to pool. Pain increases when performing respiratory toileting exercise. *Thrombophlebitis*: Pain discourages walking, leading to venous stasis and poor circulation of the femoral veins. *Interference with maternal–infant bonding*: Experiences of pain lessen tactile stimulation, which hampers the bonding process.
5. *Transcutaneous electrical nerve stimulation (TENS)*: Method of controlling pain sensation by use of electrodes on the skin to irritate or stimulate the large afferent (sensory) nerve fibers, which facilitates the gating theory. The unit is turned on and off by the patient. *Patient-controlled analgesia (PCA)*: pain control device. Patient administers precalculated dose of intravenous narcotic analgesic by pressing a button on a special pump. Pump features a "lock-out" setting to prevent drug overdose.
6. During a vaginal birth, the woman typically loses 300 to 500 mL of blood; with a cesarean birth, blood loss ranges from 500 to 1000 mL.

APPLYING YOUR KNOWLEDGE

CASE STUDY

1. Suggested answers may include but are not limited to the following: position of comfort; use of pillows to support areas; splinting incision with coughing and deep breathing.
2. Suggested answers may include but are not limited to the following: pain relief; adequate oxygenation; hemodynamic status (fluid balance and prevention of hemorrhage from lack of uterine involution); maternal–newborn bonding.
3. Suggested answers may include but are not limited to the following: blood loss from surgery; possible increased blood loss if uterine contraction ineffective; lack of fluid intake or increased fluid loss (diaphoresis, vomiting, or diarrhea) if labor prior to cesarean was prolonged; possible NPO status before cesarean.

PRACTICING FOR NCLEX

MULTIPLE-CHOICE QUESTIONS

1. b 2. d 3. c 4. a 5. a

ALTERNATE FORMAT QUESTIONS

Multiple-Answer Multiple-Choice Questions

1. a, b, d 2. a, c, d, e 3. b, c, e

CHAPTER 25

MASTERING THE INFORMATION

FILL IN THE BLANKS

1. lighter
2. perineal pads
3. Uterine inversion

MATCHING

1. e **2.** g **3.** a **4.** d **5.** f **6.** c **7.** b

TRUE OR FALSE

1. T **2.** T **3.** T **4.** F

SHORT ANSWER

1. uterine atony, lacerations, retained placental fragments, uterine inversion, or disseminated intravascular coagulation
2. Deficiency in clotting ability caused by vascular injury.
3. Premature separation of the placenta, missed early abortion, and fetal death in utero.
4. When wiping from back to front, organisms may be brought forward from the rectum to the vagina or perineal site of injury.
5. Assess lochia for color, odor, and amount. Assess uterus for tenderness, size, and consistency. Assess vital signs to support evaluation of other data.
6. Retained placental fragments keep the uterus from contracting fully, leading to possible hemorrhage. Inspection of the placenta is key to ensure that the entire placenta has been expelled. Retained fragments are common with succenturiate placenta and placenta accreta, which can be noted on inspection.

APPLYING YOUR KNOWLEDGE

CASE STUDY

1. Suggested answers may include but are not limited to the following: early rupture of membranes; retained placental fragments; postpartal hemorrhage; preexisting anemia; prolonged and difficulty labor; internal fetal monitoring; local vaginal infection present at time of birth; uterine exploration at birth.
2. Suggested answers may include but are not limited to the following: benign temperature elevation on first postpartal day with fever usually manifesting on third or fourth postpartal day (an increase in oral temperature to more than 100.4°F (38°C) for two consecutive 24-hour periods, excluding the first 24-hour period after birth); possible accompanying chills, loss of appetite, and general malaise; painful uterus not well contracted; complaints of strong afterpains; dark brown foul lochia of increased amount; possible scant or absent lochia if fever high.

PRACTICING FOR NCLEX

MULTIPLE-CHOICE QUESTIONS

1. d **2.** c **3.** c **4.** b **5.** c

ALTERNATE FORMAT QUESTIONS

Multiple-Answer Multiple-Choice Questions

1. a, c, d **2.** b, c, f **3.** b, c, e

CHAPTER 26

MASTERING THE INFORMATION

FILL IN THE BLANKS

1. blindness
2. bilirubin.
3. vitamin E
4. glycolysis

MATCHING

1. e **2.** c **3.** d **4.** a **5.** b

TRUE OR FALSE

1. T **2.** T **3.** F **4.** F

SHORT ANSWER

1. During the first few seconds of life, infant takes several weak gasps of air and then immediately stops breathing.
2. *Placenta received insufficient nutrients*: Partial placental separation leading to bleeding, infarction, fibrosis, and reduced placental surface for exchange. *Inefficient transport of nutrients to the fetus*: Systemic diseases in the mother may cause decreased blood flow to the placenta. *Lack of adequate nutrition*: Poor nutritional intake occurs in teen pregnancy.
3. Blood is removed by gravity using a venous catheter advanced into the right atrium. Blood is circulated from the catheter to the ECMO machine for oxygenation and warming, then returned to the newborn via catheter advanced through the carotid artery.
4. *Periodic apnea*: No bradycardia seen in the irregular breathing patterns. *True apnea*: Irregular breathing patterns lasting more than 20 seconds with bradycardia.
5. Small plugs of meconium may be pushed farther into the lungs if infant is ventilated before the airway is cleared.
6. Transient tachypnea of the newborn (TTN) results from slow absorption of lung fluid. Newborn respiratory rate remains between 80 to 120 after first hour of birth, mild retractions, marked cyanosis, chest radiograph reveals fluid in central lung fields with adequate aeration; syndrome peaks in 3 hours and tends to fade by 2 hours.

APPLYING YOUR KNOWLEDGE

CASE STUDY

1. Suggested answers may include but are not limited to the following: method of delivery—cesarean birth leading to slow absorption of fluids; maternal history of infection; fetal distress during labor; low APGAR score; small for gestational age and preterm status.
2. Suggested answers may include but are not limited to the following: assessing airway patency and instituting measures to ensure it including oxygen administration, intubation, and mechanical

ventilation; observing for retractions; placing new-born under infant warmer; removing clothing from chest; positioning with head of bed elevated 15°; suctioning if secretions are present; monitoring oxygen saturation levels; preventing hypoglycemia; maintaining body temperature; administering intravenous fluids; promoting newborn–parent bonding.

PRACTICING FOR NCLEX

MULTIPLE-CHOICE QUESTIONS

1. b **2.** b **3.** d **4.** d **5.** b **6.** a **7.** c **8.** a **9.** a

ALTERNATE FORMAT QUESTIONS
Multiple-Answer Multiple-Choice Questions

1. b, d, f **2.** a, d, e **3.** a, c, e

CHAPTER 27

MASTERING THE INFORMATION

FILL IN THE BLANKS

1. Anencephaly
2. Ortolani's click
3. Arnold Chiari
4. meconium plug
5. subluxation, dislocation

MATCHING

1. e **2.** f **3.** d **4.** k **5.** b **6.** q **7.** l **8.** c **9.** i
10. h **11.** j **12.** g **13.** a **14.** p **15.** r **16.** n
17. o **18.** m

APPLYING YOUR KNOWLEDGE

CASE STUDY

1. Suggested answers may include but are not limited to the following: protrusion of spinal cord and the meninges through the vertebrae with loss of motor and sensory function absent beyond this point; flaccidity and lack of sensation of the lower extremities; loss of bowel and bladder control; laxity of legs; continuous dribbling of urine and stool; often accompanying talipes (clubfoot) disorders and developmental hip dysplasia; possible hydrocephalus.
2. Suggested answers may include but are not limited to the following: priority—prevention of infection due to exposed sac; interventions—keeping sac moist with moist saline compresses or antibiotic gauze; avoiding pressure on sac; using aseptic technique when caring for sac; prone or supported side positioning with support above and below defect; towel under abdomen; protection between legs if positioned on side; prevention of fecal or urine contamination of sac; maintaining warmth; checking any leakage for glucose.

PRACTICING FOR NCLEX

MULTIPLE-CHOICE QUESTIONS

1. c **2.** a **3.** a **4.** c **5.** b **6.** d

ALTERNATE FORMAT QUESTIONS
Multiple-Answer Multiple-Choice Questions

1. b, d **2.** a, e **3.** c, d, e

CHAPTER 28

MASTERING THE INFORMATION

FILL IN THE BLANKS

1. Height, weight
2. Anticipatory guidance
3. Maturation
4. Growth
5. Development

MATCHING

1. c **2.** e **3.** f **4.** a **5.** b **6.** d

ADDITIONAL MATCHING QUESTIONS

1. c **2.** e **3.** d **4.** b **5.** a

SHORT ANSWER

1.

Stage	Childhood Division	Age Range
a. Oral stage	Infant	1 month to 1 year
b. Anal	Toddler	1 year to 3 years
c. Genital	Preschooler	3 years to 6 years
d. Latent	School-aged	5 years to 13 years
e. Genital	Adolescent	13 years to 18 years

2. **a.** Toddler (autonomy)
   b. Adolescent (identity)
   c. School-aged (industry)
   d. Infant (trust)
   e. Preschooler (initiative)

Stages of Moral Development
1. Preschooler
2. Adolescent (postconventional)
3. Infant (prereligious)
4. Toddler (punishment–obedience)
5. Young school-aged (conventional)

APPLYING YOUR KNOWLEDGE

CASE STUDY

1. Suggested answers may include but are not limited to the following: substage of preoperational thought—*intuitive thought*; ability to look at an object and see only one of its characteristics (referred to as centering); lack of conservation (the ability to discern truth, even though physical properties change) or reversibility

(ability to retrace steps); role fantasy and assimilation; magical thinking; accommodation; egocentrism.

2. Suggested answers may include but are not limited to the following: according to Freud—phallic stage in which child learning sexual identity via awareness of genital area (fondling own genitals, exploring genital areas, masturbation, exhibitionism); according to Erikson—initiative versus guilt in which child learning how to do things (basic problem solving), doing things desirable; asking questions, engaging in fantasy play, increasing motor activities.

3. Suggested answers may include but are not limited to the following: according to Kohlberg—doing good out of self-interest; egocentrism doing things only in return for things done for him or her; imitation of possible less-than-perfect role models; difficulty knowing what rules apply to new situations because they cannot judge whether a previously learned principle of right or wrong can be applied to this new situation.

PRACTICING FOR NCLEX

MULTIPLE-CHOICE QUESTIONS

1. b **2.** d **3.** c **4.** a **5.** b **6.** b **7.** a **8.** a

ALTERNATE FORMAT QUESTIONS

Multiple-Answer Multiple-Choice Questions

1. b, e **2.** c, e **3.** b, d, a, e, c

CHAPTER 29

MASTERING THE INFORMATION

FILL IN THE BLANKS

1. 2
2. 6
3. 4
4. above
5. social

MATCHING

1. a **2.** c **3.** f **4.** g **5.** d **6.** b **7.** e **8.** h

SHORT ANSWER

1. Provides parents with opportunity to ask questions; provide anticipatory guidance to parents; chart growth and development; observe for potential health problems.
2. Aspiration.
3. Ventral suspension, prone, sitting, and standing.
4. Check sources for lead paint; move furniture in front of electrical fixtures or use protective caps for outlets; store potentially poisonous substances out of infant's reach; never leave child unattended; and install gates at top and bottom of stairs.

5. Learn different textures and sensations; provides the opportunity to kick and exercise; provides parents opportunity to touch and communicate with child; allows playtime.
6. Gently wipe the gum pads with soft washcloth; brush erupted teeth with soft brush or washcloth once or twice a day.
7. Change the diaper frequently, clean the area after each diaper change and pat or air dry, and apply ointments and creams.
8. Duration of loose stools, number of stools per day, color and consistency of stools, evidence of blood or mucus in stools, associated fever, cramping or vomiting, infant's intake, number of wet diapers per day.

APPLYING YOUR KNOWLEDGE

CASE STUDY

1. Suggested answers may include but are not limited to the following: most infants doubling birthweight by age 6 months; or an average weight gain of 2 lb per month during first 6 months; doubling of birth weight of 7 lb—Stephen weighing approximately 14 lb; average weight gain of 2 lb/month—Stephen weighing approximately 17 lb at 5 months.
2. Suggested answers may include but are not limited to the following: slowing of heart rate from 120 to 160 beats per minute to 100 to 120 beats per minute by end of first year; slight elevation in blood pressure from average of 80/40 to 100/60 mm Hg; respiratory rate slowing from 30 to 60 breaths per minute to 20 to 30 breaths per minute by end of first year.
3. Suggested answers may include but are not limited to the following: risk for physiologic anemia at 2 to 3 months of age (due to life of red blood cell of 4 months; cells present at birth disintegrating and new cells not yet being produced inadequate replacement numbers); conversion of fetal hemoglobin to adult hemoglobin completed at 5 to 6 months of age; second decrease in serum iron levels at 6 to 9 months as last of iron stores established in utero used.
4. Suggested answers may include but are not limited to the following: need to assess infant to ensure loss of extrusion reflex and determine readiness (i.e., assessment of feeding [vigorously breastfeeding every 3 to 4 hours and not seeming satisfied or taking more than 32 oz of formula and not seeming satisfied]); if appropriate for Stephen, offering new foods one at a time, allowing child to eat item for 1 week before introducing another food, initiating feeding while being held in parent's arms, waiting a few days and trying again if infant resistant to taking solid food, starting out with small amounts such as two tablespoons, and using rice cereal (mixed fairly liquid) as first food. Important to ensure infant is ready for solid food to prevent overwhelming infant's kidneys with a heavy

solute load (with protein ingestion) and also possible delay development of food allergies in susceptible infants.

PRACTICING FOR NCLEX

MULTIPLE-CHOICE QUESTIONS

1. b **2.** c **3.** b **4.** d **5.** d **6.** b **7.** c **8.** c **9.** a
10. b **11.** a **12.** c

ALTERNATE FORMAT QUESTIONS

Multiple-Answer Multiple-Choice Questions

1. a, c **2.** d, e **3.** c, d, f

CHAPTER 30

MASTERING THE INFORMATION

FILL IN THE BLANKS

1. autonomy/independence
2. Poisonings
3. independence

MATCHING

1. b **2.** d **3.** a **4.** c **5.** f **6.** e

SHORT ANSWER

1. *15 months*: Walks alone, puts small pellets into small bottles, scribbles voluntarily with a pencil or crayon, speaks four to six words, stacks two blocks, enjoys being read to.

24 months: Walks up stairs alone using both feet on same step at the same time, opens doors turning knobs, unscrews lids, speaks two-word sentences (noun/pronoun and verb), parallel play.

30 months: Can jump down from chairs, makes simple lines or strokes for crosses with a pencil, can speak full name, names one color, holds up finger to show age, plays house, imitates parents, active play.

2. Head circumference increases only about 2 cm during the second year compared to about 12 cm during the first year.

3. During the toddler period, children play beside children next to them, not with them. This is called parallel play.

APPLYING YOUR KNOWLEDGE

CASE STUDY

1. Suggested answers may include but are not limited to the following: need for close supervision at all times; use of toddler-sized care seat until 40 to 60 lb; use of helmet when beginning to ride a tricycle; side rails on bed; safety gate on door of room; house windows closed or keep secure screens in place; gates at top and bottom of stairs; supervision at playgrounds; not allowing child to walk with sharp object in hand or mouth. Also

need to address other common safety issues such as drowning, animal bits, poisonings, and car safety.

2. Suggested answers may include but are not limited to the following: questions about toddler's ability to carry out activities of daily living providing information about the child's developmental progress and clues about child–parent relationship; determination of parent's level of understanding about toddler's growth and development and teaching and learning needs; focus on health promotion; evaluation for early detection of any growth and development delays; identification of areas of support needed by parents to cope with normal crises of toddlerhood.

3. Suggested answers may include but are not limited to the following: assessment providing information about areas of deficiencies or needs of the child and parents to develop individualized teaching plan for areas such as safety, promotion of autonomy, nutrition, health promotion, self care, and healthy family functioning.

PRACTICING FOR NCLEX

MULTIPLE-CHOICE QUESTIONS

1. d **2.** b **3.** a **4.** b **5.** d **6.** c

ALTERNATE FORMAT QUESTIONS

Multiple-Answer Multiple-Choice Questions

1. b, c, d **2.** b, d, f **3.** c, d

CHAPTER 31

MASTERING THE INFORMATION

FILL IN THE BLANKS

1. initiative
2. Oedipus complex
3. bruxism

MATCHING

1. e **2.** c **3.** a **4.** b **5.** d

SHORT ANSWER

1. a. Large body build.
b. Slim body build.
c. Knock-knee.
2. *Oedipus*: Preschool-aged boys have strong emotional attachment for their mother. *Electra*: Preschool-aged girls have strong attachment for their fathers. Each child competes with the same-sex parent for the love and attention of the other parent.
3. Preschoolers cannot comprehend that the same procedure can be performed in two different ways. Therefore, it is important to provide continuity when caring for this age group.

4. Seek to understand the child's fears. Monitor the child's exposure to environmental stimuli that may incite fears. Use a dim light in the bedroom at night.

5. Do not ask the child to recite or sing to strangers. Do not reward or punish the child in relationship to language fluency. Listen with patience. Do not discuss the child's difficulty in his presence. See also Box 31.8 for additional information.

APPLYING YOUR KNOWLEDGE
CASE STUDY

1. Suggested answers may include but are not limited to the following: suggesting that certain things are done in certain places but not in others; avoiding calling unnecessary attention to the act.

2. Suggested answers may include but are not limited to the following: never allowing anyone to touch his or her body unless he or she agrees that it is alright; explaining about "private parts"; never going anywhere with a stranger; telling person to stop if that person asks the child to show private part or touches private part.

3. Suggested answers may include but are not limited to the following: beginning preparation before the time child to feel the difference a new baby will make; moving child to bed about 3 months before birth of new baby and emphasizing the reason for the move as becoming a "big boy" rather than to make room for the baby; preparing child in advance if mother requires hospitalization during pregnancy; participating in birth education classes as appropriate.

PRACTICING FOR NCLEX
MULTIPLE-CHOICE QUESTIONS

1. b 2. d 3. c 4. b 5. b

ALTERNATE FORMAT QUESTIONS
Multiple-Answer Multiple-Choice Questions

1. b, e, f 2. a, c, d, e 3. c, d

CHAPTER 32

MASTERING THE INFORMATION
FILL IN THE BLANKS

1. 9
2. anovulatory, ovulation
3. nocturnal emissions

MATCHING

1. b 2. d 3. a 4. f 5. e 6. g 7. c

SHORT ANSWER

1. Gaining a sense of initiative is learning how to do things; doing them well is a step toward gaining a

sense of industry. When a child's environment does not allow this sense of accomplishment, he or she develops a feeling of inferiority and becomes convinced that he or she cannot do many things that he or she in fact is able to do.

2. *Decentering*: Ability to project one's self into other people's situations and see the world from their viewpoint rather than focusing only on their view. *Accommodation*: Ability to adapt thought processes to fit what is perceived. *Conservation*: Ability to appreciate that a change in shape does not necessarily mean a change in size. *Class inclusion*: The concept that objects can belong to more than one classification (i.e., stones and shells may be gathered on the beach but they are different objects).

3. Be flexible when approving reading materials. Select readings that allow the child to complete a topic or finish in a short period of time. See also Box 32.7 for more information.

4. School phobia is a child's resistance to attend school that may be manifested by physical illnesses. The illness may be due to fear of separation from parents, fear of the younger siblings usurping the parents' love, overdependence, or overprotection by the parents. To resolve the problem, the entire family must be counseled. The parents must be consistent and firm with the child. Initiating attendance at school gradually, such as attending school for fewer hours may prove to be beneficial.

5. a. *Drowning*: Teach child to swim; advise not to try to swim beyond capabilities.
   b. *Motor vehicle accidents*: Encourage use of seat belts; learn to cross streets safely; learn bicycle safety, parking lot, and school bus safety rules.
   c. *Sports injuries*: Wear appropriate gear; do not encourage the child to play beyond his capabilities or to the point of exhaustion.
   d. *Firearms*: Teach safe use of firearms; keep firearms in locked cabinet with bullets separated from gun.

APPLYING YOUR KNOWLEDGE
CASE STUDY

1. Suggested answers may include but are not limited to the following: timing of onset of puberty varies; length of time for passage through puberty also varies; puberty occurring increasingly earlier; breast development not always symmetrical; progression of development from elevation of papilla and breast bud development; average age of menarche; increase in sebaceous gland secretion; slight mucous vaginal discharge occurring around age 11 to 12; change in pH of vaginal secretions.

2. Suggested answers may include but are not limited to the following: competitive behaviors developing; interest in rules and fairness around age 10; importance of structured activities to strengthen sense of industry; need for strong ego strength (usually

developing around age 10); cautions related to risk of injury.

PRACTICING FOR NCLEX

MULTIPLE-CHOICE QUESTIONS

1. d **2.** d **3.** b **4.** b

ALTERNATE FORMAT QUESTIONS

Multiple-Answer Multiple-Choice Questions

1. a, b, d, e **2.** a, c, d **3.** a, c

CHAPTER 33

MASTERING THE INFORMATION

FILL IN THE BLANKS

1. three
2. decrease
3. increase
4. mature, young
5. 13,14; 15, 16; 17, 20
6. formal operational thought, 12, 13
7. sebum, comedones, bacterial
8. alcohol

MATCHING

1. a **2.** j **3.** e **4.** f **5.** b **6.** g **7.** i **8.** h **9.** c
10. d

SHORT ANSWER

1. Private history taking promotes independence and responsibility for self-care, and provides an opportunity for the youth to discuss matters he might not confide in front of a parent.
2. Inadequate diet, poor sleep patterns, busy activity schedules (also emotional problems or boredom due to understimulation).
3. *Intimacy*: Develop intimate (close) relationships with persons of the opposite and same sex; develop a sense of compassion for other persons. *Emancipation*: Must overcome their own and parental reluctance toward the adolescent's becoming an independent, responsible person. *Value system*: Determine who they are, and what kind of person they want to be (must establish values of internal origin, not just mimic others).
4. Educating adolescents against cigarettes, smokeless tobacco, alcohol, drug abuse, and violence, and acting as support people for adolescents during times of crisis.
5. *13-year-old*: Impulsive; full of self-doubt; wants to be grown-up but still looks like a child; loud and boisterous; begins to long for the opposite sex and "falls in love" for the first time. *14-year-old*: Quieter than at 13; more confident in themselves; searches for adult and older teen heroes to copy. *15-year-old*: Interested in approaching a member of the opposite sex; mainly physical attraction; "falls in love" frequently. *16-year-old*: Boys become sexually

mature, though increase in height continues; both sexes are able to trust their bodies more; are more coordinated. *17-year-old*: Quieter and more thoughtful about interactions.
6. Any seven of the following would be correct: Giving away prized possessions; organ donation questions; sudden, unexplained elevation of mood; accident proneness, carelessness, and death wishes; a statement such as "this is the last time you will see me"; decrease in verbal communication; withdrawal from peer activities or previously enjoyed events; previous suicide attempt; preference for art, music, and literature with themes of death; recent increase in personal conflicts with significant others; running away from home; inquiry about the hereafter; asking for information (supposedly for a friend) about suicide prevention and intervention; almost any sustained deviation (change) from the normal pattern of behavior.

APPLYING YOUR KNOWLEDGE

CASE STUDY

1. Suggested answers may include but are not limited to the following: need to develop trust; accept Angelique nonjudgmentally; approach Angelique at her eye level; use nonthreatening questions and demonstrate empathy; focus questions on possible issues that may be contributing to her current status; reinforce privacy of interaction.
2. Suggested answers may include but are not limited to the following: determining what she views as important; assisting with problem solving; encouraging her to speak honestly; referring for psychiatric evaluation; referring for counseling and/or drug abuse treatment; crisis intervention; if necessary, possible hospitalization if suicide is a possibility.

PRACTICING FOR NCLEX

MULTIPLE-CHOICE QUESTIONS

1. a **2.** a **3.** d **4.** c **5.** b **6.** a **7.** b **8.** b **9.** c
10. d

ALTERNATE FORMAT QUESTIONS

Multiple-Answer Multiple-Choice Questions

1. a, b, f **2.** a, b, c **3.** a, b, e

CHAPTER 34

MASTERING THE INFORMATION

FILL IN THE BLANKS

1. air
2. Geographic tongue
3. school, inspiration, expiration

MATCHING

1. d **2.** c **3.** b **4.** a

ADDITIONAL MATCHING QUESTIONS

1. b **2.** c **3.** d **4.** a

SHORT ANSWER

1. Introduction and explanation; demographic data; chief concern; history of chief concern; health and family profile; day history; past health history including pregnancy history; family health history; and review of systems.
2. The height and weight fall below the third percentile on a standard growth chart.
3. Cover test and Hirschburg's test.
4. Gently press one nostril closed and ask the child to inhale; then repeat this on the opposite side to ensure both sides are patent.
5. The tympanic membrane may be retracted; the malleus is extremely prominent; and the cone of light is missing.

APPLYING YOUR KNOWLEDGE

CASE STUDY

1. Suggested answers may include but are not limited to the following: adolescents and desire to have parent present based on privacy issues; importance of ascertaining Jennifer's desire to have parent present or not; need for appropriate draping during examination to expose only the part being assessed at that time; need for attentive listening to Jennifer's statements and complaints if any to provide clues to potential problems.
2. Suggested answers may include but are not limited to the following: division into four quadrants; need for systematic assessment, moving from one quadrant to the next; inspection first followed by auscultation, palpation (light then deep), and percussion.
3. Suggested answers may include but are not limited to the following: normal abdominal findings— scaphoid in older children, symmetrical, without scars or lesions; absence of liver or spleen enlargement.
4. Suggested answers may include but are not limited to the following: bowel sounds or high pinging sounds occurring at intervals of approximately 5 to 10 seconds; irregular vascular sounds such as bruits (swishing or blowing sound).

PRACTICING FOR NCLEX

MULTIPLE-CHOICE QUESTIONS

1. c **2.** b **3.** a **4.** c **5.** d **6.** c **7.** b **8.** a **9.** c **10.** a **11.** a **12.** a

ALTERNATE FORMAT QUESTIONS

Multiple-Answer Multiple-Choice Questions

1. a, c, d, e **2.** a, b **3.** b, c, d, e, a

CHAPTER 35

MASTERING THE INFORMATION

FILL IN THE BLANKS

1. Process recording
2. environment, family members, family functioning.
3. **a.** Psychomotor, **b.** Cognitive, **c.** Affective
4. Redemonstration
5. type, content, time
6. physical ability
7. intermixed
8. memorizing
9. stages
10. interest
11. positive

MATCHING

1. g **2.** b **3.** h **4.** d **5.** c **6.** e **7.** a **8.** f **1.** e **2.** c **3.** I **4.** a **5.** g **6.** b **7.** h **8.** d **9.** j **10.** f **11.** k

SHORT ANSWER

1. More economical; adds depth to learning; provides opportunity for shared experience.
2. Assessing the child's current level of knowledge; ability and motivation to learn new knowledge.
3. Visual aids help children see and better understand what will happen and how the procedure will affect the particular body parts
4. Children learn to a point of saturation, at which point learning stops and does not continue until that information is absorbed and understood.
5. Nurses can help by consulting with schools and health care organizations to develop health-teaching programs and by teaching such programs.

APPLYING YOUR KNOWLEDGE

CASE STUDY

1. Suggested answers may include but are not limited to the following: communication techniques such as attentive listening, open-ended questions, reflecting and clarifying, focusing; adaptations for different primary language, such as interpreter or translator if indicated; teaching methods such as gestures, pictures, puppets or dolls, avoidance of clichés, individual possible more beneficial than group initially, demonstration and redemonstration, videos in Spanish.
2. Suggested answers may include but are not limited to the following: including parents in discussion with interpreter present; using videos in Spanish for parents, having parents participate in demonstration and redemonstration with Raoul, having other parents who speak Spanish and have a child with diabetes talk with Raoul's parents, visual aids in Spanish.

3. Suggested answers may include but are not limited to the following: gaining permission from Raoul to include parents in teaching; ensuring Raoul's privacy as he wishes; including technology in teaching methods if indicated; focusing on present and how treatment will benefit him; encouraging active participation; including "what if" situations for abstract thinking; encouraging Raoul to take on responsibility; encouraging parents to "step aside."

4. Suggested answers may include but are not limited to the following: methods of teaching; nonverbal communication techniques, such as distance, eye contact, touch.

PRACTICING FOR NCLEX

MULTIPLE-CHOICE QUESTIONS

1. c   2. c   3. a   4. d   5. b

ALTERNATE FORMAT QUESTIONS

Multiple-Answer Multiple-Choice Questions

1. c, d, f   2. c, a, d, b, e   3. a, d

CHAPTER 36

MASTERING THE INFORMATION

FILL IN THE BLANKS

1. perception, support people, coping experiences
2. cognitive development, experiences, knowledge
3. stress, stress
4. favorite toy, Blanks et, or pacifier
5. unknown, abandonment, mutilation
6. factual

MATCHING

1. e   2. g   3. h   4. d   5. f   6. c   7. a   8. b

TRUE OR FALSE

1. T   2. F   3. F   4. F   5. F   6. T   7. F   8. F   9. F
10. T

SHORT ANSWER

1. (1) Harm or injury; (2) separation; (3) unknown; (4) uncertain limits; and (5) loss of control.
2. Children may misinterpret nursing procedures as punishments and may be confused by terms used in explanations that often sound alike or have double meanings.
3. a. Infants
   b. Adolescents
   c. Toddlers
   d. Older children/school-aged

APPLYING YOUR KNOWLEDGE

CASE STUDY

1. Suggested answers may include but are not limited to the following: dependent on the stage of separation

anxiety being experienced: protest, initially child exhibiting loud and demanding behavior, resisting any attempts to be comforted; despair, with the child becoming less active, crying monotonously, or wailing, turning away from parent's approach, possible weight loss, difficulty sleeping, flat facial expression; denial, with child being silent, with expressionless face and superficial responses.

2. Suggested answers may include but are not limited to the following: mother possibly feeling a loss of control, guilt over having to leave; older sister possibly feeling responsible or guilty for the mother having to leave, anger for sibling becoming sick and interrupting vacation.

3. Suggested answers may include but are not limited to the following: ways to decrease separation anxiety, such as spending one-on-one time with Devon, encouraging mother to phone frequently and having Devon talk with her on the phone; ensuring continuity of care, allowing Devon to participate in care as much as possible; ensuring opportunities for play including therapeutic play; fostering growth and development; ensuring adequate nutrition, safety, sleep, and stimulation.

PRACTICING FOR NCLEX

MULTIPLE-CHOICE QUESTIONS

1. d   2. d   3. c   4. c   5. c

ALTERNATE FORMAT QUESTIONS

Multiple-Answer Multiple-Choice Questions

1. a, d, e, f   2. a, d, e   3. b, c, d

CHAPTER 37

MASTERING THE INFORMATION

FILL IN THE BLANKS

1. 15
2. nonadhesive, waterproof
3. clean-catch

MATCHING

1. d   2. e   3. a   4. c   5. b

SHORT ANSWER

1. Obtaining an appliance small enough and skin irritation.
2. *Psychological preparation*: Familiarize the child with the techniques and equipment that are a part of the preoperative and postoperative care using an age-appropriate teaching plan. *Physical preparation*: Nothing by mouth for a designated period of time before surgery; washing the incision area; removal of items such as barrettes and bobby pins, if present; checking the mouth for loose teeth; dressing in hospital gown and underpants; checking for correct and legible identification band.

3. Any four of the following would be correct (see the text for detailed descriptions): wheelchair or cart, restraining belt, clove-hitch, jacket, elbow, or mummy. (See Table 37.1.)

4. Nurses can help by providing health counseling to aid in preventing children from becoming ill and keeping children free of disease so that they undergo a minimal number of procedures. Examples of actions may include: preventing nosocomial infection by enforcing measures such as frequent handwashing and ensuring use of sterile technique for dressing changes. They can prevent health care worker exposure by being certain they and their coworkers follow standard precautions.

APPLYING YOUR KNOWLEDGE

CASE STUDY

1. Suggested answers may include but are not limited to the following: reducing Iesha's anxiety; ensuring that Iesha's father provides consent since he is the custodial parent; explaining the procedures clearly and answering any questions of both parents; including Iesha's father in any teaching; using age-appropriate language for explanations and therapeutic play; explaining procedures close to the time of the procedure to reduce worrying time; ensuring child and parents about the need to maintain safety including restraints if necessary; providing appropriate explanations about care after procedure; reinforcing the need for verbal and non-verbal support before, during, and after the procedure.

2. Suggested answers may include but are not limited to the following: custodial parent needing instructions but including mother in discharge plan as appropriate; giving both parents explanations and written copies of instructions; encouraging consistency in care for Iesha, regardless of which parent is with the child; need for clear consistent communication between parents about the child's status or condition.

PRACTICING FOR NCLEX

MULTIPLE-CHOICE QUESTIONS

1. d **2.** c **3.** d **4.** c **5.** c

ALTERNATE FORMAT QUESTIONS

Multiple-Answer Multiple-Choice Questions

1. a, c, e, f **2.** a, b **3.** a, c, d

CHAPTER 38

MASTERING THE INFORMATION

FILL IN THE BLANKS

1. back
2. vastus lateralis muscle

3. Intravenous
4. immaturity
5. down, back

MATCHING

1. d **2.** c **3.** a **4.** b

SHORT ANSWER

1. Any four of the following routes: oral, intranasal, ophthalmic, otic, rectal, transdermal or topical, injection (subcutaneous, intramuscular, intravenous, intraosseous, or epidural), or inhalation.

2. The correct dosage of most drugs for children is based on body surface area using a nomogram.

3. An intermittent infusion device (heparin lock) can be used if frequent venous blood samples are required.

4. Automatic rate-flow infusion pump, fluid chamber, and minidropper.

5. Right medicine, right child, right dosage, right route, right time, right information, and right documentation.

APPLYING YOUR KNOWLEDGE

CASE STUDY

1. Suggested answers may include but are not limited to the following: response based on assessment of the child's ability to take the oral medication and child's past history with taking medications; determination of form of oral medication (liquid, pill, or tablet) and if child can swallow oral medication; assessment of child's cognitive level to determine the level of explanation needed; assessment of family's cultural beliefs and attitudes related to medication.

2. Suggested answers may include but are not limited to the following: determining appropriate needle size for therapy and whether an intermittent infusion device would be appropriate for the situation; evaluating appropriate site; assessing child's preference about site and advocating for the child's choice as appropriate; gathering necessary equipment including fluid for infusion and antibiotic; preparing the child and mother for actual venipuncture.

3. Suggested answers may include but are not limited to the following: assessing child's previous exposure to intravenous therapy; explaining the procedure in age-appropriate terms to the child, including pain with insertion of needle but not with infusion; explaining the procedure to the mother and the reason for intravenous administration; explaining approximate length of time for therapy, type of device to be used, and care required; describing the use of an armboard to secure the device; describing what the child can and cannot do during the infusion.

PRACTICING FOR NCLEX

MULTIPLE-CHOICE QUESTIONS

1. c **2.** d **3.** a **4.** c **5.** c **6.** b

ALTERNATE FORMAT QUESTIONS
Multiple-Answer Multiple-Choice Questions

1. a, c, d, f   **2.** a, b, c   **3.** b, c, e

CHAPTER 39

MASTERING THE INFORMATION

FILL IN THE BLANKS

1. conscious sedation
2. visual analog
3. Substitution of meaning
4. topical anesthetic

MATCHING

1. d   **2.** c   **3.** e   **4.** a   **5.** b

SHORT ANSWER

1. Any two of the following are correct: a belief that infants and young children do not experience pain; a fear of addiction to pain relief medications; and a fear of causing respiratory depression.
2. Pain assessment in children might be difficult because some will suffer pain rather than report it because of fear, some will distract themselves by play, and some will sleep from exhaustion caused by pain. In addition, infants and young children cannot verbalize what they are feeling and have the most trouble communicating how they feel. Cultural differences also influence how pain is expressed.
3. The gate control theory explains that because pain travels between the site of injury and the brain where the impulse is registered as pain, gating mechanisms in the dorsal horn of the spinal cord, when activated, can halt a pain impulse at the level of the cord. This prevents the pain impulse from being received at the brain level and interpreted as pain.

APPLYING YOUR KNOWLEDGE

CASE STUDY

1. Suggested answers may include but are not limited to the following: types of available pain medication and their routes; intramuscular injections rarely used for children due to pain caused by them; possible nonpharmacologic pain relief methods; intravenous administration as the preferred route for acute pain (most likely has an intravenous already in place due to surgery); possible epidural analgesia (if epidural catheter inserted during surgery); parental presence for support and comfort but not for "holding the child" down.
2. Suggested answers may include but are not limited to the following: assessing vital signs for changes; asking child if she has pain and having child point to area; using possible tools such as poker chip tool, FACES pain-rating scale, Oucher pain-rating scale,

or numerical or visual analog scale (if Patricia can count).

PRACTICING FOR NCLEX

MULTIPLE-CHOICE QUESTIONS

1. a   **2.** b   **3.** c   **4.** b

ALTERNATE FORMAT QUESTIONS
Multiple-Answer Multiple-Choice Questions

1. b, c, e, d, a   **2.** a, b, d   **3.** a, b, c

CHAPTER 40

MASTERING THE INFORMATION

FILL IN THE BLANKS

1. filter, warm, moisten/humidify
2. **a.** 80 to 100 mm Hg, **b.** 35 to 45 mm Hg, **c.** 95 to 100 percent, **d.** 7.35 to 7.45, **e.** 22 to 26 mEq/L.
3. first 24 hours; five; seven
4. frequent swallowing; clearing the throat; increasing restlessness
5. complete airway blockage
6. Any three of the following would be correct: dysphagia (difficulty swallowing), inspiratory stridor, high fever, hoarseness, sore throat, excessive drooling, and protruding tongue.
7. tachypnea
8. medulla; pons

MATCHING

1. d   **2.** c   **3.** h   **4.** a   **5.** b   **6.** e   **7.** f   **8.** g   **9.** k   **10.** j   **11.** i   **12.** l

APPLYING YOUR KNOWLEDGE

CASE STUDY

1. Suggested answers may include but are not limited to the following: treatment of pneumonia; chest physiotherapy; mucus clearing devices; airway clearance via nebulization or aerosol therapy; humidified oxygen; respiratory hygiene measures; prevention of respiratory acidosis and atelectasis; nutritional issues such as high-protein, high-calorie, moderate fat diet with vitamin supplementation, and medium chain triglycerides; use of pancreatic supplements before eating; emotional support; rest and comfort needs.
2. Suggested answers may include but are not limited to the following: care required by Rebecca and mother's working situation; affect of illness on family functioning; resources to care for Rebecca including those for equipment, medications; available support persons; community support resources.
3. Suggested answers may include but are not limited to the following: supplemental financial assistance; securing of necessary equipment; supportive care

providers or individuals who can provide assistance with Rebecca's care; respite care; emotional support for Rebecca (support group of other children with cystic fibrosis); emotional support for Rebecca's mother.

PRACTICING FOR NCLEX

MULTIPLE-CHOICE QUESTIONS

1. c **2.** a **3.** b **4.** b **5.** a **6.** a **7.** d **8.** d **9.** c
10. c

ALTERNATE FORMAT QUESTIONS

Multiple-Answer Multiple-Choice Questions

1. a, c, d **2.** b, d **3.** b, c, d, e

CHAPTER 41

MASTERING THE INFORMATION

FILL IN THE BLANKS

1. left; right
2. difficulty feeding
3. air; fluid
4. hyperacute, acute, chronic
5. Cardiomyopathy
6. Respiratory failure
7. a. Tetralogy of Fallot, **b.** Transposition of the great arteries, **c.** Tricuspid atresia
8. tachycardia

MATCHING

1. e **2.** d **3.** g **4.** b **5.** c **6.** o **7.** f **8.** m **9.** n
10. i **11.** j **12.** k **13.** l **14.** a **15.** h

SHORT ANSWER

1. Any three of the following are correct: bilateral congestion of ocular conjunctiva, changes in peripheral extremities, rash, swollen cervical lymph nodes, changes of mucous membrane of the upper respiratory tract such as strawberry tongue.
2. Information may include medication taken during pregnancy, nutritional adequacy, radiation exposure, vaginal or other infection, and cyanosis present at birth.
3. Information would include information about care, steps for follow-up care and how to handle emergencies.
4. Preoperative teaching includes the use of anesthesia to induce sleep, equipment used during and after surgery, such as chest tubes, ECG, oxygen therapy, ventilator, hemodynamic monitoring and other monitoring devices, cough and deep breathing exercises and incentive spirometry, positioning, and nutrition.
5. The duration of innocent murmurs is shorter than with organic murmurs. Innocent murmurs are soft and musical; organic murmurs are harsh and blowing. Innocent murmurs are of soft intensity; organic murmurs are of loud intensity.

APPLYING YOUR KNOWLEDGE

CASE STUDY

1. Suggested answers may include but are not limited to the following: use of conscious sedation and anesthesia; prevention of vomiting and aspiration during procedure.
2. Suggested answers may include but are not limited to the following: to secure blood samples or inject dye, measure blood flow pressures in all heart chambers and cardiac output or record electrical activity and diagnose arrhythmias (via electrodes introduced); diagnostic to help evaluate cardiac function, diagnose specific heart disorders prior to surgery; interventional to correct abnormality.
3. Suggested answers may include but are not limited to the following: explanations about what will happen; review of heart anatomy and path catheter will take in age-appropriate terms; review of what Harriet will see in the catheterization room and using puppets or dolls; tour of catheterization area; familiarity with equipment such as ECG electrodes; events or feelings associated with catheter insertion; need to lie still; application of pressure dressing after the procedure; need to keep affected extremity flat and unbent.
4. Suggested answers may include but are not limited to the following: lying flat to prevent oozing at insertion site; prevent postural hypotension; prevent bleeding and hematoma formation.

PRACTICING FOR NCLEX

MULTIPLE-CHOICE QUESTIONS

1. c **2.** b **3.** b **4.** c **5.** a **6.** b **7.** a **8.** b **9.** c

ALTERNATE FORMAT QUESTIONS

Multiple-Answer Multiple-Choice Questions

1. c, f **2.** d, e, f **3.** a, c

CHAPTER 42

MASTERING THE INFORMATION

FILL IN THE BLANKS

1. a. Hypogammaglobinemia, **b.** IgA deficiency
2. sexual, parental
3. Autoimmunity
4. allergen
5. reduce the child's exposure to the allergen, hyposensitize the child to produce a state of increased clinical tolerance to the allergen, modify the child's response to the allergen with a pharmacological agent
6. food diary
7. six
8. ice

MATCHING

1. c **2.** i **3.** f **4.** j **5.** h **6.** b **7.** d **8.** a **9.** e
10. g

SHORT ANSWER

1. Refer to Table 42.4; any two measures in each category would be accurate.
2. Seborrheic dermatitis has no itching, begins at birth to 6 months, rarely lasts longer than 1 year, and does not cause the child to become irritable. Infantile eczema causes severe itching, has a usual onset of 2 to 6 months, lasts from 2 to 3 years, and causes the child to be irritable and fussy.
3. Congenital immunodeficiency disorders occur because the child is born with inadequate (or totally without) essential immune substances; secondary immunodeficiency disorders occur as a result of a loss of immunity due to factors such as severe systemic infection, cancer, renal disease, radiation therapy, severe stress, malnutrition, immunosuppressive therapy, and aging.
4. Skin testing is done to detect the presence of IgE in the skin, or to isolate an antigen (allergen) to which the IgE is responding or to which a child is sensitive.

APPLYING YOUR KNOWLEDGE

CASE STUDY

1. Suggested answers may include but are not limited to the following: Jose's immunodeficiency classified as primary, therefore it is congenital; development of immunodeficiency due to being born without an essential immune substance or function or with inadequate amounts of immune substances; not contagious due to congenital nature.
2. Suggested answers may include but are not limited to the following: education for parents and siblings about the congenital nature of the disorder; Jose's increased risk for infection so he needs to be protected from infection; Jose at risk for infection from others; emphasis of teaching on prevention including immunizations up-to-date, possible antibiotic prophylaxis, and infection control precautions
3. Suggested answers may include but are not limited to the following: infection control measures; meticulous hand hygiene; possible administration of antibiotics; prevention of additional infection (including nosocomial infections).

PRACTICING FOR NCLEX

MULTIPLE-CHOICE QUESTIONS

1. c **2.** a **3.** d **4.** b

ALTERNATE FORMAT QUESTIONS

Multiple-Answer Multiple-Choice Questions

1. a, c, d **2.** a, c, d, e **3.** b, c, e

CHAPTER 43

MASTERING THE INFORMATION

FILL IN THE BLANKS

1. Incubation
2. Rocky Mountain spotted fever
3. Hookworm
4. Varicella
5. Warts
6. orchitis

MATCHING

1. b **2.** c **3.** e **4.** f **5.** g **6.** i **7.** a **8.** d **9.** j
10. k **11.** h

SHORT ANSWER

1. Five types of microorganisms: viruses, bacteria, rickettsia, helminth, and fungi.
2. Once the rabies disease process begins, it is invariably fatal.
3. Incubation period of 14 to 21 days; period of communicability shortly before or after the onset of parotitis.
4. The chain of infection must be intact, consisting of a pathogen, reservoir, a portal of exit, a means of transmission, a portal of entry, and a susceptible host.
5. Circumstances that cause a child to be susceptible to infection include a lack of natural antibodies or immunization against infection, young age, gender, the virulence of invading organisms, poor body defenses (physical, chemical), and immune type.
6. Any time the health care worker comes in contact with bodily fluids or blood, gloves should be worn. A gown, mask, and goggles should be worn if splattering of blood or body fluids is likely. Hands should always be washed before and after contact with clients. Sharp objects should be handled carefully. Refer to Box 43.4 in the text for reference to blood spills, specimens, and resuscitation.
7. Signs and symptoms of scarlet fever are abrupt and include fever, sore throat, headache, rash, chills, increased pulse rate, and malaise.

APPLYING YOUR KNOWLEDGE

CASE STUDY

1. Suggested answers may include but are not limited to the following: age (most commonly occurring in adolescents); close contact with others increasing risk of transmission (readily spread from one to another, often by kissing).
2. Suggested answers may include but are not limited to the following: explanation of the need for rest; increased risk for splenic rupture with splenomegaly during acute stage.
3. Suggested answers may include but are not limited to the following: increased fluid intake to prevent

dehydration from fever and decreased intake due to anorexia and sore throat; cool nonacidic fluids due to sore throat; small frequent meals; soft nonirritating food.

PRACTICING FOR NCLEX

MULTIPLE-CHOICE QUESTIONS

1. c **2.** c **3.** b

ALTERNATE FORMAT QUESTIONS

Multiple-Answer Multiple-Choice Questions

1. b, d, e **2.** a, c, d **3.** b, d

CHAPTER 44

MASTERING THE INFORMATION

FILL IN THE BLANKS

1. stem cell transplantation
2. Hemolysis
3. Graft-versus-host disease
4. Platelets/thrombocytes
5. Erythrocytes

MATCHING

1. c **2.** g **3.** a **4.** e **5.** b **6.** i **7.** d **8.** j **9.** h
10. f

APPLYING YOUR KNOWLEDGE

CASE STUDY

1. Suggested answers may include but are not limited to the following: fever; anemia; local pain; swelling of the hands and feet (a hand–foot syndrome); slight build and characteristically long arms and legs; protruding abdomen because of an enlarged spleen and liver.
2. Suggested answers may include but are not limited to the following: pain management/relief; hydration/fluid balance; oxygenation; child and parental support and education.
3. Suggested answers may include but are not limited to the following: possible decreased kidney function (urine specific gravity testing and observation for hematuria to detect extent or presence of kidney damage from infarcts); need for adequate hydration without overloading the workload of the kidneys; intravenous therapy to restore hydration and reduce sickling; strict intake and output.
4. Suggested answers may include but are not limited to the following: oxygen saturation levels below 95%; arterial blood gases with low Po_2 level; signs and symptoms of respiratory distress; signs and symptoms of acute chest syndrome (hypoxia, decreased hemoglobin, chest pain, fever, tachypnea, wheezing, or cough and persistent diffuse pneumonia).

PRACTICING FOR NCLEX

MULTIPLE-CHOICE QUESTIONS

1. b **2.** a **3.** d **4.** d **5.** c

ALTERNATE FORMAT QUESTIONS

Multiple-Answer Multiple-Choice Questions

1. a, b, f **2.** b, c, d **3.** a, c, e

CHAPTER 45

MASTERING THE INFORMATION

FILL IN THE BLANKS

1. acidosis
2. alkalosis
3. insensible

MATCHING

1. c **2.** b **3.** g **4.** a **5.** d **6.** e **7.** h **8.** f

SHORT ANSWER

1. The spitting up associated with achalasia is described as effortless and nonprojectile.
2. The most common cause of abdominal surgery in children is appendicitis.
3. Fiberoptic endoscopy is the most reliable diagnostic test to confirm peptic ulcer disease.

APPLYING YOUR KNOWLEDGE

CASE STUDY

1. Suggested answers may include but are not limited to the following: major fluid loss sources: urine and feces (infants with greater fluid loss via kidneys due to immaturity of kidneys and inability to concentrate urine as well as adults); minor fluid loss sources: evaporation from the skin and lungs, and from salivaluid intake (greater body surface area to body mass in infants leading to greater insensible fluid losses).
2. Suggested answers may include but are not limited to the following: history —previous history of problems: onset of problems; observation of any weight loss; evidence of vomiting or diarrhea; usual oral intake including amount and frequency of feedings; any change in feedings (such as change in type of formula); usual solid food intake and any change in foods being given (such as more fruits or vegetables); number of wet diapers per day; number of stools per day and any changes; any other family members ill. Physical assessment—weight and comparison to baseline, skin turgor, consistency and temperature; fontanels (if still open); level of alertness; status of mucous membranes; urine color and concentration; appearance of stool; laboratory testing such as electrolyte levels, urine output, and specific gravity; signs and symptoms of metabolic acidosis or alkalosis.

PRACTICING FOR NCLEX

MULTIPLE-CHOICE QUESTIONS

1. a **2.** b **3.** b **4.** c

ALTERNATE FORMAT QUESTIONS

Multiple-Answer Multiple-Choice Questions

1. a, d, e, f **2.** a, d, e **3.** b, c, d

CHAPTER 46

MASTERING THE INFORMATION

FILL IN THE BLANKS

1. antigen–antibody
2. edema, hypoalbuminemia, hyperlipidemia, proteinuria
3. pale, oliguria, hematuria
4. polycystic
5. creatinine
6. Vesicoureteral reflux

MATCHING

1. h **2.** j **3.** d **4.** e **5.** f **6.** c **7.** i **8.** g **9.** a
10. b

SHORT ANSWER

1. The urethra is closer to the vagina in girls, and shorter and closer to the anus than in boys, allowing organisms to spread to the bladder.
2. Nephrotic syndrome occurs insidiously with rare hematuria, marked hyperlipidemia, extreme edema, and mild hypertension, whereas glomerulonephritis occurs abruptly with profuse hematuria, mild hyperlipidemia, mild edema, and marked hypertension. The treatment for nephrotic syndrome involves a high-protein, low-sodium diet, whereas glomerulonephritis commonly involves a diet normal for the age of the child; however, protein supplement or restrictions may be individually required.
3. The acute form of renal insufficiency usually occurs from a sudden body insult, whereas the chronic form of renal failure results from extensive kidney disease.
4. Salt restriction needs to be individualized: some children need less sodium, some need no restriction, and some children need additional sodium.

APPLYING YOUR KNOWLEDGE

CASE STUDY

1. Suggested answers may include but are not limited to the following: most likely acute renal failure due to recent insult (dehydration and infection); possible acute glomerulonephritis as underlying mechanism leading to acute renal failure; if glomerulonephritis not treated, then possible development of chronic renal failure. Other assessment findings: oliguria, azotemia, uremia, fixed urine-specific gravity, hyperkalemia (weak, irregular pulse, abdominal cramps, decreased blood pressure, muscle weakness), acidosis, elevated serum phosphorus level and low-calcium level.
2. Suggested answers may include but are not limited to the following: underlying mechanism due to insult to kidneys from dehydration and possible infection; reaction of body to stress; treatment focusing on support of body systems with correction of underlying condition.
3. Suggested answers may include but are not limited to the following: initially bed rest to minimize metabolic demands; as recovery occurs, gradual increase in activity as tolerated; need for quite play; play therapy for activities that can be done at bedside, such as blocks, toys that can be manipulated; gradual resumption in usual activities as child recovers.

PRACTICING FOR NCLEX

MULTIPLE-CHOICE QUESTIONS

1. c **2.** c **3.** a **4.** b **5.** d

ALTERNATE FORMAT QUESTIONS

Multiple-Answer Multiple-Choice Questions

1. b, c, e **2.** a, c, d, e **3.** a, c, d, f

CHAPTER 47

MASTERING THE INFORMATION

FILL IN THE BLANKS

1. varicocele
2. Gynecomastia
3. Cryptorchidism
4. scrotum, rare (or painless), metastasizes
5. Mittelschmerz, abdomen
6. Balanoposthitis

MATCHING

1. f **2.** j **3.** c **4.** h **5.** k **6.** b **7.** d **8.** g **9.** i
10. e **11.** a

APPLYING YOUR KNOWLEDGE

CASE STUDY

1. Suggested answers may include but are not limited to the following: signs and symptoms—evidence of chancre or lesion; swollen lymph nodes; rash on soles and palms; generalized illness; serologic testing such as VDRL, ART, ROR, or FTA-ABS.
2. Suggested answers may include but are not limited to the following: description of syphilis and progression of disease if not treated; measures to reduce the risk of transmission including safe sex

practices; treatment; need to report to the local health department; need to identify sexual contacts.

3. Suggested answers may include but are not limited to the following: checking state regulations related to minors and whether or not parents must be informed (most states allow treatment for pregnancy, contraception, and STIs without parental notification); informing Peter of requirement to report syphilis to local health department; reinforcing nurse's legal, professional, and ethical responsibility to maintain confidentiality.

PRACTICING FOR NCLEX

MULTIPLE-CHOICE QUESTIONS

1. c 2. d 3. a 4. c 5. b

ALTERNATE FORMAT QUESTIONS

Multiple-Answer Multiple-Choice Questions

1. a, c, d, e 2. a, b, c, e 3. b, c

CHAPTER 48

MASTERING THE INFORMATION

FILL IN THE BLANKS

1. insulin, glucose, hyperglycemia, ketoacidosis
2. 30
3. goiter

MATCHING

1. d 2. f 3. a 4. h 5. b 6. e 7. g 8. c

SHORT ANSWER

1. The endocrine system acts to regulate and coordinate body systems.
2. a. Thyroid gland
   b. Pituitary gland
   c. Pancreas
   d. Pituitary gland
   e. Adrenal gland
   f. Pituitary gland
3. The onset of Humulin N occurs in 1 to 2 hours with peak effect occurring in 4 to 12 hours.

APPLYING YOUR KNOWLEDGE

CASE STUDY

1. Suggested answers may include but are not limited to the following: education for the mother about the underlying etiology of diabetes; explanation of immunologic damage to insulin producing cells in susceptible individuals; possible effects of environment on stimulating this immunologic response; increased frequency of human leukocyte antigen; need for environmental trigger dysfunction; possible familial pattern.

2. Suggested answers may include but are not limited to the following: routine application of topical anesthetic cream to site; use of intermittent infusion device; nonpharmacologic methods such as distraction, guided imagery, and thought stopping.

PRACTICING FOR NCLEX

MULTIPLE-CHOICE QUESTIONS

1. b 2. d 3. a 4. c 5. b

ALTERNATE FORMAT QUESTIONS

Multiple-Answer Multiple-Choice Questions

1. a, b, e 2. b, c, e 3. a, b, c

CHAPTER 49

MASTERING THE INFORMATION

FILL IN THE BLANKS

1. central, peripheral
2. balance, coordination
3. disorientation or confusion
4. arterial
5. streptococcal
6. supportive care
7. preschool
8. a. Cerebellar, b. Motor, c. Sensory
9. a. Tonic–clonic, b. Simple partial, c. Psychomotor, d. Absence

MATCHING

1. d 2. c 3. e 4. a 5. b 6. g 7. h 8. f 9. i 10. j

APPLYING YOUR KNOWLEDGE

CASE STUDY

1. Suggested answers may include but are not limited to the following: signs and symptoms such as seizure with fever; analysis of Cerebrospinal fluid via lumbar puncture (increase WBC count and protein levels; lowered glucose level); blood cultures to rule out septicemia; CT, MRI, or ultrasound to rule out abscesses.

2. Suggested answers may include but are not limited to the following: antibiotic therapy based on culture and sensitivity testing, usually given intravenous but possibly intrathecally; corticosteroid or osmotic diuretic possibly to decrease intracranial pressure and prevent hearing loss; standard precautions; droplet precautions for 24 hours after start of antibiotic therapy. Complications such as neurologic sequelae (learning problems, seizures, hearing and cognitive changes, inability to concentrate urine); possible septicemia; fulminant possibly fatal case.

3. Suggested answers may include but are not limited to the following: easily transmitted; concern for immediate family members and others in close contact with child; prophylactic antibiotics for immediate family members and others in close contact.

PRACTICING FOR NCLEX

MULTIPLE-CHOICE QUESTIONS

1. a **2.** a **3.** d **4.** d **5.** a **6.** d **7.** b **8.** d **9.** d
10. d

ALTERNATE FORMAT QUESTIONS

Multiple-Answer Multiple-Choice Questions

1. b, c, d **2.** a, b, c, e **3.** a, b, f

CHAPTER 50

MASTERING THE INFORMATION

FILL IN THE BLANKS

1. Stereopsis
2. orthoptics
3. Hyperopia
4. Coloboma

MATCHING

1. h **2.** i **3.** f **4.** g **5.** q **6.** b **7.** j **8.** d **9.** a
10. c

APPLYING YOUR KNOWLEDGE

CASE STUDY

1. Suggested answers may include but are not limited
to the following: present at birth; possibly a dominantly inherited condition; galactosemia, or inability to metabolize the lactose in milk; result of
steroid use or radiation exposure; trauma to the eye
if the lens is injured; due to birth injury or possibly
contact between the lens and the cornea during
intrauterine life; nutritional deficiency during
intrauterine life, such as rickets or hypocalcemia;
prenatal contracting of rubella.
2. Suggested answers may include but are not
limited to the following: close monitoring to
determine that child is fully alert and awake
after conscious sedation; slow introduction of
fluid to prevent nausea and vomiting that
could lead to increased IOP; use of fluids child
prefers.
3. Suggested answers may include but are not limited
to the following: instructions related to patching
(if appropriate); allowing parent and child to practice with eye patches; need to speak slowly and
clearly; favorite toy within reach; fluid intake but
gradual increase to prevent nausea and vomiting;
not allowing child to cry which would increase
intraocular pressure; procedure for eyedrop
administration; importance of adhering to
follow up.

PRACTICING FOR NCLEX

MULTIPLE-CHOICE QUESTIONS

1. b **2.** a **3.** c **4.** b **5.** d **6.** c **7.** a **8.** a

ALTERNATIVE FORMAT QUESTIONS

Multiple-Answer Multiple-Choice Questions

1. a, b, d **2.** a, b, e **3.** a, c, d

CHAPTER 51

MASTERING THE INFORMATION

FILL IN THE BLANKS

1. epiphyseal plate, periosteum
2. 1, 1.5, 20
3. thickening, enlargement, adolescent, preadolescent
4. adolescents, lift
5. rested, isometric
6. strain, sprain

MATCHING

1. j **2.** f **3.** d **4.** g **5.** e **6.** l **7.** a **8.** k **9.** h
10. c **11.** b **12.** i

SHORT ANSWER

1. The leg brace would cause the child, particularly
an adolescent, to feel different from peers; the mobility limitations would also decrease opportunities for socialization with other children, resulting in isolation and decreased opportunity for
development.
2. Encourage contact with school friends; arrange the
bed to permit visualization of unit activities;
arrange for visits from friends; maintain activity by
involving the child in age-appropriate activities; tu-
toring may be needed.
3. *Positive measures*: Massage the area under the cast
edge with hand; apply lotion to the cast edge area;
when possible blow cool air through the cast.
Negative measures: Avoid using coat hangers,
knitting needles, or any sharp objects for scratch-
ing.
4. Walk on tiptoe for 5 to 10 minutes; practice picking
up marbles with the toes; an older child could
stand pigeon-toed and throw-weight forward into
the lateral aspect of the feet.
5. Functional scoliosis is caused by secondary
physical or visual problems and is treated by
correcting the underlying problem and
encouraging good posture and spinal-stretching
exercises. Structural scoliosis is an idiopathic, often
inherited, permanent spine curvature requiring
long-term bracing or traction, or both. Slight curva-
tures may require no treatment except observation
until age 18.
6. *Milwaukee brace*: A torso brace with one anterior
and two posterior rods, leather pads, and a torso
piece; used to improve spinal alignment. *Halo traction*: Involves a metal ring attached to the skull
with pins; used to stabilize cervical spine and
reduce spinal curves. *Bryant's traction*: Skin traction
used for fractured femurs and for congenital developmental defects; used in children less than 2 years

old. *Buck's traction*: Skin traction used to immobilize fractured femurs in children older than 2 years old. *Skeletal traction*: The child's body serves as the counter-pull; used to reduce dislocation and immobilize fractures.

APPLYING YOUR KNOWLEDGE

CASE STUDY

1. Suggested answers may include but are not limited to the following: emphasis on avoiding any type of trauma, regardless of how small; close supervision of activities to avoid falls; possible limitation of activity to reduce risk of trauma or use of protective devices to avoid injury; gentle lifting with avoidance of lifting by a single arm or leg; underlying problem associated with condition (brittle bones); use of prescribed therapy to stimulate growth, increase bone mass, or aid bone healing.

2. Suggested answers may include but are not limited to the following: encouragement of age-appropriate activities with safety measures (important but risk for injury not as severe); routine cast care; education about safety measures related to cast and injury; medications primarily for pain relief (not for growth stimulation, bone healing, or increased bone mass); braces or intermedullary rod insertion not necessary.

PRACTICING FOR NCLEX

MULTIPLE-CHOICE QUESTIONS

1. b **2.** c **3.** c **4.** c **5.** b **6.** b **7.** c

ALTERNATIVE FORMAT QUESTIONS

Multiple-Answer Multiple-Choice Questions

1. b, c, d **2.** b, c **3.** a, b, e

CHAPTER 52

MASTERING THE INFORMATION

FILL IN THE BLANKS

1. the injuring agent, the part of the body, the immediate care
2. third
3. sterile
4. open

MATCHING

1. b **2.** j **3.** g **4.** c **5.** a **6.** h **7.** k **8.** e **9.** f **10.** d **11.** i

SHORT ANSWER

1. Responses are: eye opening, motor, and verbal.
2. Provide written instructions regarding the child's care at home; provide a telephone number for the parent to call if questions arise; schedule a return appointment for follow-up care.

3. The body proportions of infants and children differ from the adult proportions on which the rule of nines was based.

4. These burns are often accompanied by respiratory tract problems related to airway trauma due to heat, carbon monoxide, and smoke inhalation.

5. Aseptic technique and appropriate barriers are necessary to reduce the risk of infection.

6. *First-degree burn*: Apply ice to cool the skin and prevent further burning; cleanse the area with an antiseptic; apply an analgesic and antibiotic ointment and a gauze bandage. Keep dressings dry. *Second- or third-degree burn*: Do not break blister; cover with a topical antibiotic and bulky dressing; debride broken blisters. Some measures include prophylactic antibiotics; daily debridement and whirlpool; overextend joints with splints; pain management with analgesics (see toddler nursing care plan). *Electrical burns*: Unplug the electric cord and control bleeding with pressure to site; monitor for airway obstruction.

APPLYING YOUR KNOWLEDGE

CASE STUDY

1. Suggested answers may include but are not limited to the following: education about safety issues in and outside the home; typical growth and development of 3-year-olds (preschoolers); importance of child's development of initiative through activities; emphasis on exposure to experiences and creative play but with the need for continued supervision and limits; redirecting Jay's activity level to safer outlets; ensuring all potentially injurious items such as cleaning products are out of Jay's reach (childproofing the home). Further assessments including: typical day and activities of Jay and parents (preschoolers imitate what they see); degree of supervision of activities; home environment and degree of childproofing; parental knowledge level of safety, preschooler growth and development; knowledge of cast care and follow up.

2. Suggested answers may include but are not limited to the following: use of imagination for play; imitation; exposure to wide ranging experiences (trips to zoo or amusement park) and creative play materials (clay, soapy water, bubbles, sand, finger paint); play with other children.

PRACTICING FOR NCLEX

MULTIPLE-CHOICE QUESTIONS

1. c **2.** b **3.** c **4.** d

ALTERNATIVE FORMAT QUESTIONS

Multiple-Answer Multiple-Choice Questions

1. a, b, d, e **2.** d, e **3.** a, c, d, e

CHAPTER 53

MASTERING THE INFORMATION

FILL IN THE BLANKS

1. nausea, vomiting
2. Ewing's sarcoma
3. Retinoblastoma
4. Enucleation

MATCHING

1. c 2. d 3. f 4. g 5. a 6. i 7. b 8. j 9. h
10. e

SHORT ANSWER

1. The three phases are induction, sanctuary (or consolidation), and maintenance.
2. Hodgkin's disease is confirmed by a lymph node biopsy.
3. Any five of the following would be accurate: alkylating agents interfere with DNA synthesis, antibiotics impair DNA synthesis and destroy malignant cells, antimetabolites interfere with cell function, plant alkaloids interfere with cell mitosis, nitrosourea compounds interfere with DNA synthesis;, enzymes remove substances needed to grow, steroids inhibit mitosis in cells, or immunotherapy stimulates the immune system to attempt destruction of foreign or malignant cells.
4. Malignant cells take more than their share of nutrients from normal cells; nausea and vomiting from chemotherapy make it difficult for the child to maintain an adequate oral intake; stomatitis causes difficulty eating; and gastrointestinal ulcers and changes in fatty acid metabolism may interfere with absorption of nutrients. Some medications may alter taste sensations, which will affect appetite.

APPLYING YOUR KNOWLEDGE

CASE STUDY

1. Suggested answers may include but are not limited to the following: enema not given due to risk of increasing intracranial pressure; possible stool softener administered preoperatively to prevent straining with bowel movements; bowel preparation possibly dependent on the facility and/or surgeon preference.
2. Suggested answers may include but are not limited to the following: positioning (side opposite incision) with bed flat or only slighted elevated and degree of neck movement allowed; neurologic status (level of consciousness, facial or eye swelling, pupil reaction, muscle strength, sensory capabilities); cardiopulmonary status (respiratory status, ability for spontaneous ventilation, vital signs); fluid balance/hydration (intravenous fluids, use of mannitol, or hypertonic dextrose); nutritional status (oral intake); surgical site (dressings, drainage); safety measures; seizure

precautions; monitoring for increased intracranial pressure.

PRACTICING FOR NCLEX

MULTIPLE-CHOICE QUESTIONS

1. c 2. d 3. b 4. b 5. b 6. d 7. c

ALTERNATIVE FORMAT QUESTIONS

Multiple-Answer Multiple-Choice Questions

1. a, e, f   2. c, d, e   3. a, c, d

CHAPTER 54

MASTERING THE INFORMATION

FILL IN THE BLANKS

1. Pica
2. Autism
3. coprolalia, palilalia

MATCHING

1. c 2. a 3. e 4. d 5. b

SHORT ANSWER

1. Subaverage general intellectual functioning—an intelligence quotient (IQ) of 70 or lower with onset before 18 years of age—and concurrent deficits in adaptive functioning.
2. Crying, suddenly followed immediately by giggling or laughing.
3. *Graphesthesia*: Ability to recognize a shape that has been traced on the skin. *Stereognosis*: Ability to recognize an object by touch. *Choreiform*: Aimless movements of arms.
4. Flat.

APPLYING YOUR KNOWLEDGE

CASE STUDY

1. Suggested answers may include but are not limited to the following: most likely autistic disorder due to impaired social and communication skills and display of stereotypical behaviors (hand gestures). Additional symptoms such as bizarre responses to the environment (intense reactions to minor changes in the environment [screaming] and attachment to odd objects such as always carrying a string or a shoe; repetitive hand movements, rocking, and rhythmic body movements; intense preoccupation by objects that revolve; hitting, head banging, and biting; abnormal responses to sensory stimuli; decreased sensitivity to pain; inappropriate or decreased emotional expression; limited intellectual problem solving abilities; stereotyped or repetitive use of language; impaired ability to initiate or sustain conversation.
2. Suggested answers may include but are not limited to the following: providing support so parents do

not reject child; encouraging adherence to therapy such as behavior modification therapy; use of supportive services; use of day care program to promote social awareness.

PRACTICING FOR NCLEX

MULTIPLE-CHOICE QUESTIONS

1. d **2.** a **3.** b **4.** c **5.** d **6.** b

ALTERNATIVE FORMAT QUESTIONS

Multiple-Answer Multiple-Choice Questions

1. a, b **2.** a, d, e **3.** a, b, d

CHAPTER 55

MASTERING THE INFORMATION

FILL IN THE BLANKS

1. The nurse
2. alcohol
3. repeat or support

MATCHING

1. d **2.** e **3.** a **4.** g **5.** h **6.** c **7.** i **8.** b **9.** j
10. f

SHORT ANSWER

1. Special triad of circumstances includes: parent has the potential to abuse a child (special parent); child is seen as "different" in some way by the parent (special child); an event or circumstance brings about the abuse (special circumstance).
2. The family is a disrupted one; family members are reluctant to seek medical assistance for medical problems due to fear of discovery of abuse.
3. Abusive behavior is often the only role-modeling for parenting the child has been exposed to; abuser becomes a learned behavior.
4. Place the infant on an age-appropriate diet, and if the child gains weight the problem is probably nonorganic.
5. Findings: below the fifth percentile for standard weight and height; motor and social developmental delays; lethargy, poor muscle tone; reluctance to initiate human contact, few comfort-seeking behaviors.

APPLYING YOUR KNOWLEDGE

CASE STUDY

1. Suggested answers may include but are not limited to the following: determining who Alissa is referring to as "he"; assessing onset and duration (first time or something that has been going on for a while), and family living situation; assessing the child looking for signs and symptoms of abuse (See Box 55.8.); engaging the child to describe events such as by using dolls or having child draw a picture; ensuring the child's safety.

2. Suggested answers may include but are not limited to the following: reporting of abuse with follow up interview of suspected perpetrator by police; providing physical care for Diasy's condition; psychological counseling of all involved; follow up treatment for possible sexually transmitted infections; counseling for parents as appropriate; teaching related to rules to avoid sexual abuse.

PRACTICING FOR NCLEX

MULTIPLE-CHOICE QUESTIONS

1. b **2.** d **3.** a **4.** d **5.** d **6.** c **7.** d **8.** d **9.** a

ALTERNATE FORMAT QUESTIONS

Multiple-Answer Multiple-Choice Questions

1. c, d, f **2.** c, d, e **3.** a, b, c, e

CHAPTER 56

MASTERING THE INFORMATION

FILL IN THE BLANKS

1. fear
2. know/are aware of
3. denial

MATCHING

1. c **2.** e **3.** b **4.** a **5.** d

ADDITIONAL MATCHING QUESTIONS

1. i **2.** d **3.** e **4.** g **5.** j **6.** h **7.** a **8.** c **9.** f
10. b

SHORT ANSWER

1. Their perception of the event, the type and kind of support they receive from people around them, and the ways they have found successful in coping with stressful situations.
2. With a nondisabling chronic illness, the child and family feel they have some control over the course of the illness. The illness would likely have minimal effect on family functioning, although some adjustments may be needed. A disabling illness will likely have a great effect on a family due to many role changes, feelings of helplessness and powerlessness, and lack of control or ability to alter the course of the disease.
3. Youth may impair the ability of parents to care for a child due to lack of experience and problem-solving ability, making all phases of parenting more difficult than for older parents. However, youth may be an advantage to parents because young parents tend to be more flexible and creative in parenting than older parents.
4. Should the child's parents die, the disabled or chronically ill child will need a designated caretaker; the will would provide for this care, should it be needed. It also would identify sources for economic support for the child.

5. Determining the effectiveness of the plan of care might help the nurse to better plan assistance for the next terminally ill child and family.

6. Any three of the following would be accurate: continue active conversation, use silence therapeutically, use the words "dying", and "death" when appropriate, preserve the dying child's defenses, sit with the child at night and allow the child to talk about dying if desired, be supportive, be aware that not all people's beliefs are the same as yours. (See also Box 56.7.)

APPLYING YOUR KNOWLEDGE

CASE STUDY

1. Suggested answers may include but are not limited to the following: parents' reaction: initial shock; disbelief; denial; then progressing through grief response. Factors including severity of illness, relationship with own parents, onset of illness (sudden versus gradual or chronic), effect of parental

experience (first-time parents or more experienced parents), availability of support people, life events (achievement of developmental milestones).

2. Suggested answers may include but are not limited to the following: response influenced by personal attitude and temperament, self-concept, age and development, understanding of condition (usually aware of what is happening), and degree of disorder; initially possibly fear, anger; influenced by reaction of family, peers, other support persons; possible feelings of being different, socially excluded; responses changing over time.

PRACTICING FOR NCLEX

MULTIPLE-CHOICE QUESTIONS

1. c 2. c 3. c 4. b 5. b

ALTERNATE FORMAT QUESTIONS

Multiple-Answer Multiple-Choice Questions

1. b, d 2. e, d, c, a, b 3. c, e